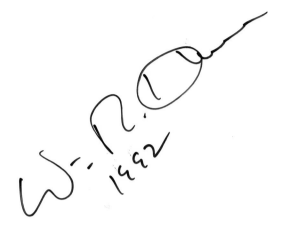

VETERINARY LABORATORY MEDICINE

Interpretation and Diagnosis

VETERINARY LABORATORY MEDICINE

Interpretation and Diagnosis

D. J. MEYER, DVM

Diplomate, ACVP and ACVIM
Associate Director of Clinical Pathology
Smith Kline Beecham Pharmaceuticals
King of Prussia, Pennsylvania

EMBERT H. COLES, DVM, PhD

Professor Emeritus
Department of Laboratory Medicine
Kansas State University
Manhattan, Kansas

LON J. RICH, DVM, PhD

Diplomate, ACVP
President Professional Animal Laboratory, Inc.
Irvine, California

W.B. SAUNDERS COMPANY
Harcourt Brace Jovanovich, Inc.

Philadelphia   London   Toronto   Montreal   Sydney   Tokyo

W. B. SAUNDERS COMPANY
Harcourt Brace Jovanovich, Inc.

The Curtis Center
Independence Square West
Philadelphia, PA 19106

Library of Congress Cataloging-in-Publication Data

Meyer, Dennis J.
   Veterinary Laboratory Medicine: Interpretation and Diagnosis / by Dennis J. Meyer.
Embert H. Coles, and Lon J. Rich.
      p.   cm.
   ISBN 0-7216-2654–8
   1. Veterinary clinical diagnosis.   2. Veterinary medicine—
Diagnosis, Differential.   I. Coles, Embert H.   II. Rich, Lon J.
III. Title.
SF772.6.M49   1992
636.089′6075—dc20   91-28796
                                                            CIP

Editor: Linda Mills

Veterinary Laboratory Medicine—*Interpretation and Diagnosis*   ISBN   0-7216-2654-8

Printed in MEXICO.

Last digit is the print number: 9   8   7   6   5   4   3   2   1

What we learn in life, we learn from others.

GRACIAN

Dedicated to veterinary practitioners, the cornerstone of our profession, and veterinary students, our profession's future—continue your pursuit of excellence . . .

. . . and my parents (Denny's) who struggled to give me the opportunity to be what I am. I hope you are proud.

ACKNOWLEDGMENTS

If I have seen further, it is by standing on the shoulders of giants.

SIR ISAAC NEWTON

We wish to thank all the veterinary practitioners whose cases and phone calls provided the material for this book. We wish we could list all of you by name.

Denny is especially grateful to the faculty, residents, students and staff at the College of Veterinary Medicine-University of Florida who facilitated his investigative efforts over the years. Thank you to Vic Perman, Bob Hardy, Carl Osborne, Gerry Ling, Ira Gorley, Niels Pedersen and Don Strombeck for their influence during those "formative" years. He wishes to affectionately thank his family (Jae, Chris, Jeni) for putting up with his absence during many weekends and his coming home late at night so that one more page could be written, then rewritten. Pam Miller and Anna Maxwell, he thanks you for helping develop the schematics, each of which replace, thankfully, a thousand of his words. His appreciation goes to SmithKline Beecham, especially Bill Kerns, for allowing him the opportunity to complete the project; Leon Saunders, thanks for your guidance.

Embert is obliged to students and veterinary practitioners who continue to provide the stimulus for an "old timer" to strive to remain up-to-date. They prevent him from losing perspective of what is most important in our profession and our life—an inquiring mind that continues to ask "What? When? Where? Why?" Special applause for the dedicated professionals whose continual search for the truth prompted the development of this book.

We appreciate the helpful suggestions from Drs. David Williams, Sharon Center, Grant Guilford, Dave Twedt and Dr. Mike Schaer in the preparation of parts of the book.

We are indebted to the staff at W.B. Saunders, especially Linda Mills, for seeing that this project, years in preparation, finally came to fruition.

DENNY MEYER, EMBERT COLES, *and* LON RICH

PREFACE

We know that one-half of what we teach will be proved false
in ten years; the hard part is that we do not know which half.
WISE MEDICAL PEDAGOGUE

Since the mid-1950's when SGOT (now AST) was introduced as a "marker" for myocardial infarction, there has been a profuse effort to develop new tests and add to our understanding of the existing tests in order to broaden and improve the clinician's diagnostic armamentarium. We have arbitrarily restricted the material to the clinicopathologic parameters which we believe are the more useful in veterinary practice. We have, undoubtedly, forgotten to include some and omitted others. Except for the case illustrations, the book is purposely devoid of history and physical examination and assumes that clinical pathology results have already been obtained on the patient.

Our objectives are simple, yet complex: (1) to indicate the more clinically useful tests and suggest their diagnostic application and interpretation, (2) provide differential diagnostic considerations in two formats (tables and algorithms) to serve as a guide and/or quick reminder for the practitioner or student, (3) develop a quickly accessed supplement to other veterinary texts, and (4) introduce the use of the systeme international (SI) units. We wish to emphasize that "numbers" (abnormal test results) do not make a diagnosis; they should be considered as "markers" reflecting the pathophysiologic consequences of disease.

Some will criticize the use of algorithms as a mindless task which uses a restrictive maze-like structure. It is true that they cannot cover all diagnostic possibilities; however, we hope that some will perceive them as a thought-provoking pathophysiologic conduit toward a diagnosis—an adjunctive "tool" in the complex process of differential diagnoses.

It is inevitable that conversion to the use of SI units will occur soon. Our country is the final holdout. SI units are already beginning to appear in some medical journals and in veterinary articles submitted by authors outside of our country, and are being encouraged by the medical profession (N Engl J Med 1990; 323:1075–1077). To facilitate the change, which is always uncomfortable, we include a conversation table, **a table of SI normal values,** and list the clinical pathology parameters associated with case illustrations with both units. Some commercial clinical pathology laboratories already provide reports in SI units. We encourage our readers to actively request their laboratory to report values in both units and begin assessing the results with the use of the SI reference table included in this book.

We have chosen to discuss the clinical pathology parameters in the common veterinary species—dog, cat, horse, and ruminant. While the majority of the discussions are oriented to the dog and cat, species variations are emphasized, we hope, in a cohesive manner, in order to meet the broad needs of our profession. Furthermore, there is material covered in the figure legends and case discussions which is not repeated in the chapters.

It is our hope that the book facilitates the daily investigative efforts of the veterinary practitioner who must be a master of many disciplines and, by the veterinary student, is perceived as a lucid guide linking the diagnostic utility of clinical pathology to the underlying pathophysiologic consequences of disease. Achievement of this goal will be reflected by the book's placement near the "in-file" for the daily clinical pathology reports and in the pocket of the student's lab coat.

Dr. Watson: **This is indeed a mystery. What do you imagine it means?** Sherlock Holmes: **I have no data yet. It is a capital mistake to theorize before one has data. Insensibly one begins to twist facts to suit theories, instead of theories to suit facts.**

Scandal in Bohemia
DENNY MEYER

CONTENTS

Part I

General Discussions

LABORATORY TESTS CLINICAL ENZYMOLOGY

Sources of Variation

The quality and reliability of laboratory test results begin with selection and preparation of the patient, continue with collection and handling of the specimen, and terminate in an analytical report. Each step must be undertaken with care as variations from established procedures may affect results.

Patient Variables

The veterinarian should attempt to standardize sample collection by minimizing as many variables as possible.

Exercise can dramatically influence hematology results, particularly in those animals such as the horse which have a responsive spleen. Blood samples taken immediately after exercise will have an increased packed cell volume. The accelerated blood flow and stress hormones cause an increased total leukocyte count. These changes usually disappear within several hours after exercise.

If exercise is prolonged, increased activity of muscle enzymes (creatine kinase [CK], aspartate aminotransferase [AST], lactate dehydrogenase [LD]) will appear in the serum.

Emotional stress is common in animals presented to a veterinarian. They are transported from a home environment into a situation in which there are strange people, noises, smells, and other animals. Such changes can induce release of epinepherine which causes an increase in blood glucose and lymphocytes (especially in the cat) and leukocytosis as neutrophils shift from the marginal peripheral blood pool into the circulating peripheral blood pool. If the stress is accompanied by endogenous release of glucocorticoids a "stress leukogram" characterized by a mature neutrophilia, lymphopenia, and eosinopenia may be noted, especially in the dog.

Diet may also influence laboratory results. A patient should be fasted overnight (8 to 10 hours) before a sample is collected for chemical analysis. Samples collected soon after a patient (monogastric animal) has eaten may be lipemic. Such samples are difficult to analyze (as we will see later) and may have increased concentrations of glucose and lipids and affect other analytes such as a factitious increase in bilirubin. Lipemia may also predispose to *in vitro* hemolysis which causes an increase in certain enzymes such as AST and LD. Certain foods may also influence laboratory results. Pets that are fed diets consisting principally of "leftovers" often have a high serum cholesterol whereas those receiving a diet high in animal protein may have an elevated urea nitrogen.

Starvation may influence the results of serum chemistry analyses. Urea nitrogen levels may be decreased, serum albumin levels may fall, and, in horses (especially ponies), lipemia may develop.

Drugs. Some drugs directly influence laboratory results, for example, certain cephalosporins cause factitiously increased creatinine concentrations in some analytical systems, and tetracycline interferes with glucose determination. Some substances secreted in urine interfere chemically with tests on urine. Endogenously produced (dog) or exogenous administration of ascorbic acid will bias the glucose and nitrate test negatively.

Therapeutic agents given prior to sampling may alter the physiologic activity of a patient, resulting in changes in the concentration of substances being measured. For example, the administration of glucocorticoids alters total and differential leukocyte counts, may increase liver tests such as serum alkaline phosphatase (ALP) and alanine aminotransferase (ALT) activities in dogs, cause an increase in urea nitrogen, alter serum electrolytes, and affect the results of tests to detect immune-mediated diseases. Exogenous insulin administration decreases serum glucose, phosphate, and potassium concentrations. Even when one knows alterations are likely to occur, it is difficult to determine whether the change is entirely as a result of drug action or is being influenced by the disorder being evaluated.

The veterinarian should ascertian if the results are appropriate for the patient. For example, if the total bilirubin is 2.1 mg/dL (35.91 μmol/L) on a profile but no bilirubin is noted in the urine one of the results is factitious (lipemia possibly increasing the bilirubin result).

Collection and Handling the Specimen

Variations in laboratory data may be the direct result of specimen handling.

Collection

The selection of the proper container and the presence of the proper anticoagulant (if needed) must be made prior to specimen collection. The container must be identified carefully with the owner's name, pet's name, and, if the specimen is submitted to an outside laboratory, information that will identify the hospital or veterinarian submitting the sample. Some of the effects of anticoagulants on blood tests are listed in Table 1–1.

Most commercial laboratories will provide appropriate vials for blood collection, if not, the use of commercially prepared containers is recommended. Tubes containing the appropriate amount of the preferred anticoagulant are readily available for routine hematologic and biochemical examinations. Most of these tubes are evacuated and are identified by the color of their rubber stopper. Using a proper size holder, blood can be drawn directly into the tube. This is the preferred method for collection. However, many veterinarians prefer to collect blood in a syringe and transfer it into the appropriately prepared container. If this method is used, care must be taken ensure that the blood is transferred quickly from the syringe into the anticoagulant to prevent initiation of the clotting mechanism. Care must be taken to handle the blood gently in order to avoid red blood cell (RBC) destruction which might result in enough hemolysis to interfere with laboratory

TABLE 1–1. Effect of Anticoagulants on Laboratory Results[a]

Test Affected	Anticoagulants	Alteration
Differential WBC count	Heparin	Poor staining quality
Calcium	EDTA, oxalate, citrate	Decrease
Potassium	Potassium heparin	Increase
Urea nitrogen	Ammonium oxalate, ammonium heparin	Increase
Alkaline phosphatase	EDTA, oxalate, citrate	Decrease
Creatine kinase	EDTA, oxalate, citrate	Decrease
Lipase and amylase	EDTA, oxalate, citrate	Decrease
SD	EDTA, oxalate, citrate	Decrease
Glucose	Sodium fluoride	Decrease if glucose oxidase method used
LD	Oxalate	Decrease
Amylase	Sodium fluoride	Increase

[a] WBC, white blood cell; SD, sorbitol(iditol) dehydrogenase; EDTA, ethylenediaminetetraacetic acid.

determinations. Vacuum tubes should be filled until the vacuum is gone. Failure to fill purple topped tubes can result in falsely decreased packed cell volumes (PCVs) and total proteins (measured on refractometer) and invalidate the erythrocyte parameters. Overfilling predisposes to a clotted specimen.

Specimen Handling

Specimen handling is just as important as collection. The majority of the chemical analyses are conducted on the extracellular (plasma or serum) portion of the blood so that anything that enters this phase from an intracellular source may influence results. Some substances present in plasma or serum are present within blood cells in a much higher concentration. Thus if hemolysis is present as a result of RBC lysis or leakage it will influence laboratory results. The consequences of hemolysis are summarized in Table 1–2.

In vitro hemolysis may occur when blood is placed into vacuum tubes too quickly, the blood is agitated too vigorously while mixing it with anticoagulant, the blood specimen is allowed to freeze, or the blood is kept at room temperature for a long period of time or at too high an ambient temperature. Of course, *in vivo* hemolysis is a critical sign of a disease process. When hemolysis is noted, a second specimen may be *collected carefully* and the plasma in the microhematocrit tube examined after centrifugation. Since the binding capacity of haptoglobin is overwhelmed rapidly by free hemoglobin, urine collected at the same time as the suspect blood specimen can be checked for the presence of hemoglobin (occult blood positive).

Lipemia most frequently occurs in samples taken too soon after a patient (monogastric animal) has eaten. The presence of lipemia causes apparently increased concentrations of substances whose measurements are based on absorbance at the same wavelengths at which lipids absorb light. The effects of lipemia on various laboratory analyses are summarized in Table 1–3. Postprandial lipemia can be avoided by fasting patients a minimum of 6 to 12 hours (overnight) prior to sampling. Persistence of lipemia beyond 24 hours suggests an underlying metabolic disorder.

Holding samples will affect most tests. Most analytes are stable for 3 to 4 days at refrigerated temperature; exceptions are listed in Table 1–4.

TABLE 1–2.   Effect of Hemolysis on Laboratory Results[a]

Test	Effect of Hemolysis
Hematology	
RBC count	Decrease
Hemoglobin	Increased in relation to RBC count and PCV
MCHC	Increase
MCV	Decrease
Plasma protein	Increase
von Willebrand antigen	Decrease
Serum analytes	
AST	Increase
ALT	Increase
LD	Increase
CK	Increase
Amylase	Decrease
Lipase	Increase
ALP	Increase or decrease (depending on method used)
Total protein	Increase
Albumin	Increase
Calcium	Increase (cresolphthalein complex method)
Phosphorus	Increase
Creatinine	No change/increase (Jaffe method)/decrease (depends on method)
Potassium	Increase (horse, cow, Akita dog)
Bilirubin	Slight increase

[a] Effects may vary according to the method used in the analysis and the severity of the hemolysis. Each laboratory should establish the effect of hemolysis on the results of chemical analysis. MCHC, mean cell hemoglobin concentration; MCV, mean cell volume.

TABLE 1–3.   The Effects of Lipemia on Laboratory Results

Test	Change Caused by Lipemia
Hematology	
Hemoglobin	Increase
MCHC	Increase
Plasma protein (refractometer)	Increase
Serum chemistry	
Enzymes	
Amylase	Decrease in severe lipemia
Other analytes	
Albumin	Decrease
Total protein	Decrease
Calcium	Increase
Glucose	Increase
Phosphorus	Increase
Bilirubin	Increase
Potassium, sodium, chloride	Decrease if method involves dilution

TABLE 1-4. Constituent Stability[a]

Constituent	Temperature	Stability and Other Conditions
ACTH	Ice immediately	Must be collected in cold and kept frozen
Ammonia	Use lithium heparin, store at 4° C	Values increase on standing, lithium heparin will prevent some changes Best assayed within 2 hr, hold in crushed ice
Bilirubin	In dark	Stable if not exposed to ultraviolet light; short exposure ultraviolet causes degradation
	24° C	In dark, stable for 2 days
	4° C	In dark, stable for 4–7 days
Carbon dioxide (total)	24° C in air	Significant drop in 1 hr
	24° C in stoppered tube	No significant loss for 12 hr
Creatine kinase	24° C	Rapid loss after 2–4 hr
	4° C	12 hr
Glucose	24° C	Rapid decrease (7% hr); this loss increased by presence of leukocytosis or erythrocytosis. Can be prevented by use of impermeable separator tube that is centrifuged as soon as possible after collection. Stable in sterile cell-free serum or plasma but drops rapidly if any bacterial growth.
	24° C in NaF	Sodium fluoride tube, stable for 8 hr
	4° C	Some loss but not as great as at room temperature
	4° C in NaF	Sodium fluoride tube, stable for 3 days
Insulin	Ice immediately	Must be collected in cold and maintained frozen if possible
Potassium	4° C	Increase in species with high K^+ in RBC (horse, cow, Akita breed of dog
	24° C	No change in 8–12 hr if serum separated from RBC; rapid increase in animals with high RBC potassium concentration
Sorbitol(iditol) dehydrogenase	24° C	Unstable
	4° C	Relatively stable for 24 hr
Complete blood count	24 or 4° C	Stable for 24 hours
MCV	24 or 4° C	Tends to increase with time
MCHC	24 or 4° C	Tends to decrease with time
Platelet count	24 °C	5 hr
	4° C	24 hr

[a] Most routine analytes are stable at refrigerated temperature for at least 3–4 days. The exceptions are listed in this table. ACTH, adrenocorticotropic hormone.

PRINCIPLES OF ENZYMOLOGY

For the past several decades, serum enzymes have been measured to diagnose, monitor, and prognose the disease process. Despite our familiarity with the empirical clinical use of serum enzymes, the pathophysiologic reasons for the observed changes are poorly understood. Further studies to determine the manner in which the serum changes reflect disturbances in organs, cells, and subcellular organelles will result in more meaningful diagnostic interpretation.

Location of Enzyme in Cell

The location within the cell impacts on the release of the enzyme into the blood (Fig. 1–1 and Table 1–5). *Cytoplasmic* enzymes are usually soluble, easily re-

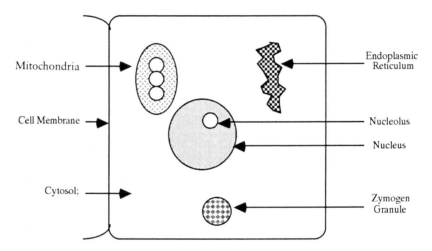

FIGURE 1–1. Cellular components involved in enzyme production and escape.

TABLE 1–5[1]. **Distribution in the Cell of Some Clinically Used Enzymes**

Cellular Location	Enzyme
Cytoplasm	ALT
	AST_1 (cytosolic isoenzyme)
	SD
	CK (isoenzymes 1–3)
	LD (isoenzymes 1–5)
Mitochondria	AST_2 (mitochondrial isoenzyme)
Endoplasmic reticulum	GGT
Membrane	ALP
	GGT
Zymogen (intracytoplasmic) granules	Amylase
	Lipase
	Immunoreactive trypsin

(Boyd, J. W.: The mechanism relating to increases in plasma enzymes and isoenzymes in disease in animals. Vet. Clin. Pathol., 12: 9–24, 1982.)

leased, and readily pass through the cell membrane (even when it appears microscopically intact). This property makes them *sensitive* diagnostic markers. *Mitochondrial* enzymes usually appear in blood after a *severe* insult since they are attached and must cross two or more membranes. *Lysosomal* enzymes are attached to intracellular granules and appear in the blood only after the organelle is injured. They usually have a greater rate of autodigestion as well. *Membrane enzymes* are not soluble, are firmly attached to the cell membrane, and may be shed after severe damage. However, their appearance in the blood usually follows a stimulation for *increased production*.

Factors Affecting Enzyme Activity in the Serum

The intracellular enzyme activity is usually thousands of times greater than in the serum. The "normal" serum enzyme activity probably reflects a balance between physiologic cell death (release) and degradation/inactivation by the macrophage system or, less commonly, excretion. Cell regeneration may also contribute to the enzyme activity in serum. The released enzyme usually passes into the interstitial fluid and then into the lymphatics before appearing in the blood; this is a complex series of events.

When there is tissue injury there is increased release of some enzymes. The *magnitude* of increase is dependent on several factors: the tissue concentration of the enzyme (which is *tissue and species variable*) (Table 1–6), the cellular location of the enzyme (Table 1–5), the amount of tissue injured, the type of tissue injury, and the rate of enzyme removal from the serum (Fig. 1–2). Injury may range from overt cell death (damaged membrane and organelles) to metabolic alterations without microscopically visible cell changes. For example, in the case of an acute anemia or heart failure, anoxia may cause the hepatocellular membrane to become "leaky" while remaining viable. The serum enzyme is a useful marker of tissue injury as long as the etiologic agent or resulting pathologic process does not damage or destroy the enzyme.

Most increases in serum enzyme activity appear to be the result of an increased release of the highly concentrated tissue enzyme; followed by an increased pro-

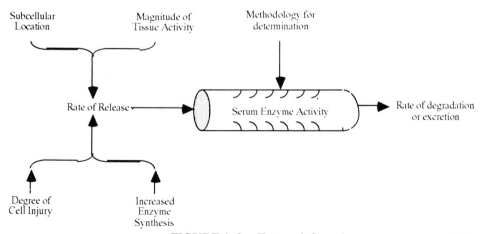

FIGURE 1–2. Factors influencing serum enzyme activity.

TABLE 1–6.   Enzyme Activities in Tissues

Enzyme	Dog	Cat	Horse	Cow	Pig
Alanine aminotransferase			IU/g		
Liver	32	29.8	0.9	0.3	0.9
Heart	8.7	1.4	1.7	1.7	3.1
Muscle	1.8	1.0	4.4	2.0	1.3
Kidney	2.9	3.7	0.4	0.3	0.5
Intestine	0.4	0.5	0.03	0.3	
Pancreas	1.5	0.9	0.7		
Sorbitol dehydrogenase					
Liver	11.7	0.60	5.2	9.7	9.5
Heart	1.0	0.20	0.2	0.1	0.00
Muscle	0.4	0.05	0.0	0.1	0.03
Kidney	6.5	0.10	1.0	3.0	3.70
Intestine	0.7	0.04	0.1	0.4	0.20
Pancreas	0.4	0.06	0.2		0.00
Glutamate dehydrogenase					
Liver	6.8	125	10.4	19.0	1.3
Heart	2.3	10.0	0.1	2.1	0.1
Muscle	0.6	2.0	0.1	0.7	0.01
Kidney	5.1	40	0.7	8.5	0.3
Intestine	2.0	3.0		1.2	
Pancreas	0.5		0.3		
Aspartate aminotransferase					
Liver	53	59	33	70	57
Heart	67	69	32	48	115
Muscle	46	22	54	70	44
Kidney	24	17	7	30	47
Intestine	12	7	6	6	
Pancreas	22	10			
Lactate dehydrogenase					
Liver	130	127	82	57	25
Heart	320	89	354	97	60
Muscle	169	259	155	336	591
Kidney	256	40	122	69	30
Intestine	58	47	18	20	29
Pancreas	52	16	52		12
Creatine kinase					
Liver	50	1	7		
Heart	1150	518	1710		
Muscle	2500	692	4300		
Kidney	50	1	97		
Intestine	200	20	254		
Pancreas		15			
Alkaline phosphatase					
Liver	0.3	0.30	0.74	0.09	0.3
Heart	0.8	0.05	0.07	0.01	0.1
Muscle	0.1	0.05	0.10	0.02	0.1
Kidney	6.4	3.79	10.20	0.80	13.0
Intestine	220	7.98	2.24		10.1
Pancreas	1.3	0.19	2.15	0.07	
γ-Glutamyltransferase					
Liver	0.90		2.40	4.97	2.69
Heart			0.12	0.31	0.02
Muscle	0.00		0.28	0.01	0.02
Kidney	86.10		38.66	60.50	16.45
Intestine	1.50		0.59	0.59	1.47
Pancreas	41.70		6.80	22.18	8.58

(Boyd, J. W.: The mechanism relating to increases in plasma enzymes and isoenzymes in disease in animals. Vet. Clin. Pathol., 21: 9–24, 1982.)

duction during the reparative process subsequently contributing to the serum enzyme activity. However, certain enzymes (most notable hepatic ALP and γ-glutamyltransferase [GGT]) are present in very low tissue concentration. Their increased serum activity is associated with an increased tissue synthesis secondary to a stimulus. There are two stimuli most commonly involved in the induction of the *de novo* protein synthesis: impaired bile flow and drugs/hormones.

Enzyme activity is determined indirectly, as opposed to the direct measurement of enzyme mass, primarily through the use of kinetic assays. These reactions are affected by a number of factors such as temperature, pH, substrate concentration, cofactors, inhibitors, and reagent stability. Consequently, the serum enzyme activity value may vary between laboratories assaying the same serum sample. The determination of a normal reference range for enzymes must be done for every laboratory. Furthermore, the reference range should be validated periodically since the laboratory may change methodology.

Different molecular forms of the same enzyme occur for some enzymes. These *isoenzymes* or *isozymes* have different physical and chemical properties. Separation of isozymes is usually performed by electrophoresis based on their differences in charge; however, the recent development of immunoprecipitation methodologies provides greater specificity and speed. Since certain isozymes are unique or in greater concentration in a particular tissue, they offer the potential for increased diagnostic sensitivity.

2

ERYTHROCYTIC TESTS
AND DISTURBANCES*

Production of the formed elements of blood proceeds in an orderly fashion in which production equals utilization plus loss. A disorder that accelerates cell utilization and/or destruction or which impairs production will result in changes in the cellular elements in peripheral blood. Figure 2–1 provides an overview of hematopoiesis.

The following two chapters are designed to review briefly the factors that influence cell counts and morphology.

PRODUCTION

Erythrocyte production (Fig. 2–2) is regulated by erythropoietin, a hormone that is secreted by the kidney (Fig. 2–3). The bone marrow can increase its rate of production as much as six to eight-fold. The magnitude of this stimulation as reflected by changes in the peripheral blood may take 48 to 72 hours. For the marrow to respond there must be an adequate supply of protein, iron, copper, cobalt, and certain vitamins. A deficiency in one or more of these nutrients may be manifested clinically by an impaired erythrogenic response.

The destruction of senescent erythrocytes by the macrophage system is a continual process. In humans it is estimated that two to three million erythrocytes per second are removed, an enormous metabolic load. After erythrocytes are removed from the blood the hemoglobin is metabolized into iron, globin, and bilirubin. Iron is stored temporarily for reuse, globin goes to the amino acid pool, and bilirubin is excreted by the liver (Fig. 2–4). One manifestation of accelerated erythrocyte destruction can be jaundice as a result of increased bilirubin production.

EVALUATION OF ERYTHROCYTES

The erythron (circulating red blood cells [RBCs] plus marrow erythropoiesis) is evaluated by determining the number of RBC per μL of blood, the hemoglobin content (g/dL), the packed cell volume (per cent) and using this information to calculate mean cell volume (MCV) and mean cell hemoglobin concentration (MCHC). Since the packed cell volume (PCV), RBC count, and hemoglobin concentration generally parallel each other with change, the PCV is the pragmatic

---

* See Algorithms 1, 2, and 3.

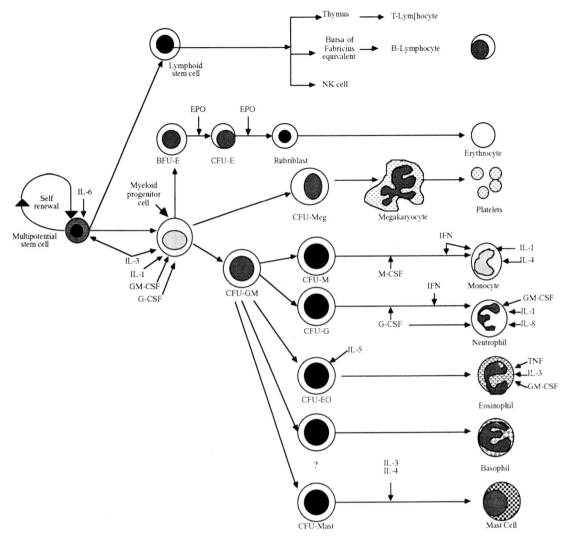

FIGURE 2–1. Cytokines and hematopoietic development. A self-renewing multi-potential stem cell gives rise to a myeloid stem cell and a lymphoid stem cell. The latter circulates either to the thymus or to the bursa of Fabricius equivalent for committed development to either a T-lymphocyte or a B-lymphocyte, respectively. The circulating lymphoid cell without T- or B-markers is referred to as an NK cell. The myeloid stem cell gives rise to a number of committed stem cells including the megakaryocyte colony forming unit (*CFU-MeG*), the precursor of platelet formation. The erythroid burst forming unit (*BFU-E*) differentiates into the erythroid colony-forming unit (*CFU-E*) giving rise to the erythroid series; both BFU-E and CFU-E are influenced by erythropoietin (*EPO*). The granulocyte/macrophage colony forming unit (*CFU/GM*) differentiates further into the granulocyte colony forming unit (*CFU-G*) and macrophage colony forming unit (*CFU-M*) with the ultimate development of neutrophils and monocytes, respectively. The myeloid stem cell appears also to form committed stem cells for eosinophils, identified as the eosinophil colony forming unit (*CFU-EO*), mast cells, identified as mast cell colony forming unit (*CFU-Mast*), and basophils. The influence of cytokines, interleukins (*IL*), and colony stimulating factors (*CSF*) on hematopoiesis and cell function is indicated. The differentiation of the multipotential cell into the myeloid stem cell is stimulated by IL-3 and IL-6. Further differentiation into selected cell lines is facilitated by GM-CSF (granulocyte/macrophage), G-CSF (granulocyte), IL-1, and IL-3. Interferon (*INF*) and G-CSF stimulate the development of neutrophil with IL-1 and IL-9 activating the mature neutrophil. Monocyte development is stimulated by M-CSF (macrophage) and interferon whereas IFN, IL-1, and IL-4 affect the mature monocyte/macrophage. Eosinophil development is enhanced by IL-5 while the mature cell is activated by IL-3, GM-CSF, and tumor necrosis factor (*TNF*). Mast cell development is facilitated by IL-4 and IL-3.

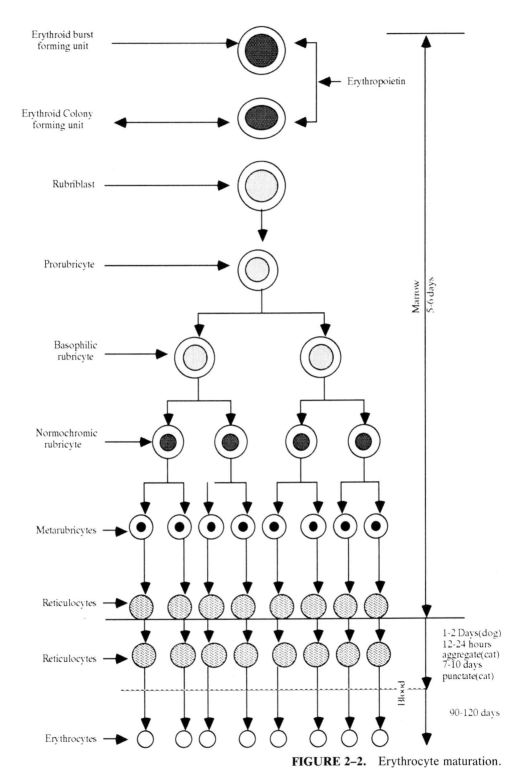

FIGURE 2–2. Erythrocyte maturation.

15

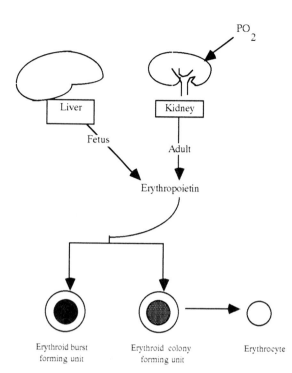

FIGURE 2–3. Erythropoietin is formed by the liver in the fetus and by the kidney in the adult. Renal tubule/peritubular tissue sensitive to the partial pressure of oxygen is the stimulus of erythropoietin production.

choice clinically. The routine reporting of all three parameters is traditional because the RBC count and hemoglobin concentration are determined to calculate the erythrocyte indices. Adjunct information is gained by evaluating the morphology of the erythrocytes on a stained blood film and by a reticulocyte count. Additional information relative to the interpretation of the PCV can be obtained by comparing it with the plasma protein concentration (Table 2–1).

Measurement of Cell Numbers, Size, and Hemoglobin Content

The most common method for determining PCV is with the microhematocrit centrifuge. Previously published normal values for PCV, MCV, and MCHC are based on a spun hematocrit. Modern automated counters, however, calculate PCV (hematocrit-Hct) based on total erythrocyte count and the erythrocyte size as measured electronically. These electronic measurements avoid the problem of trapped plasma in the column of packed RBCs, and as a consequence, the spun PCV will be 1 to 3% higher. Normal values for each species should be established for the particular automatic cell counter being used.

Total erythrocyte counts are accurate if counted electronically. These techniques are, however, subject to error unless the laboratory has adjusted its counter to accommodate the variable sized erythrocytes of animals. With the exception of the dog, erythrocytes are smaller in animals than in the human. Electronic counters adjusted for human blood may err in evaluating animal RBC numbers, determination of the MCV, and consequently the calculated PCV.

The MCV and the MCHC are the most clinically useful erythrocyte indices. The MCV refers to cell size which may be normal (*normocytic*), smaller than normal (*microcytic*), or larger than normal (*macrocytic*). The MCHC is the average con-

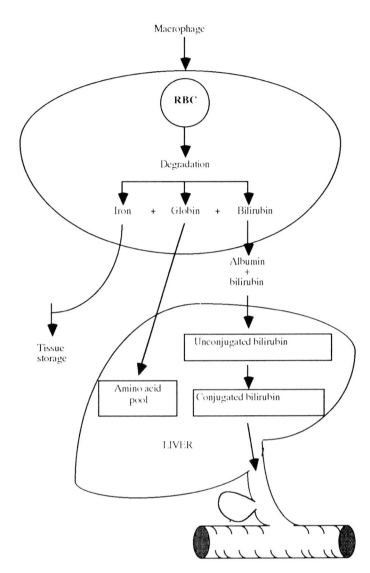

FIGURE 2–4. RBC destruction occurs in the macrophage, in which it is cleaved into iron, globin, and bilirubin. Bilirubin combines with albumin in the plasma and is carried to the liver, in which it is conjugated and eliminated into the biliary system. Other products of erythrocyte metabolism join the body reserves for reuse.

centration of hemoglobin in a given volume of packed erythrocytes. Normal values are referred to as *normochromic* and, if less than normal, *hypochromic*. Erythrocytes cannot be produced with increased hemoglobin content. Since an MCHC greater than normal is physiologically impossible, an increased value is always an *artifact*. Free hemoglobin, lipemia, or Heinz bodies are the most common causes. *Erythrocyte indices can be used as one means to classify anemia. It should be emphasized that erythrocyte indices are crude markers of erythrocyte change and, when abnormal, direct further investigation.*

The red cell distribution width (RDW) is an electronically calculated parameter available on some laser cell counters. The RDW can be thought of as a numeric representation of erythrocyte anisocytosis. It is a much more sensitive reflection of erythrocyte volume variation than visual inspection for size variation of erythrocytes on a blood smear. An *increased* RDW indicates the presence of an increased number of an erythrocyte subpopulation: larger, smaller, or a combination. If the printout representing the bell-shaped erythrogram is viewed, a *shift to*

TABLE 2–1. Relationship Between Packed Cell Volume and Plasma Protein

Packed Cell Volume	Plasma Protein	Interpretation
Increased	Increased	Dehydration
	Normal	Splenic contraction (especially horse Primary or secondary polycythemia Dehydration masked by hypoproteinemia
	Decreased	Hypoproteinemia with splenic contraction
Normal	Increased	Anemia masked by dehydration Increased globulins
	Normal	Normal
	Decreased	Increased protein loss (kidney, gastrointestinal tract) Decreased production (liver disease)
Decreased	Increased	Anemia associated with dehydration
	Normal	Increased RBC destruction Decreased RBC production Chronic blood loss (iron deficiency)
	Decreased	Overhydration External blood loss

the right indicates a subpopulation of larger erythrocytes, for example, macrocytosis associated with a regenerative response. A *shift to the left* indicates a subpopulation of smaller erythrocytes, for example, microcytosis secondary to iron deficiency. Since the MCV is related to the RDW, an increased MCV may be noted in the former example and a decreased MCV in the latter. However, since the RDW is a more sensitive reflection of erythrocyte volume variability, the MCV could still be in the normal range when the RDW is abnormal in the two examples given. Therefore, the combined use of the RDW and MCV can be helpful in classifying anemia numerically. This can be particularly valuable in assessing a regenerative response in the horse since a reticulocytosis does not develop.

Hemoglobin is determined spectrophotometrically and will provide an accurate estimation of hemoglobin concentration. The determination is affected by substances that are not lysed by the hemoglobin reagent or which increase the optical density causing a factitiously high hemoglobin value. Lipemia and the presence of

Heinz bodies are common causes. Hemolysis *in vivo* or *in vitro* will increase the total hemoglobin value of a sample as well as the MCHC value. A rule of thumb is that hemoglobin value is approximately *one third of the PCV*.

Erythrocyte Morphology

Erythrocyte morphology is assessed by microscopic examination of a blood film. The more common abnormalities detected include anisocytosis (variation in size), poikilocytosis (variation in shape), variation in tinctoral properties) (polychromasia and hypochromia), and the presence of erythrocyte inclusions and infectious agents (Table 2–2).

Anisocytosis occurs to a small degree in almost all species of domestic animals but is most common in normal cattle blood. Anisocytosis will be accentuated in animals with a regenerative anemia when immature macrocytic RBCs (polychromatophils) are being released into the blood. Conversely, a microcytosis secondary to iron deficiency will also give an overall impression of anisocytosis. However, the MCV tends to be increased in the first example and decreased in the latter.

Reticulocytes are commonly demonstrated by incubating blood with new methylene blue. Reticulocytes in most species have an aggregate staining pattern. However, two types of reticulocyte patterns have been identified in the cat and are referred to as *punctate* and *aggregate*. Punctate cells are thought to represent those that have been in the blood for some time (delayed maturation) whereas the aggregate are those that have been most recently released. *Feline aggregate reticulocytes are the best indicator of erythrogenesis* whereas punctate reticulocytes

TABLE 2–2. Morphologic Abnormalities of Erythrocytes

Acanthocytes: Erythrocytes in which the cell membrane forms spike-like projections
Anisocytosis: Variation (heterogeneity) of erythrocyte size
Basophilic stippling: Fine bluish inclusions scattered throughout cytoplasm of erythrocyte
Double population: Coexistence of two erythrocyte populations on same smear (e.g., normochromic and hypochromic cells)
Elliptocytes: Erythrocytes of oval or elliptic shape
Heinz bodies: Hemoglobin precipitates visible in fresh blood by phase microscopy or by supravital staining
Howell-Jolly bodies: Chromatin residues in polychromatic or normochromic erythrocytes
Hypochromia: Erythrocytes with decreased hemoglobin content and decreased staining intensity
Leptocyte (target cells): Cells with "Mexican hat" or "bull's-eye" appearance
Macrocytosis: Erythrocytes with increased volume and diameter
Microcytosis: Erythrocytes with decreased volume and diameter
Normochromia: Normal color intensity on a Romanowsky stain
Normocytes: Erythrocytes that are normal in size and shape
Poikilocytosis: Variation in erythrocyte shape on the same blood film
Polychromasia: Variation in staining color of erythrocytes on the same blood film (cells that stain bluish or purple represent RNA-rich cells)
Schizocytes: Fragmented erythrocytes of varied size and shape (usually angular in appearance)
Spherocytes (dogs only): Small erythrocytes of spherical shape and lacking normal central pallor (homogeneous staining of cells)

suggest a response weeks earlier (see Cases 7 and 8). Reticulocytes are not found in the blood of healthy horses, sheep, goats, or cows. A maximum of 0.5 to 1.0% of aggregate reticulocytes may be present in the blood of the healthy cat and dog, respectively. In the pig there may be up to 2% reticulocytes. Aggregate reticulocytes may be recognized in blood films by their larger size and polychromatophilic staining characteristics with Romanowsky stains. If present in large enough numbers the MCV will increase indicating macrocytosis.

The reticulocyte count should be corrected for the degree of anemia. The correction can be done in two ways:

$$\text{Corrected \% reticulocytes} = \text{\% reticulocytes} \times \frac{\text{patient's PCV}}{\text{normal PCV [45 = dog, 37 = cat]}}$$

or

$$\text{Absolute reticulocyte count}/\mu L = \text{\% reticulocytes} \times \text{patient's RBC count.}$$

For example, a dog has a PCV of 28, RBC count of $4.4 \times 10^6/\mu L$, and reticulocyte count of 15%, the formulas would be

$$\text{Corrected \% reticulocytes} = 15\% \times \frac{28}{45} = 9.3\%$$

or

$$\text{Absolute reticulocytes}/\mu L = 15\% \times 4.4 \times 10^6 = 660,000/\mu L.$$

In humans, it has been shown that with the increasing severity of an anemia, the immaturity of the reticulocytes released increases, and they remain in the circulation longer as reticulocytes. Correction factors have been developed to account for this phenomenon. Although some veterinary authors have empirically applied identical correction factors to the dog, there has been no validation of their applicability. We feel that one correction method should be used consistently, and we recommend the absolute reticulocyte count at this time.

Basophilic stippling is characterized by the presence of punctate aggregations of dark blue staining material in Romanowsky-stained erythrocytes. Basophilic stippling may be seen in responsive anemias of cattle and sheep and occasionally in cats. Basophilic stippling also occurs in most animals with lead poisoning, sometimes in association with nucleated erythrocytes out of proportion to the degree of anemia.

Howell-Jolly bodies, remnants of nuclear material, appear as single or multiple bluish spheric bodies of varying size and location within the cell in Romanowsky-stained smears. These bodies commonly appear in responsive anemia and in patients without a spleen. About 1% of the erythrocytes of cats normally have an eccentric Howell-Jolly body. They are occasionally seen in normal dog blood and are common in young pigs to 3 months of age.

Heinz bodies are small round inclusions within an erythrocyte and represent oxidized hemoglobin. They are not readily visible in Romanowsky-stained preparations but are easily identified with reticulocyte stains and new methylene blue wet preparations. Although healthy cats may have up to 10% Heinz bodies, some cats with gastrointestinal disease or fed semimoist food have been observed to have increased numbers of Heinz bodies. Certain hemolytic anemias produced by agents toxic to erythrocytes cause Heinz body formation; phenothiazine, onions, kale, methylene blue, and acetaminophen have been reported in cats and in dogs receiving daily doses of prednisolone. Heinz bodies should be suspected in animals with high MCHC values when hemolysis or lipemia is not present (see Case 8).

Nucleated erythrocytes (NRBC) are rarely observed normally in any species of domestic animal with exception of the suckling pig up to 3 months of age. If there has been an excessive demand for erythrocyte regeneration, NRBC may appear. Release of NRBC from the marrow may also occur after an anoxic insult or in association with toxemia or myelophthisic disorders. Nucleated erythrocytes may be noted in dogs with hemangiosarcoma, lead toxicity, and inflammatory liver disease. Some miniature schnauzers and dachshunds with no evidence of underlying disease have been observed to have NRBC in the peripheral blood.

A *leukoerythroblastic reaction* has been described in the dog. It is characterized by the presence of NRBC and immature myeloid cells in the peripheral blood. There is usually a leukocytosis, but anemia may be variable. The significance is not well established.

ANEMIA

Anemia occurs because of excessive blood loss (hemorrhage) or destruction (hemolysis) or decreased erythrocyte production.

The causes of an anemia are summarized in Table 2–3.

Classification of Anemia

Stage of Regeneration

Regeneration is indicated by reticulocytosis (polychromasia). Anemias resulting from increased RBC destruction show a more dramatic reticulocytosis than blood loss anemias of equal severity. The horse is an exception because reticulocytes are not released from the marrow. At this time, sequential PCVs or bone marrow examination is the only practical way to confirm a regenerative anemia in the horse. An increased MCV is occasionally noted in some equine responsive anemias.

Morphology

Anemias may be classified with erythrocyte indices. The terms used for size are *normocytic* (normal), *macrocytic* (larger) or *microcytic* (smaller) and for hemoglobin-related tinctoral properties are *normochromic* (normal) or *hypochromic* (pale). For all practical purposes anemias are not classified as hyperchromic. Morphologic and etiologic classifications of anemia are compared in Table 2–4.

Diagnosis of Causes of Anemia

Blood Loss Anemia

Blood loss anemias may be acute or chronic.

Acute. Initially (within hours) all laboratory findings remain normal as blood elements and plasma are lost in equal proportion. If there is splenic contraction

TABLE 2–3. Causes of Anemia

Responsive Anemias

Acute blood loss
1. Trauma
2. Ulcers of the gastrointestinal tract
3. Primary hemostatic defects
4. Ingestion of substances that result in a hemostatic defect (warfarin, moldy sweet clover, bracken fern)

Chronic blood loss
1. Parasitism (fleas, hookworms, coccidiosis, strongylosis)
2. Ulcers (especially secondary to neoplasia) of the gastrointestinal tract and hematuria
3. Thrombocytopenia
4. Vitamin K deficiency

Hemolytic anemia
   Intravascular destruction of erythrocytes
1. Immune-mediated RBC destruction
2. Erythrocyte parasites such as *Babesia* sp.
3. Bacterial infections such as leptospirosis, *Clostridium perfringens* type A, and *Clostridium hemolyticum*
4. Chemicals (phenothiazine, onions, kale, methylene blue)
   Extravascular destruction of erythrocytes
1. Immune-mediated RBC destruction
2. Parasites of the RBC such as *Anaplasma* sp., *Haemobartonella* sp., *Eperythrozoon* sp., *Trypanosoma* sp.
3. Pyruvate kinase deficiency, phosphofructose kinase deficiency, porphyria, hereditary stomatocytosis, and with drug sensitivities
4. Disseminated intravascular coagulation in which fragmented erythrocytes are removed by the reticuloendothelial system

Poorly Responsive Anemias

Reduced erythropoiesis
1. Lack of erythropoietin as in renal disease
2. Endocrine diseases (hypopituitarism, hypothyroidism, hypoadrenocorticism, hyperestrogenism)
3. Chronic disease (inflammation, neoplasia)
4. Myelophthisis (granulocytic leukemia, lymphocytic leukemia, metastatic neoplasia, myelofibrosis)
5. Cytotoxic damage to the marrow (bracken fern poisoning, leukemia chemotherapy, radiation)
6. Infections (feline leukemia virus, feline immunosuppressive virus, panleukopenia virus, parvovirus, *Ehrlichia canis,* trichostrongyles (non-blood sucking)

Defective erythropoiesis
1. Deficiencies that interfere with synthesis of heme (iron, copper, pyridoxine) and lead poisoning
2. Abnormal maturation as with erythremic myelosis and erythroleukemia
3. Drugs such as estrogens, phenylbutazone, meclofenamic acid, trimethoprim-sulfadiazine, fenbenadole, quinidine, and chloramphenicol (cats)

there may be a temporary increase in PCV. As blood volume is restored by fluids entering the vascular system the PCV, hemoglobin, and RBC counts decrease. Hypoproteinemia (albumin and globulin both decreased) may be present, and its severity will depend upon the quantity of blood lost. Polychromasia and reticulocytosis occur in 48 to 72 hours. If polychromasia/reticulocytosis persist and the PCV does not gradually increase, one should suspect continued loss.

Chronic. Blood loss is gradual, and there is no hypovolemia. Hypoproteinemia may be present, and initially there is a mild reticulocytosis. If chronic blood loss is external, iron stores will be progressively depleted, and eventually erythro-

TABLE 2–4. **Comparison of the Morphologic and Etiologic Classifications of Anemia**

Morphologic Classification	Etiologic Classification

Normocytic normochromic	Depression of erythrogenesis
	  Chronic inflammation
	  Chronic renal insufficiency
	  Endocrine deficiencies
	  Neoplasia
	  Marrow hypoplasia as with bracken fern poisoning, radiation, ehrlichiosis, chloramphenicol toxicity, excess estrogens, phenylbutazone
	  Acute hemorrhage after fluid volume has been restored and before regeneration occurs
	  Feline leukemia virus infection
	  Early (days to weeks) iron deficiency

Macrocytic normochromic (no reticulocytosis)	Dietary deficiencies a. Cobalt deficiency in ruminants Poodle macrocytosis (healthy miniature poodles, no anemia) Feline leukemia virus-related dyscrasias (no reticulocytosis) Regenerative anemias
Macrocytic hypochromic	Markedly responsive anemias (with reticulocytosis)

Microcytic normochromic/hypochromic	Iron deficiencies (months)
	  Lack of dietary iron
	  Chronic blood loss to exterior (mild reticulocytosis may be initially present)
	Defect in utilization of iron stores
	  Copper deficiency
	  Molybdenum poisoning
	Congenital portosystemic shunts (may not be anemic)

cyte parameters change (takes weeks to months). At first, the parameters are normocytic/normochromic with a mild reticulocytosis. Then the erythrocytes become microcytic/normochromic with a mild reticulocytosis (see Case 9). The combination of *microcytosis plus mild reticulocytosis* should stimulate investigation for gastrointestinal ulceration, especially secondary to leiomyosarcoma and blood-sucking parasites. Eventually the reticulocytosis dissipates, and the parameters progress to microcytic/hypochromic. If chronic blood loss has been within tissues or into a body cavity, such as with a hemangiosarcoma, iron will be recycled, and the erythrocyte parameters are usually normocytic and normochromic with a mild reticulocytosis.

Hemolytic Anemia (Responsive)

Hemolytic anemias are usually reflected by a moderate to marked reticulocytosis and macrocytic/normochromic to macrocytic/hypochromic erythrocyte parameters (see Case 3). Remember that it takes at least several days for changes in these indices to become apparent.

Intravascular Destruction.   Anemias resulting from intravascular destruction are of sudden onset and are characterized by hemoglobinemia and hemoglobinuria and, if severe enough, icterus. A search for the cause of intravascular destruction should include examination of blood films for parasites and Heinz bodies, and a direct Coombs' test (see Cases 7 and 8). Spherocytes may be observed in the dog if the anemia is immune mediated, and within 2 to 3 days there is a dramatic regenerative response in most cases. A concomitant leukocytosis with a left shift may develop (see Cases 3 and 5).

Extravascular Destruction.   In the dog extravascular destruction is more common than intravascular and usually is less dramatic in onset. Blood films should be examined for spherocytes, a direct Coombs' test is indicated, and, if there is erythrocyte fragmentation disseminated intravascular coagulation should be ruled out (see Case 25).

There is an immune-mediated, occasionally Coombs'-positive, poorly responsive anemia in which erythrocyte precursors are phagocytized in the bone marrow. This variant may be detected when a bone marrow examination is performed to investigate a poorly responsive anemia (see Case 4).

Most blood parasite-induced hemolytic anemias are the result of extravascular RBC destruction and in the cat with haemobartonellosis may be Coombs' positive (see Case 7).

Poor Responsive (Nonresponsive) Anemia, Ineffective Erythropoiesis

There are numerous causes of poorly (non)regenerative anemias. Potential bone marrow insults include neoplasia, antibiotics, chemicals, radiation, ehrlichiosis, myelofibrosis, hyperestrogenism, feline panleukopenia virus infection, feline leukemia virus, and feline immunodeficiency virus infection. The feline leukemia virus can cause a unique poorly responsive anemia characterized by macrocytic/normocytic erythrocyte parameters with no reticulocytosis (polychromasia) (see Case 6). A macrocytic normochromic ineffective erythropoiesis secondary to vitamin B_{12} and folic acid deficiencies occurs in humans but has not been documented in domestic animals even though folate deficiency may occur secondary to chronic malabsorption diseases. Poorly regenerative anemia accompanied by abnormal morphology of the erythrocytes occurs with myelodysplasia, erythremic myelosis, and erythroleukemia and is most common in cats (see Case 1).

ERYTHROCYTOSIS (POLYCYTHEMIA)

Erythrocytosis (polycythemia) refers to an increase in the PCV (hematocrit) out of the reference range. The erythrocyte count and hemoglobin concentration will, by default, parallel the PCV value and provide no additional information in the differential diagnosis. Likewise, the erythrocyte indices do not contribute to the differential considerations. The approach to the differential diagnosis of erythrocytosis is to consider first whether the disorder is absolute or relative.

Absolute erythrocytosis refers to an accelerated production of erythrocytes by the bone marrow. Increased erythrogenesis may or may not be erythropoietin driven, and this difference can be used to divide the absolute classification further into primary and secondary erythrocytosis. *Primary erythrocytosis* (formerly polycythemia vera) results from an autonomous (erythropoietin-independent) proliferation of erythroid precursors; consequently, it is considered a myeloproliferative disease. As expected, plasma erythropoietin concentrations in this uncommon disorder are depressed or undetectable. *Secondary erythrocytosis* is stimulated by an increased concentration of erythropoietin. Therefore, the plasma erythropoietin concentration is increased. The differential considerations for secondary erythrocytosis can be subdivided into causes of increased erythropoietin production which are physiologically *appropriate* or *inappropriate*. Hypoxia, resulting from cardiac insufficiency or chronic pulmonary disease, is the most common physiologic drive of an appropriate acceleration of erythropoietin production. Congenital methemoglobinemia may also cause an increased PCV as an appropriate response to the decreased oxygen carrying capacity of the ferric state of methemoglobin. Dark colored blood and cyanotic mucous membranes in an apparently healthy patient are indicative of the disorder. An inappropriate accelerated production of erythropoietin has been associated with renal neoplasia-carcinoma, lymphosarcoma, fibrosarcoma; extrarenal fibrosarcoma (nasal, pulmonary); and nonneoplastic renal pathology (cysts, hydronephrosis). The plasma protein concentration is usually normal attendant to the increased PCV of absolute erythrocytosis.

Relative erythrocytosis, the most common cause for an increased PCV, results from a decrease in the fluid compartment of blood, for example, secondary to dehydration. The plasma protein concentration is usually *increased* in parallel to the increased PCV resulting from the relative erythrocytosis unless there is a concurrent protein-losing pathologic process. Acute splenic contraction, usually an epinepherine-driven event (excitement) will "inject" a concentrated volume of blood PCV (approximately 80%) into the peripheral circulation. However, this cause for a temporary increase in the PCV (hours) is uncommon in a clinical situation, the potential being greatest in the "hot-blooded" horse because of the relatively large smooth muscle component of the spleen of the species. The plasma protein does not parallel the increase in the PCV after splenic contraction.

The *approach* for the differential diagnosis of erythrocytosis is usually a process of elimination. Cytologic/histologic examinations of the bone marrow are not helpful. Remembering that common things occur commonly, one should first broach relative erythrocytosis by considering the hydration status of the patient and noting a decrease in the PCV *and* the plasma protein concentration subsequent to the appropriate administration of intravenous fluids. In certain diseases, such as acute hemorrhagic gastroenteritis, the return of the PCV to normal may be accompanied by a notable hypoproteinemia, the protein-losing process masked by the dehydration.

The persistence of an increased PCV suggests absolute erythrocytosis. The erythrocyte mass can be quantitated by the use of an isotope dilution technique employing radioactive chromium. However, the procedure is restricted to research facilities. The next practical step is to measure the partial pressure of oxygen in the arterial blood. Arterial oxygen saturation less than 90% is suggestive of underlying cardiac insufficiency or pulmonary disease or both (causing physiologically appropriate increased erythropoietin production).

Normal blood gases focus the investigation toward the kidneys. Plain and contrast radiographic studies and ultrasonography are used to detect renal pathology. Negative renal studies direct the differential toward primary erythrocytosis. At this time, it is worth the effort of finding a laboratory (usually a research facility) that has a validated assay for the determination of erythropoietin. As mentioned earlier, the plasma erythropoietin concentration is decreased to not measurable in primary erythrocytosis since the accelerated production of erythrocytes is autonomous, and the resulting erythrocyte mass shuts off normal erythropoietin production.

3

LEUKOCYTIC TESTS
AND DISORDERS*

Under normal conditions production and release of leukocytes, particularly of the granulocytic series, is equal to utilization.

KINETICS AND FUNCTIONS OF LEUKOCYTES

Granulocyte Kinetics

Granulocytopoiesis progresses in an orderly fashion beginning with the myeloblast and advancing through progranulocyte → myelocyte → metamyelocyte → band → and mature granulocyte (segmenter) (Fig. 3–1). Granulocyte proliferation is stimulated by a family of glycoprotein hormones (granulopoietins, probably of macrophage origin).

Bone marrow granulocyte compartments include: (1) a stem cell pool; (2) a proliferating pool; and (3) a nonproliferating (maturation-storage) pool.

The proliferating compartment consists of myeloblasts and progranulocytes, and the nonproliferating (maturation-storage) pool is composed of metamyelocytes, bands, and segmenters. The nonproliferating granulocyte pool represents a proportionately larger component, with the segmented neutrophil the most abundant.

The production and release of granulocytes is dependent upon two factors: (1) the normal production and maturation of granulocytes; and (2) the peripheral utilization of granulocytes.

Neutrophils in the peripheral blood are either circulating or adhered to the endothelium and are referred to as the circulating granulocyte pool (CGP) and the marginated granulocyte pool (MGP), respectively. Combined these two pools are known as the total granulocyte pool (TGP). Margination facilitates tissue migration as well as providing a reserve that can be quickly released into the circulating pool. There is a continual exchange between the CGP and the MGP. The size of the marginated pool is species variable. The CGP to MGP ratio is approximately 1 : 1 for the dog and 3 : 1 for the cat.

Granulocytes have a short stay in the circulation (approximately 10 hours) and do not return from tissues. Most granulocyte loss in a healthy animal occurs in the digestive and respiratory tracts. Components of the complement system are important chemotactic stimuli for neutrophil migration. It has been estimated that 8 to 10 times the number of cells in the circulating pool can be released in 6 to 7

---

* See Algorithms 4, and 5.

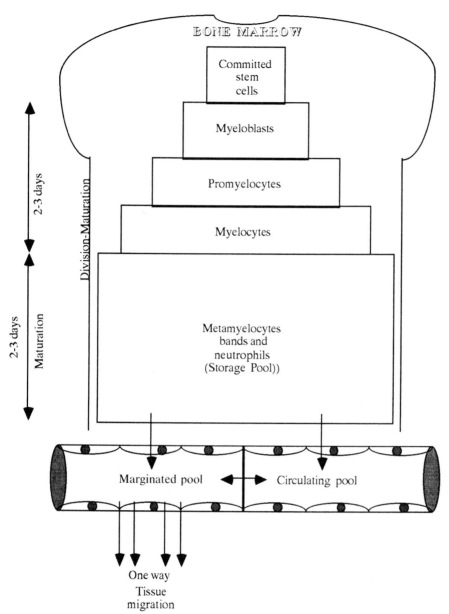

FIGURE 3–1. Stages of granulopoiesis.

hours. If the bone marrow reserve pool cannot meet the tissue demands it may require 2 to 3 days or longer in some animals to make up the depletion of the reserve.

Granulocyte Functions

Neutrophils

The principal function of the neutrophil is phagocytosis of bacteria (Fig. 3–2). Neutrophils are associated with inflammatory reactions secondary to bacteria,

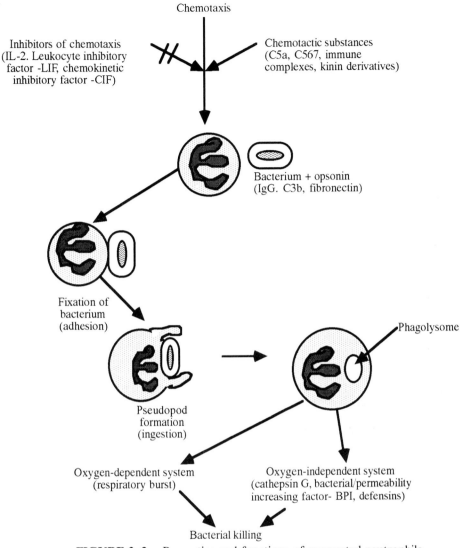

FIGURE 3–2. Properties and functions of segmented neutrophils.

immune-mediated disease, and nonspecific tissue necrosis. Powerful proteolytic enzymes and superoxide radicals that destroy phagocytosed organisms may also escape and cause tissue damage.

Eosinophils

Eosinophils moderate reactions that occur when tissue mast cells and basophils degranulate. The eosinophil chemotactic factor of anaphylaxis (ECF-A) is present in basophils and mast cells. Eosinophils contain substances that inactivate factors released by mast cells and basophils such as histamine, leukotrienes, and platelet-activating factor. When mobilization occurs it may or may not be accompanied by an increase in the number of eosinophils in blood.

Basophils

The precise function of basophils has not been determined although it is known that granules contain heparin, histamine, ECF-A, and a platelet-activating factor. They appear to be involved in immediate hypersensitivity reactions. Immunoglobulin E (IgE) binds readily to basophil as well as mast cell membranes, and when specific antigens react with the membrane-bound IgE, degranulation occurs with release of the mediators of immediate hypersensitivity. At the time of stimulation, basophils will synthesize and release leukotrienes and probably platelet-activating factor. These mediators activate platelets, attract eosinophils, cause smooth muscle contraction, initiate edema formation, and may affect coagulation.

Lymphocyte Formation and Function

Lymphocyte Formation

During fetal life lymphocyte precursors originate in bone marrow and are then influenced toward a particular function by either the thymus gland for T-lymphocytes or the "bursal equivalent" for B-lymphocytes. In late fetal and postnatal life most lymphocytes are produced in the spleen, lymph nodes, and intestine-associated lymphoid tissue. Lymphopoiesis in the secondary lymphoid organs depends on antigenic stimulation.

The life span of a lymphocyte varies from several days to months/years. The types are morphologically indistinguishable in the blood.

Lymphocytes are in a constant state of recirculation. Thoracic duct lymphocytes recirculate from the blood via postcapillary venules into lymph nodes and efferent lymphatics and then back into the thoracic duct. Recirculation occurs at a relatively constant rate so the numbers of lymphocytes entering and leaving blood are approximately equal, which results in a fairly constant level of blood lymphocytes in a healthy animal.

Lymphocyte Function

The principal functions of lymphocytes are related to immunologic activity. T-lymphocytes and their progeny function in cell-mediated immunity, which includes graft rejection, graft-*versus*-host reactions, delayed hypersensitivity, defense against intracellular organisms, and in defense against neoplasia. B-lymphocytes and their progeny are important in the production of antibodies either as lymphocytes or after being transformed into plasma cells.

Monocyte Formation and Function

Monocyte Formation

Monocytes arise in the bone from the same committed progenitor cell as granulocytes. Monocytes in the blood are distributed into circulating and marginal monocyte pools similar to granulocytes.

Monocyte Functions

The monocyte *migrates into tissues where it transforms into a fixed tissue macrophage*. This mononuclear phagocytic system (macrophages and blood monocytes) plays an important role in the defense against intracellular microorganisms (fungi, viruses, and certain bacteria such as mycobacteria and brucella) and in antigen processing for presentation to lymphocytes. Macrophages play an important role in inflammation because they contain or secrete many biologically active substances including proteolytic enzymes, interferon, interleukin-1, complement components, prostaglandins, and carrier proteins. Macrophages are responsible for removal and processing of senescent cells and debris and for filtration of bacteria and toxins from portal blood.

INTERPRETATION OF LEUKOCYTE RESPONSES

Neutrophil kinetics (Fig. 3–3) are primarily responsible for changes in the total leukocyte counts. The differential count of other leukocytes may provide diagnostic information.

Physiologic Leukocytosis

Physiologic leukocytosis refers to an increase in *mature* neutrophils and, less consistently, *mature* lymphocytes (Fig. 3–4). The neutrophilia is the result of an epinepherine-induced demargination which is temporary, lasting only a few hours. The cause of the lymphocytosis is speculated to result from an alteration in

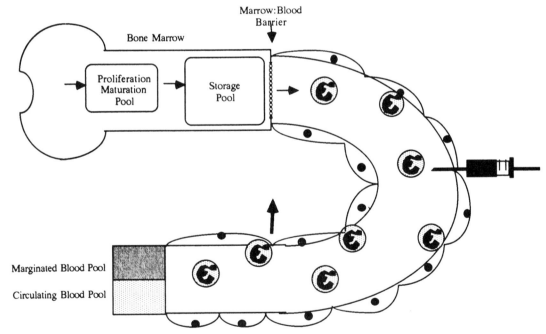

FIGURE 3–3. Normal neutrophil kinetics. The kinetics of neutrophils in the peripheral blood is usually the most consistent reflection of pathology in most species. Neutrophils progress through proliferation and maturation stages before entering the temporary (days) storage in the bone marrow. In the peripheral blood neutrophils are either marginated (the magnitude is species variable) or circulating. The leukocyte count only enumerates those in circulation at that point in time.

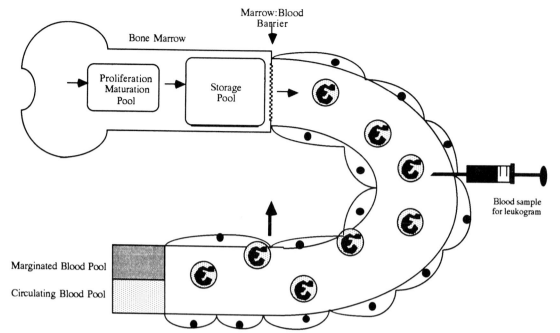

FIGURE 3–4. Physiologic leukocytosis. The acute release of epinepherine stimulates a number of systemic events which cause demargination resulting in a temporary (hours) neutrophilia; there is no left shift. A temporary lymphocytosis (hours) may contribute to the leukocytosis.

recirculation kinetics, and it likewise returns to normal within hours (Fig. 3–5). The cat most commonly demonstrates the lymphocytosis component with counts as high as 10,000/μL. Fear and exertion, for example struggling during restraint, are responsible for the epinepherine release and increased blood flow. *No immature neutrophils* appear in the blood as an effect of epinepherine.

Corticosteroid-induced Leukocytosis

Corticosteroids, exogenous and increased endogenous secretion, cause changes in the leukogram, most predictable for the dog and cat, less predictable for the horse and cow (Fig. 3–6). The leukocyte response is classically characterized by *neutrophilia, lymphopenia, monocytosis,* and *eosinopenia* (see Cases 18, 24, 29, 33, 40, 44, and 58). The dog demonstrates these leukocyte responses most consistently. The cat occasionally has a monocytosis. Horses and cattle usually show no monocyte change although occasionally cattle will have a monocytopenia.

Corticosteroids cause endothelial demargination of neutrophils, resulting in a temporary increase in neutrophils. If bone marrow release contributes to the neutrophilia a left shift does not occur.

The mechanism for lymphopenia is only speculative. Although some lymphocytes are susceptible to corticosteroid-induced lysis, others are resistant. It has been proposed that corticosteroids alter lymphatic recirculation, contributing to the lymphopenia.

The eosinopenia appears to be associated with sequestration and inhibition of eosinophil release from the bone marrow.

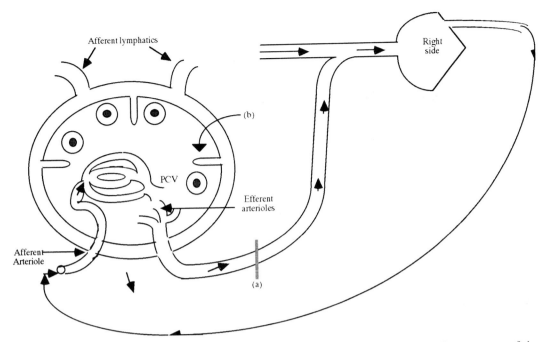

FIGURE 3–5. Lymphocyte recirculation. Only a small percentage of the lymphocytes circulate in the peripheral blood. Lymphocytes reenter the lymph node by crossing the wall of the postcapillary venules (*PCV*). Glucocorticoids may temporarily impair the return of lymphocytes to the circulation (*a*) or (*b*) chronically cause the depletion of lymphoid tissue.

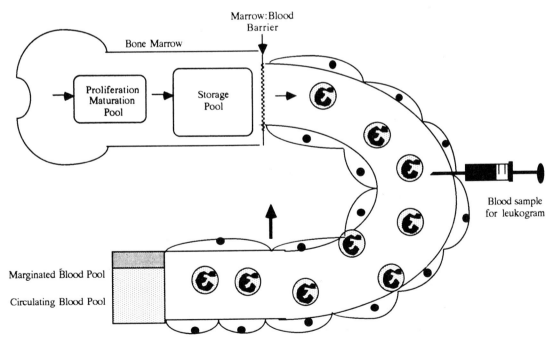

FIGURE 3–6. Glucocorticoid response. Exogenous or endogenous glucocorticoids cause demargination of neutrophils resulting in a neutrophilia. A slight stimulus for release from the bone marrow may contribute to the neutrophilia; there is no left shift.

Corticosteroid-induced *leukocytosis can be observed within 6 hours of increased corticosteroid concentration* in the blood. Stress (i.e., stimulation of the pituitary-adrenal axis) is a common cause of this leukocyte response (Fig. 3–7).

Neutrophils and Inflammation

The leukogram is commonly used to detect and monitor inflammatory processes (Figs. 3–8 and 3–9). The neutrophil responds quickly (hours) to numerous chemotactic stimuli associated with the inflammatory process (Fig. 3–7). The neutrophil response is associated with infections, tissue necrosis and immune-mediated diseases (Table 3–1) (see Cases 3, 7, 16, 22, 24, and 42).

The neutrophil response represents a balance between extravascular tissue demand and the rate of bone marrow release. Acute inflammation (Fig. 3–8) causes increased neutrophil margination and migration with an immediate decrease in

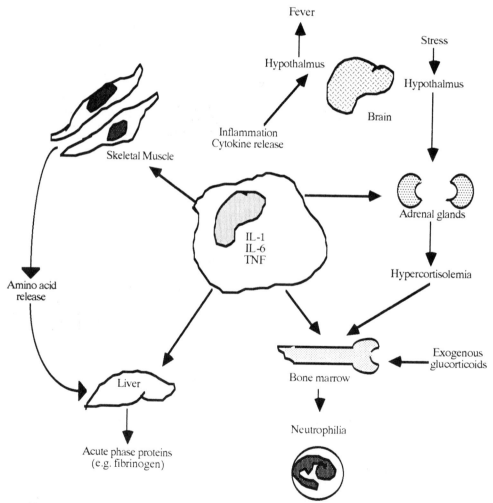

FIGURE 3–7. The systemic effects of stress and inflammation. Nomenclature for the cytokines and direct effects on inflammatory cells are covered in Figure 2–1.

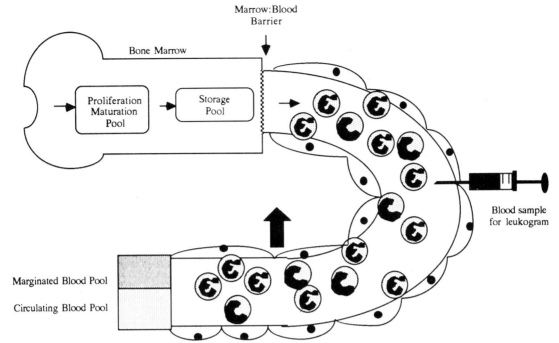

FIGURE 3–8. Acute inflammation. Cytokines associated with an acute inflammatory process stimulate the bone marrow proliferation/maturation pool and storage pool to increase the release of mature and immature neutrophils resulting in a neutrophilia with a left shift. The neutrophilia may persist for a period of time (days) after the inflammatory process has resolved because of the accelerated kinetics in the bone marrow. If the demand for neutrophil exceeds the storage a neutropenia with a left shift develops (see Fig. 3–10).

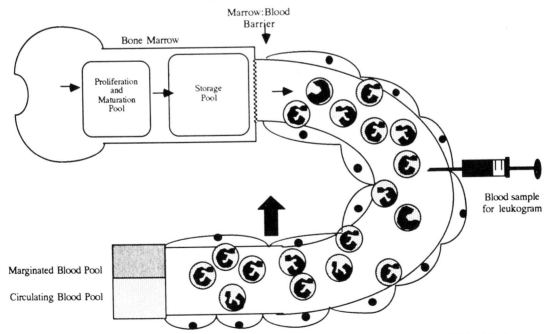

FIGURE 3–9. Chronic inflammation. A persistent (established) inflammatory process causes expansion of the proliferation, maturation, and storage pools in the bone marrow to match the accelerated needs of peripheral tissue. A neutrophilia with a slight to no left shift is reflected in the peripheral blood. The neutrophilia may persist (days) after resolution of the pathologic process.

TABLE 3–1. Neutrophilia

Cause	Neutrophil Response	Other Leukocytes	Mechanism
Physiologic, exercise, hypoxia, excitement	Mature-moderate absolute ↑	Lymphocytosis, particularly in cats	MGP → CGP (neutrophils), altered recirculation (lymphocytes)
Increased glucocorticoids (endogenous, exogenous)	Mature-moderate absolute ↑	Lymphopenia, eosinopenia, monocytosis (dogs, sometimes cats)	Decreased migration of neutrophils from blood, increased removal from marrow storage pool; altered recirculation of lymphocytes, sequestration of eosinophils in bone marrow
Early inflammation	Left shift with increase in absolute neutrophil count	Variable	Increased tissue demand with excess release from storage pool of bone marrow
Acute, intense inflammation	Marked left shift neutrophilia; often toxic neutrophils	Variable	Continued stimulation and tissue demand for same
Established inflammation	Increase in absolute neutrophil count, slight to no left shift	Variable	Increased neutrophil production and release to meet established tissue demand

circulating neutrophils. The decrease is rapidly compensated for by increased bone marrow release (hours) and production (days) (Fig. 3–9). A neutrophilic *leukocytosis with a left shift* results when release and production exceed the demand of the inflammatory process. The left shift is orderly, for example, more bands than metamyelocytes than myelocytes.

The *magnitude of the neutrophilic response* is an approximate reflection of the magnitude of the inflammatory process. Furthermore, a localized inflammatory process, for example, pyometra, elicits a greater neutrophil response than generalized inflammation. Pyogenic bacteria stimulate a more intense neutrophil response than other types of infectious agents. The *severity of the inflammatory process* is reflected by the degree of the left shift.

Neutropenia

Neutropenias (see Cases 1, 4, 6, 13, 15, 20, and 23) can be grouped as follows: (1) reduced survival of mature neutrophils (Fig. 3–10); (2) reduced production by the bone marrow (Fig. 3–11); and (3) ineffective neutrophil production (Table 3–2 and

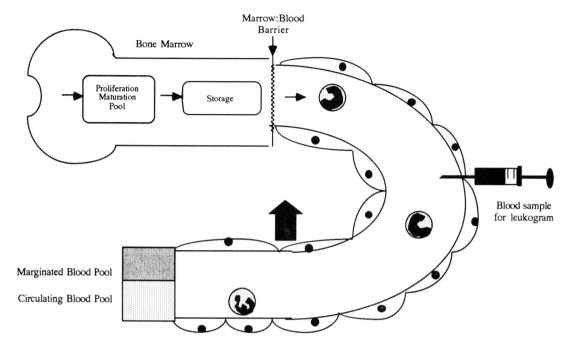

FIGURE 3–10. Reduced survival. A peracute, severe inflammatory process which rapidly depletes the storage without allowing time for input from the proliferation maturation pool results in a neutropenia with a left shift (immature outnumber mature neutrophils).

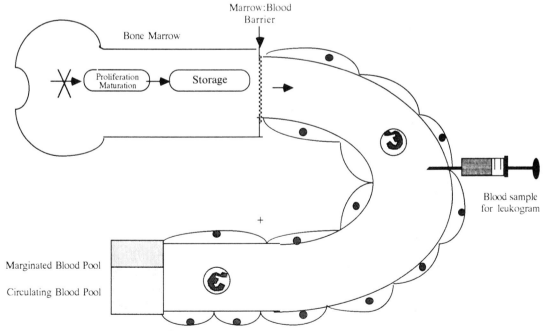

FIGURE 3–11. Reduced production. An insult that injures the proliferation/maturation pool terminates the input into the storage pool for release, resulting in a mature neutropenia; no left shift is present. Examination of the bone marrow reveals sparse granulocytic precursors.

TABLE 3–2. Neutropenia

Cause	Neutrophil Response	Other Leukocytes[a]	Mechanism
Overwhelming bacterial infection	Neutropenia usually with left shift (immatures exceed matures)	Normal	Increased tissue demand with depletion of peripheral blood and marrow pools
Decreased production of neutrophils	Neutropenia, no left shift	Normal	Decreased marrow production
Sequestration	Sudden neutropenia, no left shift	Normal	CGP → MGP (as in shock)
Ineffective	Neutropenia, no left shift	Increased marrow granulopoiesis	Abnormal maturation and release from marrow pools

[a] A stress pattern may be present.

Fig. 3–12). A fourth classification, termed *sequestration,* is less clearly defined. *Neutropenia from reduced survival* occurs when there is an acute massive tissue demand that depletes the blood neutrophil pool rapidly. A continued excessive demand will exhaust the bone marrow storage pool and exceed production, resulting in a *degenerative left shift,* that is, more immature neutrophils than mature (see Case 1). The total neutrophil count may be normal or decreased. A degenerative left shift indicates an unfavorable systemic situation; *toxic morphologic changes* are often observed in the neutrophils. These changes include cytoplasmic basophilia and vacuolization and Döehle bodies; the horse neutrophil may also show eosinophilic granularity in the cytoplasm.

Immune-mediated neutropenia resulting in reduced survival occurs in animals but has not been well documented. There is no left shift, and the bone marrow storage pools appear normal on examination. Tests to determine antineutrophil antibody are necessary to confirm this diagnosis.

Neutropenia secondary to reduced production is associated with a primary bone marrow failure (see Cases 6 and 20). Other cell lines may also be affected. The neutropenia is not accompanied by a left shift. Known causes include infections (canine and feline parvo virus, *Ehrlichia canis,* feline leukemia virus, feline immunosuppressive virus) and drugs (trimethoprim-sulfa, phenylbutazone, estrogens, chemotherapeutic agents) and cyclic hematopoiesis of blue collies.

Neutrophil sequestration occurs with anaphylaxis and endotoxemia by causing a rapid shift to the marginating pool. Endotoxins are known to cause some of their effect via complement activation, resulting in the aggregation and sequestration of neutrophils (and platelets) in pulmonary capillaries.

Leukemoid Response

A leukemoid response refers to a total leukocyte count of 50,000 to 100,000 or more, comprised predominantly of granulocytes that may be shifted back to the

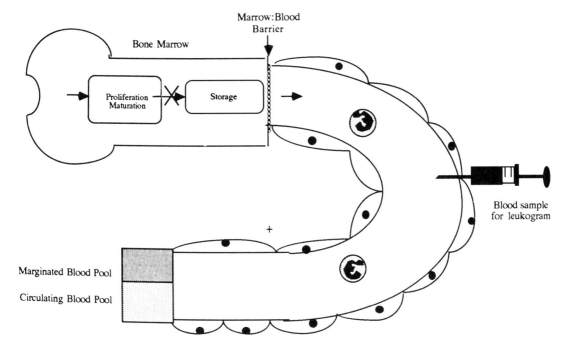

FIGURE 3–12. Ineffective production. An insult that impairs the maturation process but not proliferation causes a build-up of immature precursors in the bone marrow. Examination of bone marrow indicates an overwhelming predominance of one immature cell type. There is no progression to formation or release of mature neutrophils resulting in a nature neutropenia; there is no left shift.

myelocyte stage. The left shift is orderly with predominantly segmenters and sequentially lesser numbers of bands, metamyelocytes, and myelocytes. When nucleated erythrocytes are also present, the term *leukoerythroblastic response* is used. Neither response is specific for the type of underlying pathology. A leukemoid pattern has been occasionally associated with neopasms (*e.g.*, renal carcinoma, fibrosarcoma) and is thought to represent a paraneoplastic process.

Other Leukocyte Alterations

Causes of other changes in leukocytes are summarized in Tables 3–3 through 3–8.

Fibrinogen

Fibrinogen is one member of a group of proteins referred to as acute phase reacting proteins produced by the liver. Fibrinogen has been traditionally deter-

TABLE 3–3. Causes of Monocytosis

Inflammation and tissue necrosis
Increased glucocorticoids (dog)
Suppuration (body cavity)
Granulomatous disorders
Monocytic or myelomonocytic leukemia

TABLE 3–4.   Causes of Lymphocytosis

Physiologic (cats, uncommon other species)
   Increased epinepherine activity, e.g., exercise, anxiety
   Temporary after some vaccinations (reactive lympho-
     cytes frequently present)
Pathologic
   Autoimmune disease
   Lymphosarcoma (not in all patients)
   Bovine leukemia virus (not in all cases)
   Hypoadrenocorticism (rarely an absolute increase but
     counts are normal in an obviously ill patient)

TABLE 3–5.   Causes of Lymphopenia

Excess glucocorticoids
   Endogenous
     Stress
     Debilitating disease
     Hyperadrenocorticism
     Surgery
     Shock
     Trauma
     Heat or cold exposure
   Exogenous
     Glucocorticoid therapy

Lymphocytes loss
   Protein losing enteropathy (lymphangectasia)
   Chylothorax with repeated drainage

Reduced lymphopoiesis
   Prolonged corticosteroid therapy
   Congenital T-cell immunodeficiency (combined
     immunodeficiency (CID), horse)

Viral infections (acute stages)
   Canine distemper
   Feline panleukopenia
   Infectious canine hepatitis
   Coronavirus enteritis
   Feline leukemia virus (thymic atrophy)

TABLE 3–6.   Causes of Eosinophilia

Hypersensitivity
   Parasitism in sensitized hosts
   Immediate hypersensitivity reactions
Specific eosinophilic diseases
   Eosinophilic enterocolitis
   Eosinophilic granuloma (cat)
   Eosinophilic pneumonitis (dog, cat)
   Eosinophilic leukemia (rare)
Other associations
   Carcinoma
   Lymphosarcoma
   Mast cell tumor
   Myeloproliferative disease (cat)
   Hypoadrenocorticism; normal numbers
     in a stressed patient (inappropriate)

es

m

tress

apy

**of Basophilia
3lood)**

ally also present)
ally also present)
in hypersensitivity

methodology involved. More recently, C-reative protein have been evaluated in the medical and more sensitive reflection of an underlying inflammatory process. The stimulus initiating increased acute phase reactive protein production by the liver is linked to the production of cytokines by the cells involved in the inflammatory process, most specifically the monocyte/macrophage cell component. These cytokines, most notably *interleukin-1*, cause a variety of systemic responses including fever, neutrophilia, stimulation of the release of corticotropin-releasing factor, activation of lymphokine production (interleukin-2), and last and most pertinent, stimulation of the hepatic production of acute phase reacting proteins which we determine clinically to reflect an underlying inflammatory process.

Two points should be emphasized relative to the determination of fibrinogen. The ease of methodology of fibrinogen determination is offset by the test sensitivity. The test should not be used as the salient reflection of inflammation but should be combined with interpretation of the leukogram. In the carnivora and marsupialia a neutrophilia is more frequent than hyperfibrinogenemia as a reflection of inflammation. In the perissodactyla (horse/rhinoceros), the proboscidea (elephant), and artiodactyla (camel) hyperfibrinogenemia occurs with greater frequency than do alterations of the leukogram as a reflection of inflammation. Using the heat precipitation method for determination of plasma fibrinogen concentration, normal values in the canine, feline, and equine species range between 100 and 400 mg/dL (1 to 4 g/L) and in the bovine 100 to 600 mg/dL (1 to 6 g/L). Increased values support an inflammatory process whereas decreased values support a coagulation-consumptive process, most notably disseminated intravascular coagulopathy.

In herbivorous animals fibrinogen is a sensitive indicator of inflammation and may be a more consistent indicator of an inflammatory process than is the leukogram (see Cases 18, 30, and 31). Fibrinogen is a less sensitive indicator of inflammation in carnivorous animals.

EVALUATION OF HEMOSTASIS AND COAGULATION DISORDERS*

FACTORS INVOLVED IN HEMOSTASIS

There are three principal components of hemostasis: (1) vascular integrity; (2) platelets; and (3) blood coagulation (Fig. 4–1).

Vascular Factors

The vascular component of hemostasis depends upon the integrity of the endothelium. There are no laboratory techniques that measure the functional status of blood vessels directly. If there is a diffuse cutaneous discoloration suggestive of hemorrhage or subcutaneous edema and if all coagulation, platelet, and protein measurements are normal a vascular disorder should be suspected. Rickettsial infection and, less commonly, immune-mediated vasculitis should be included in the differential diagnosis.

Platelets

Blood platelets are derived from megakaryocytes located in the bone marrow.

Adequate platelet numbers are required for a number of important physiologic activities related to hemostasis. Platelets aggregate to form the initial hemostatic plug. Platelets initiate the coagulation cascade and clot retraction (Fig. 4–2).

Platelets aggregate after exposure to vascular collagen and release serotonin, histamines, and adenosine diphosphate (ADP). Serotonin and histamines act as vasoconstrictors while ADP causes aggregation and adherence of additional platelets.

Clot retraction is, in part, dependent upon the presence and action of platelets. There is a quantitative relationship between platelet numbers and clot retraction. Adequate platelet numbers with normal function are required for clot retraction. The platelet substance responsible for clot retraction is thomboesthenin, a contractile protein. Clot retraction is also dependent on fibrinogen concentration and normal fibrinogen structure.

---

* See Algorithm 6.

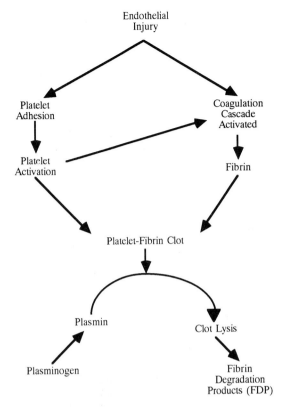

FIGURE 4–1. There is a continual physiologic balance between repair of damaged vascular endothelium and clot lysis to maintain patency. Three important imbalances include: (1) thrombocytopenia, often manifested clinically with petechial hemorrhages, blood will still clot; (2) deficiency of coagulation factor(s) manifested by overt hemorrhage as a result of the inability of platelets to plug large vascular defects; and (3) DIC, manifested clinically with overt hemorrhage because of a combination of accelerated clot formation in small vessels with simultaneous enhancement of fibrinolysis resulting in an increase of FDPs.

Blood Coagulation

Blood coagulation is a complicated sequence of interrelated factors. These factors have been characterized and assigned numbers and names (Table 4–1).

The mechanism for blood coagulation consists of *intrinsic, extrinsic,* and *common* systems. (Fig. 4–3). The intrinsic system is assessed by the activated partial

TABLE 4–1. International Nomenclature of Blood Clotting Factors

Factor	Synonym	Coagulation Function
I	Fibrinogen	Converted to fibrin
II	Prothrombin	Converted to thrombin
III	Tissue thromboplastin	Activates factor VII
IV	Calcium	Cofactor
V	Labile factor, Ac-globulin, proaccelerin- - - - -	Accelerates factor X action Binds factor Xa to platelets Endothelial cell receptor
VII	Proconvertin, stable factor	Activates Factor X
VIII	Antihemolytic factor, thromboplastinogen	Cofactor in activation of factor X
IX	Plasma thromboplastin component (Christmas factor)	Cofactor in activation of factor X
X	Stuart-Prower factor, Stuart factor	Formation of thrombin
XI	Plasma thromboplastin antecedent	Activates factor IX Binds to injured endothelium
XII	Hageman factor, glass-activation factor- - - - - -	Activates Factor XI Formation of kallikrein
XIII	Fibrin-stabilizing factor, fibrinase, Laki-Lorand factor	Facilitates fibrin cross-linking and impairs plasmin degradation

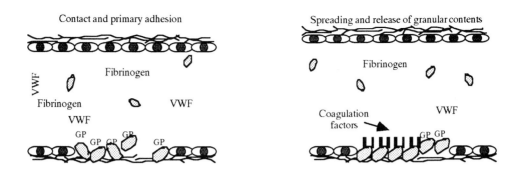

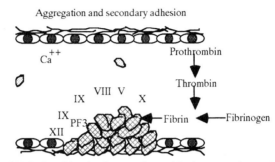

FIGURE 4–2. Platelet interaction with the vascular endothelium and coagulation cascade. Unactivated platelets come in contact with damaged
endothelium and attach = *primary adhesion*. The attachment, which is
facilitated by the exposure of glycoproteins (GP-I, GPIIb-IIIa complex) on
the platelet surface in conjunction with other adhesive molecules such as
von Willebrand factor (*VWF*) and fibrinogen, results in shape changes and
bonding of platelets to each other and the endothelial surface = *spreading*.
The continued *aggregation* of the platelets causes the release of the granular contents which activates other platelets prior to encountering the damaged surface = *secondary adhesion*. Platelet activation, along with confor-
mational changes in factor XII after exposure to the injured endothelial
surface, is involved in initiating the intrinsic coagulation cascade. The damaged tissue also releases thromboplastin, which activates factor VII and
initiates the extrinsic coagulation pathway. The coagulant activity of factor
VII is enhanced by the activated factor XIIa or IXa. This myriad of events
demonstrates the integral relationship of the endothelium, platelets, and
coagulation factors in the clotting process.

thromboplastic time (APTT). A simplified variation of the APTT is the activated
coagulation test (ACT). Blood is collected in a special gray-topped tube containing
surface contact agent (diatomaceous earth). This is a good test for the initial
evaluation of a bleeding patient or as a presurgical screen.

The extrinsic system is evaluated with the prothrombin time (PT). The next to
last step forms thrombin, which converts fibrinogen into a monomer and, in the
presence of factor XII and calcium, converts it into an insoluble fibrin clot. The
latter step can be evaluated with the thrombin clot time (TCT).

The liver is the major site of production of all plasma coagulation factors; factor
VIII is also produced by extrahepatic vascular endothelium. Factors II, VII, IX,
and X are vitamin K dependent.

There is a system of inhibitors that destroy an activated factor soon after it
appears. Without this protective mechanism massive thromboses could occur.

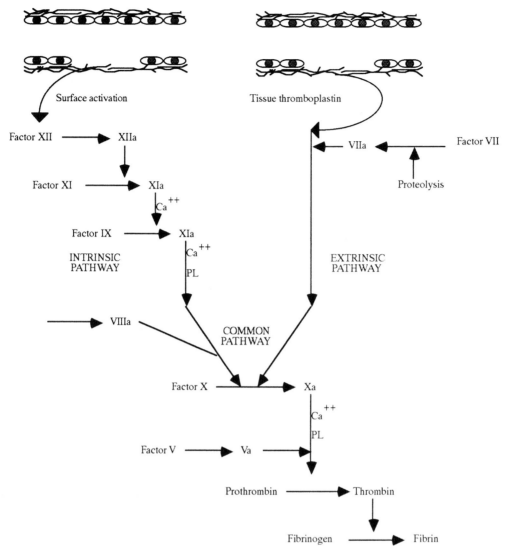

FIGURE 4–3. Waterfall diagram representing the interaction of coagulation factors, tissue factors, Ca^{++}, and phospholipid (*PL*) culminating in the formation of a clot. The APTT and ACT assess the intrinsic plus common pathways (factors XII, XI, IX, VIII, plus X and V). The PT assesses the extrinsic plus common pathways (factors VII plus X and V). One notes that the vitamin K-dependent factors (II, VII, IX, and X) are involved in all pathways.

The coagulation system is moderated by a fibrinolytic enzyme system consisting of the inactive precursor plasminogen (profibrinolysin) and the active component plasmin (fibrinolysin). Products generated are referred to as fibrin degradation products (FDPs) or fibrin split products (FSPs) (Fig. 4–4). Increased concentrations are associated with disorders of accelerated clot formation and breakdown such as disseminated intravascular coagulation (DIC).

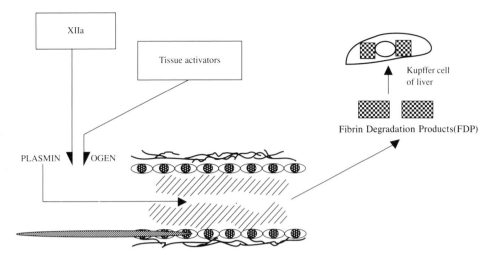

FIGURE 4–4. Physiologic clot dissolution is dependent on the functions of *plasmin* formed from the plasma protein *plasminogen*. Tissue activators such as urokinase and tissue activator, released from the endothelium and hepatocytes, along with factor XIIa, activate plasminogen. Clot lysis results in the formation of FDP, some having potent anticoagulant activity, which are removed by the liver. Plasminogen activation is regulated by the proteolytic enzyme inhibitors α_2-plasmin inhibitor and plasmin α_2-macroglobulin.

TESTS FOR COAGULATION DEFECTS

Sample Collection

Trisodium citrate is the anticoagulant used. It is used as 1 part of a 3.8% solution to 9 parts of blood. Blood is collected and handled as follows.

1. One part of the 3.8% trisodium citrate anticoagulant is used for 9 parts of blood (1 : 10) dilution.

2. The required amount of citrate anticoagulant is placed in a *plastic* syringe (*e.g.*, 0.4 mL).

3. The proportional amount of blood (*e.g.*, 3.6 mL for 0.4 mL of anticoagulant for a total volume of 4 mL) is drawn by *clean venipuncture* through the anticoagulant. The blood should not be drawn first and then add to the anticoagulant as coagulation will be activated prior to contact with citrate, and results will be compromised.

Alternatively a small (4-mL draw) *blue-topped* Vacutainer tube containing the required citrate anticoagulant can be used. The tube should be filled completely as dictated by the amount of vacuum.

If venipuncture (by either of the methods above) does not yield a clean flow of blood or if the flow is very slow, the procedure should be repeated using a *new needle* and another blood vessel.

4. The anticoagulated sample should be mixed immediately and the needle removed. The sample is then transferred to an empty *plastic* test tube for centrifugation.

5. Centrifugation should be at 2,500 to 3,000 rpm or higher for 12 to 15 minutes and *should be completed within 30 minutes of sampling.*

6. The supernatant plasma is then aspirated off carefully with a *plastic* pipette or small *plastic* syringe such as a tuberculin syringe. Care should be taken not to aspirate any RBCs or any part of the buffy coat.

7. The specimen should be refrigerated or frozen for the transfer to the laboratory.

Bleeding Time

The easiest method of measuring bleeding time is to clip the quick of a toenail and measure the time required for the bleeding to stop. The nail should *bleed freely* (*undisturbed*) and the time until the bleeding stops recorded. In normal dogs bleeding will stop within 5 minutes and in cats 2½ to 3 minutes. Although it is a simple but crude evaluation of hemostasis, additional tests should be completed if the time is prolonged. Bleeding times measured by this method are sensitive to defects in vascular contraction, platelet function, and coagulation. Thrombocytopenia, von Willebrand's disease, and hyperglobulinemia (plasma cell myeloma) are some of the more common differentials to consider. Prior aspirin administration may result in an abnormal bleeding time. A method using the oral mucous membrane and a lancet has been reported to be a more sensitive procedure for assessing bleeding time.

LABORATORY TESTS

Laboratory tests for coagulation defects that are most commonly used are: (1) one-step prothrombin time (PT); (2) activated partial thromboplastin time (aPTT); (3) thrombin clot time (TCT); (4) platelet count; and (5) von Willebrand's factor (measured as factor VIII-related antigen).

Prothrombin Time

PT measures the extrinsic (EF) and common (factor V, factor X, prothrombin [factor II], and fibrinogen) pathways. One or more of these factors may be involved when the PT is prolonged.

Activated Partial Thromboplastin Time

APTT measures the intrinsic (factors VIII, IX, XI, and XII) and common (factors V, X, II, and fibrinogen) pathways. The common pathway is common to both PT and APTT.

Thrombin Clot Time

TCT is measured by determining the length of time required for a fibrin clot to form in citrated plasma after the addition of thrombin. It is a measure of functional fibrinogen and will be increased when fibrinogen concentration is low if fibrinogen degradation products are elevated or heparin is present.

Activated Coagulation Test

Special tubes containing diatomaceous earth are used. Blood is added to the tubes that have been heated to 37° C. Platelet counts less than $10,000/\mu L$ may cause falsely prolonged ACT. Normal results are: dog, less than 120 seconds; cat, less than 65 seconds; horse, less than 40 seconds.

Platelet Count

Platelets can be counted directly or an estimate can be made by examination of a stained peripheral blood film (10–15 per oil immersion field (Fig. 4–5). Absolute direct counts are desired. Platelet morphology should be evaluated from a Romanowsky stained blood film for granularity and size variation.

A preponderance of large platelets with sparse granularity suggests increased platelet turnover.

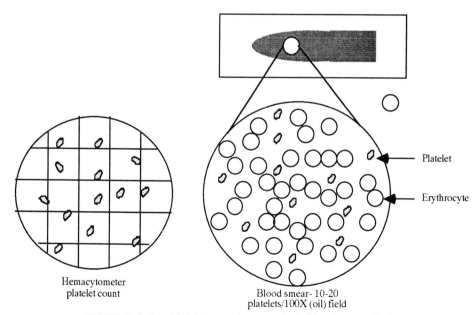

Hemacytometer
platelet count

Blood smear- 10-20
platelets/100X (oil) field

Platelet

Erythrocyte

FIGURE 4–5. Platelets can be quantitated by the use of a hemacytometer or microscopically semiquantitated on a thin, evenly spread, air-dried blood film. A wet preparation made by placing a drop of *new methylene blue* directly on the dried blood film and adding to coverslip is an ideal stain for assessing platelet or neutrophil numbers quickly. Platelets and nuclei appear blue, and only the outline of the erythrocytes is visible. *Haemobartonella,* Heinz bodies and Howell-Jolly bodies can also be identified with this preparation. Less than 20 neutrophils/10X suggests neutropenia.

LABORATORY FINDINGS IN COAGULATION DISORDERS

Hereditary Coagulation Defects

Deficiency of Factor VIII (Hemophilia A)

Hemophilia A is a lack of factor VIII activity which results in a *prolonged APTT* with a *normal PT* (see Case 24). The bleeding time is normal.

Hemophilia A has been reported in horses, cats, and in the following breeds of dogs: Shetland sheepdog, beagle, English setter, Irish setter, Labrador retriever, German shepherd, collie, greyhound, weimaraner, Chihuahua, Samoyed, vizsla, English bulldog, miniature poodle, miniature schnauzer, Saint Bernard, and in mixed breeds.

Deficiency of Factor IX (Hemophilia B, Christmas disease)

Hemophilia B is an X chromosome-linked recessive trait that occurs with less frequency than hemophilia A. It has been reported in the cairn terrier, American cocker spaniel, Labrador retriever, French bulldog, black-and-tan coonhound, Saint Bernard, Alaskan malamute, Scottish terrier, English sheepdog, Shetland sheepdog, bichon frise, Airedale terrier, and a family of British shorthair cats.

As with hemophilia A, hemophilia B results in a prolonged APTT and a normal PT and bleeding time. The disorder can be tentatively differentiated from hemophilia A by the addition of fresh normal serum to plasma and completion of an APTT. Fresh serum contains factor IX but not factor VIII. If there is a factor IX deficiency, fresh serum will usually correct the prolonged APTT of the patient plasma. The PT is normal.

Factor VII Deficiency

This uncommon autosomal dominant trait is characterized by a prolonged PT. It has been reported in the beagle, Alaskan malamute, boxer, miniature schnauzer, and bulldog. Affected animals do not usually have serious overt bleeding tendencies, but excessive hemorrhage can occur during surgery. Because factor VII is a vitamin K-dependent product of the liver and has a short half-life (6 hours), it may be deficient in advanced liver disease or with vitamin K deficiency such as that associated with warfarin toxicity or malabsorption.

Factor XI Deficiency

This deficiency has been detected in cattle and dogs. In dogs it is characterized by autosomal inheritance, minor bleeding problems, and protracted bleeding after surgery. It has been diagnosed in the springer spaniel, Great Pyrenees, Kerry blue terrier, and weimaraner. This deficiency does not occur commonly and rarely is a clinical problem.

Factor X Deficiency

A factor X deficiency has been described in a family of cocker spaniels. It may cause hemorrhagic problems in newborns and young pups but does not seem to cause any problem in adults unless they are subjected to surgery. Hemorrhage into the thoracic and abdominal cavity and hemorrhage from the umbilical cord are common findings in affected newborns. In young adults hematuria, hemorrhage of the gums, prolonged bleeding during estrus, and intrathoracic hemorrhages have been reported. Both the PT and APTT are prolonged.

Factor II (Prothrombin) Deficiency

This is a rare coagulation defect that has been reported in a family of boxer dogs and a cocker spaniel. Affected animals have epistaxis, umbilical bleeding in newborns, and mucosal bleedings in young adults. The APTT and PT are prolonged.

Factor XII Deficiency

Factor XII deficiency has been reported in cats, standard poodle, and German shorthair pointer. The APTT is prolonged, but the PT is normal. Affected animals do not usually have any clinical signs and are usually detected during presurgical screening.

von Willebrand's Disease (VWD)

von Willebrand's (VWD) disease (see Case 28) is a heritable coagulopathy that is detected by measuring factor VIII-related antigen. The disease occurs in many (54) breeds of dogs. It is most prevalent in the Doberman pinscher, Scottish terrier, miniature schnauzer, golden retriever, Shetland sheepdog, basset hound, standard poodle, miniature poodle, Pembroke Welsh corgi, German shepherd, rottweiler, standard Manchester terrier, Manchester toy terrier, keeshond, dachsund, and miniature dachsund. Breeds with a lower or unknown prevalence of the VWD gene are the Greate Dane, Chesapeake Bay retriever, Afghan hound, cairn terrier, Samoyed, American cocker spaniel, English cocker spaniel, English springer spaniel, vizsla, Lhasa apso, Shih Tzu, Irish setter, English setter, boxer, Airedale terrier, Kerry blue terrier, Lakeland terrier, fox terrier (smooth), fox terrier (wire), soft-coated wheaten terrier, Yorkshire terrier, Tibetan terrier, papillon, Great Pyrenees, Akita, bearded collie, Irish wolfhound, Labrador retriever, collie, Swiss mountain dog, Siberian husky, Alaskan malamute, German shorthair pointer, Kuvasz, bichon frise, greyhound, and whippet.

The diagnostic considerations in the confirmation of von Willebrand's disease are summarized in Table 4–2.

Abnormal Platelet Function

Abnormal platelet aggregation is a hereditary abnormality that occurs in the basset hound. It is characterized by normal platelet morphology; counts and aggregation are normal with thrombin, but aggregation is abnormal with other agents (see Case 26).

Acquired Coagulation Defects

The veterinarian is more likely to encounter hemostatic problems associated with acquired rather than a congenital defect.

TABLE 4–2. Diagnosis of von Willebrand's Disease

Bleeding Time	Factor VIII-Related Antigen %	Interpretation
Normal	60 or greater	Normal range, 60–172%
Normal[a]	60–69	Lower end of normal range; caution advised for breeding stock; males should have higher levels and pups should be checked
Normal or prolonged[a]	50–59	Borderline normal (equivocal result) or heterozygous carrier of VWD gene Recommend retesting or breeding only to higher testing mates; pups should be checked
Normal or prolonged[a]	Less than 50	Heterozygous carrier of VWD gene, if asymptomatic; carriers can revert to VWD affected status if bleeding problem develops subsequently Breed only to VWD normal mates and test pups
Prolonged[a]	Less than 50	Type I VWD; clinically affected heterozygote; should not be used for breeding This is the most common form of VWD
Normal or prolonged[a]	Less than 7 (undetectable)	Severe penetrant heterozygous carrier of VWD gene, if asymptomatic; generally not advisable to breed such animals
Prolonged[a]	Less than 7 (undetectable)	If clinically affected, has severe (penetrant) form of type I VWD (an affected heterozygote); homozygosity is lethal in this form of VWD; affected animals should not be used for breeding
Prolonged[a]	Less than 7 (undetectable)	If clinically affected, Scottish terrier or Chesapeake Bay retriever, the patient is a true homozygote (zero antigen level) for type III VWD; this animal is the product of two asymptomatic, heterozygous carrier parents and should not be used for breeding
Normal	200 or greater	Probably reflects stress, an improper sample, or activation from disease Recommend retesting

[a] Concomitant thyroid dysfunction or hypothyroidism alone will aggravate existing VWD and increase the risk for bleeding with or without VWD being present.

Liver Disease

Hemostatic problems associated with liver disease result from the diminished synthesis of proteins, from metabolic abnormalities, and from diminished clearance of fibrin degradation products; they are not common. Abnormal platelet function and prolonged bleeding times have been demonstrated in icteric dogs (see Case 33), cats, and horses.

Because factors of both the intrinsic and extrinsic system may be deficient, one or both of the coagulation tests (PT and APTT) may be prolonged. If liver disease is severe, fibrinogen production can be affected, in which case the TCT may be prolonged. Thrombocytopenia may also occur with some liver diseases if associated with DIC.

Rodenticide Toxicity

Coumarin derivatives and several chemical analogs used to poison rodents are known to cause bleeding problems in domestic animals. These substances interfere with vitamin K metabolism and therefore prevent synthesis of those coagulation factors dependent upon vitamin K (see Case 11).

Thrombocytopenia

The *most common cause of hemostatic problems* encountered by the veterinarian is thrombocytopenia (see Cases 19 and 27). It is clinically suggested by finding petechial and ecchymotic hemorrhages on the mucous membranes or skin and is confirmed by a low platelet count. The bleeding time may be prolonged. Clot retraction is abnormal, and occasionally the APTT is slightly prolonged.

Thrombocytopenia may occur as a result of *lack of production, consumption,* or *destruction.*

Because platelets are produced by megakaryocytes in the bone marrow, anything that causes overall marrow hypoplasia will produce thrombocytopenia.

Platelet destruction may be associated with immune-mediated hemolytic anemia (Evans's syndrome), systemic lupus erythematosus, and certain drugs such as trimethoprim-sulfa antibiotics.

Platelets are consumed when there is hypercoagulability as in DIC.

Disseminated Intravascular Coagulation

Fibrinolytic activity is normally kept under control by circulating plasmin inhibitors. However, increases in fibrinolytic activity do occur in association with a variety of conditions including heatstroke, snakebite, incompatible blood transfusions, neoplasia, surgery, endotoxemia, gastric torsion, heartworm disease, severe hepatic necrosis, diaphragmatic hernia, pancreatitis, hemorrhagic enteritis, and polycythemia. This condition is known as DIC, consumption coagulopathy, or intravascular coagulation-fibinolysis syndrome. DIC is not a primary condition but occurs as a secondary phenomenon in association with one of the above conditions (see Case 25).

DIC is a paradox as there is both *hypercoagulation* and *increased fibrinolytic activity.* The simultaneous activation of these two processes initially causes intravascular formation of fibrin in small blood vessels in multiple organs. Massive amounts of coagulation factors, platelets, and fibrinogen are consumed. The fibrinolytic system is activated immediately to remove these thrombi. The fibrinolytic removal of fibrin and fibrinogen produces fibrin degradation products (FDP) with potent anticoagulant activity potentiating the hemorrhage diathesis.

Clinical/clinopathologic findings are variable depending on the organ most severely affected and at what point in time the animal is first seen. DIC is characterized initially by hypercoagulability, but the veterinarian rarely encounters an animal in this early phase of DIC. The consumptive phase is characterized by thrombocytopenia, prolonged APTT and PT with a low fibrinogen or a prolonged TCT. Misshaped and fragmented erythrocytes (poikilocytes, schistocytes) along with variably sized platelets are observed frequently on a blood smear. Increased concentration of FDP further supports the presence of this ominous disorder.

FIBRINOLYTIC DEGRADATION PRODUCTS.

5

HEPATIC TEST ABNORMALITIES*

The liver is an integral component of the digestive system anatomically and functionally interposed between the gastrointestinal tract and the systemic circulation. For our purposes, the liver is composed structurally of hepatocytes, a biliary ductular system, and a rich blood supply, both venous (portal) and arterial. Clinicopathologic parameters used to evaluate the liver reflect these structural components and can be divided into serum enzyme tests and function tests. It is critical to appreciate that abnormal results of these tests may reflect either a *primary* or *secondary* hepatic disturbance. Metabolic, cardiovascular, and gastrointestinal diseases are examples of extrahepatic organ systems in which disorders can cause abnormal test results. It is prudent to consider the possibility of extrahepatic disease in addition to primary disease of the liver when interpreting abnormal liver test results (see Cases 29 through 36).

1. Serum enzyme tests
   a. *Leakage enzymes* are alanine aminotransferase (ALT) (also called ALAT; formerly GPT); aspartate aminotransferase (AST) (also called ASAT; formerly GOT); sorbitol dehydrogenase (SD) (formerly SDH); lactate dehydrogenase isoenzyme 5 (LD_5) (formerly LDH_5); glutamate dehydrogenase (GLDH).
   b. Enzymes increased subsequent to *accelerated production* stimulated by bile retention or dugs are alkaline phosphatase (ALP) and γ-glutamyltransferase (GGT, also referred to as GGTP).
2. Function tests
   a. *Substances produced* are albumin, urea, coagulation factors, and glucose.
   b. Substances dependent on *uptake and metabolic processing or excretion* are bilirubin, bile acids, ammonia, cholesterol, and dyes.

HEPATIC ENZYME TESTS

These tests can be divided into those that reflect hepatocellular *injury* and those that reflect *increased enzyme production* consequent to cholestasis or drug induction.

---

* See Algorithms 7, 8, and 9.

Injury Enzymes

The cytoplasm of the hepatocyte is rich in alanine aminotransferase in the dog, cat and primate; horses and ruminants are notable exceptions (Fig. 5–1). An insult (toxin, hypoxia) to the hepatocellular membrane results in an increase in serum ALT activity. Acutely (hours to days), the magnitude of increase roughly parallels the number of hepatocytes with altered membrane permeability.

The highest tissue activities for aspartate aminotransferase are located primarily in the skeletal muscle cells and hepatocytes. Based on studies in humans, approximately 60 to 80% of the AST within the hepatocyte is associated with the mitochondria and the remainder as a soluble form in the cytosol (Fig. 5–1). Although it is inappropriate to extrapolate the exact percentages, we do know that both forms of AST exist in the dog. Studies have shown that a more severe insult is required to cause the release of the mitochondrial form of AST than one which alters only cell membrane permeability. Consequently, the serum ALT activity will more readily increase and usually be higher than the serum AST activity. The occurrence of an increased serum AST value in association with a higher serum ALT value is suggestive a severe hepatocellular injury when both values are moderately to markedly increased. Although uncommon, occasionally the serum AST activity is noted to be higher than the serum ALT activity, especially in the cat, early (hours) following a severe hepatic insult but will rapidly decrease to less than the ALT value.

The specific mechanisms responsible for the increase in serum ALT and AST activities (as well as for other serum enzyme activities) remain a mystery. In the past, we have used terms such as *leakage* and *altered permeability* of the damaged cell membrane in an attempt to conceptually explain the transfer of enzyme from cell to blood. Recent studies demonstrate that the hepatic activities of ALT and AST actually increase for a period of time following an insult. This implies that the remaining viable hepatocytes and regenerating hepatocytes contribute to the increase in the serum enzyme activities (perhaps, in part, by increased production during the reparative stage). We may be able to use this concept to our interpretive advantage. Markedly increased serum ALT and AST activities suggest a severe diffuse hepatic insult, especially if jaundice is present. This is followed by a gradual decrease (days) in the values; the AST decreasing faster, in part, because

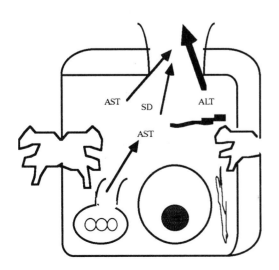

FIGURE 5–1. Injury to hepatic tissue results in release of cytoplasmic ALT (except horses and ruminants) and AST to the blood. Accelerated production and release by viable and regenerating hepatocytes may contribute to the serum aminotransferase activity. Injury to the mitochondria results in additional AST release to the blood. Increased serum SD activity is associated with hepatic injury in all species. (Modified from Meyer, D. J.: The liver. Part 1: Biochemical tests for the evaluation of the hepatobiliary system. Comp. Contin. Educ. Small Anim. Pract. 4:663, 1982.)

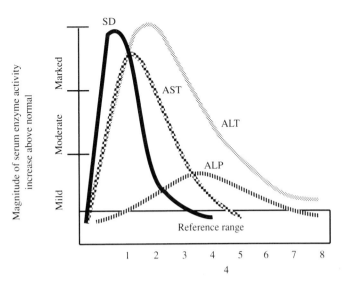

FIGURE 5–2. Serum enzyme activity after liver injury in the *dog* and *cat*. Initially, following a severe injury, the serum AST activity may temporarily exceed the ALT value. Note: the GGT will remain normal or show a slight increase day 3 to 5. Feline ALP may remain normal.

of a shorter half-life. In contrast, moderate increases in serum ALT and AST activities in a jaundiced patient subsequent to an acute insult with a precipitous decrease (hours to days) in these serum enzymes activities suggest a more severely damaged liver with fewer viable and regenerating hepatocytes.

In chronic hepatic disease, especially as the end-stage (cirrhosis) is approached, the serum ALT and AST values may be normal or only mildly increased. The attenuation of their magnitude is probably a reflection of the decreased viable parenchymal mass, altered intrahepatic architecture and the limited magnitude of the on-going injury. Studies have shown that as the hepatocyte undergoes degeneration, there is a temporary persistence of the mitochondrial AST. During the final stage of necrobiosis, this component of AST appears in the blood. Consequently, the documentation of mild to moderated increases in serum ALT and AST activities of similar magnitude on multiple occasions over time (weeks to months) implies a smoldering pathologic process in the liver; abnormal hepatic function (jaundice or increased serum bile acid concentration) may or may not be present.

Since we now appreciate that ALT may be increased secondarily to severe skeletal muscle injury, a *caveat* regarding the diagnostic use of the ALT and AST combination is prudent. *Coexistent* skeletal muscle injury should be ruled out by measuring the skeletal muscle specific enzyme *creatine kinase* (CK, formerly CPK) (Fig. 5–3). *Severe* skeletal muscle injury may result in a mild increase in the ALT; however, the increase in AST and CK will be dramatically greater.

The activity of ALT and AST requires the cofactor pyridoxal 5′-phosphate, the active metabolite of vitamin B_6. A *deficiency* of this vitamin results in decreased enzyme activity. Pyridoxine appears to be activated in the liver by the zinc-containing metalloenzyme alkaline phosphatase. The differential considerations for *decreased* (less than the reference range) aminotransferase and alkaline phosphatase values should include the state of nutrition (zinc or vitamin B_6 deficiency) and chronic liver disease (impaired activation).

Sorbitol dehydrogenase is a liver-specific cytosolic enzyme that can be used in the differential diagnosis of hepatic injury in those species in which measuring the ALT is not useful (Fig. 5–1). The increased serum SD activity is short lived (Fig. 5–2). One limitation is that the assay is not readily available.

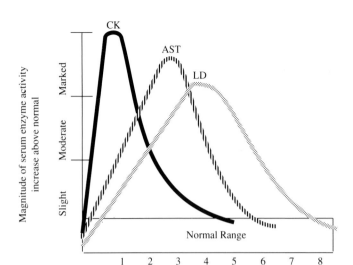

A

Days Following Muscle Injury

FIGURE 5–3. Muscle injury will result in increased serum activities of AST, and LD. Serum ALT activity will remain normal (or increase slightly) if there is concurrent liver injury.

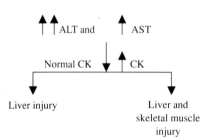

B

Lactate dehydrogenase is a cytosolic enzyme located in many tissues including hepatocytes, skeletal and cardiac muscle; consequently, total serum LD activity has no diagnostic advantage over AST. However, LD is composed of five isoenzymes, some of which can be determined spectrophotometrically, allowing diagnostic application. LD_1 and LD_2 are located primarily in cardiac muscle and can be determined as *α-hydroxybutyrate dehydrogenase*. LD_5 can also be measured spectrophotometrically and is located primarily in hepatocytes and skeletal muscle. If the LD_5 is increased and the CK is normal, altered hepatocellular membrane permeability is suggested (Fig. 5–4).

Glutamate dehydrogenase is a mitochondrial bound enzyme that is liver specific for all species. Even though its determination is not readily available in this country, clinical and experimental studies in Europe suggest that it is a sensitive marker of hepatocellular injury. Increased serum GLDH activity appears to show a time-related parallel to serum SD activity.

When considering plasma enzyme kinetics, the plasma half-life affects the duration of increase and ultimately, its window of diagnostic utility. Most half-lives are minutes to hours when determined subsequent to parenteral administration. Since a pathologic event causes tissue injury that does not resolve immediately we have chosen to illustrate graphically the time course of increased leakage enzyme activities after a pathologic insult as a closer approximation of the clinical situation (Figs. 5–2, 5–4, 5–5 and 5–6).

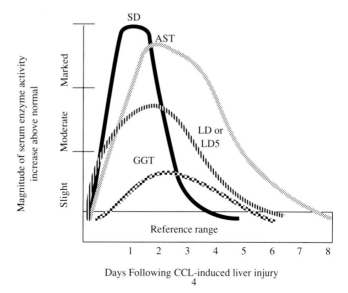

FIGURE 5–4. Serum enzyme activity following chemically-induced liver injury in the *horse*. Note: the ALT, CK and ALP are unchanged or show only slight increases days 1 to 3 (ALT, CK) and 3 to 5 (ALP).

Increased Enzyme Production Consequent to Cholestasis or Drug Induction

Certain enzymes normally have minimal tissue activity yet become remarkably increased in the serum subsequent to impaired bile flow or drug induction subsequent to *increased enzyme production*. The increased production starts within hours with subsequent appearance in the plasma. Likewise, after resolution of the stimulus, enzyme production will continue for a period of time. These enzymes, which are usually *membrane bound,* show minimal increase after an acute insult (as opposed to ALT and AST); any initial increase is probably a reflection of enzyme activity on membrane fragments released directly to the plasma as a result of the cell damage.

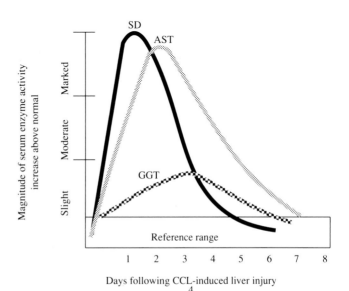

FIGURE 5–5. Serum enzyme activity after chemically induced liver injury in the *ruminant*. Note: The ALT, CK, and ALP are unchanged.

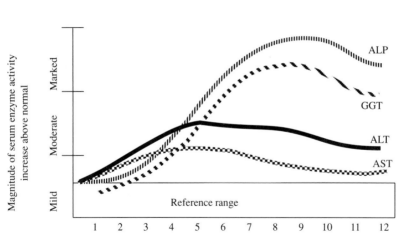

FIGURE 5–6. Serum enzyme activity after *ligation* of the common bile duct in the *dog, cat,* and *horse*. Note: Relative magnitude of ALP increase is greatest for the dog, then the cat, then the equine.

Alkaline phosphatase is a membrane-associated enzyme located in a variety of tissues, but only two are diagnostically important; bone and hepatobiliary. Each tissue has an isoenzyme form that can be separated with electrophoresis. With the exception of the growing animal or patient with bone disease, increased serum ALP activity is usually of hepatobiliary origin. There is considerable species variation with regard to the diagnostic usefulness of ALP. Impaired bile flow (*cholestasis*) results in increased ALP production in all species (Fig. 5–6). Increased serum ALP activity occurs before the development of hyperbilirubinemia. The magnitude of ALP increase is not helpful in differentiating intrahepatic from extrahepatic cholestasis. The reference range for ALP is wide for horses and ruminants, which limits the test's diagnostic impact. The hepatobiliary tissue of the cat has a limited capacity for accelerated ALP production, so any increase is suggestive of cholestasis. The magnitude of increase of serum ALP activity in the cat is further attenuated by a half-life of approximately 6 hours. In contrast, the dog has a robust capacity for ALP production, and, with a half-life approximately 3 days, dramatic increases in serum ALP values can develop. Even though increased ALP activity precedes the development of icterus, a low renal threshold* for bilirubin in the dog allows the presence of marked *bilirubinuria* to support further the differential consideration of a cholestatic process.

The dog also appears uniquely sensitive to increased ALP production secondary to *drug induction*. *Glucocorticoids* and *anticonvulsant* drugs are the most common inducers (Fig. 5–7). There is a remarkable individual variation in the magnitude of increase ranging from minimal to marked. It is noteworthy that in contrast to ALP associated with hepatic disease, *no* concomitant hyperbilirubinemia develops. Corticosteroids appear to cause the production of a novel isoenzyme that can be differentiated electrophoretically from the cholestatic-induced hepatobiliary isoenzyme. The procedure potentially should be helpful in the differential interpretation of increased serum ALP activity in the dog; however, the

---

* *Low renal threshold* refers to the plasma equilibrium between albumin-bound and unbound conjugated bilirubin. As the concentration of conjugated bilirubin increases, there is an increase in the unbound component that enters the glomerular filtrate.

FIGURE 5–7. Glucocorticoids (exogenous or endogenous) and anticonvulsant drugs may cause an increase in serum ALP and ALT activities in dogs. (Modified from Meyer, D. J.: The liver. Part 1: Biochemical tests for the evaluation of the hepatobiliary system. Comp. Contin. Educ. Small Anim. Pract. *4*:663, 1982.)

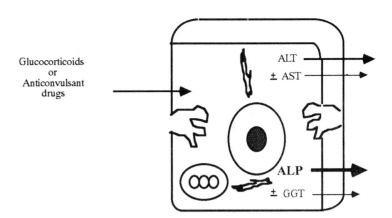

appearance of both isoenzymes in hepatic and extrahepatic diseases as well as consequent to increased endogenous production (hyperadrenocorticism) and exogenous corticosteroid administration limits the diagnostic applicability.

Occasionally, dogs receiving *corticosteroids* will also have mild increases in serum ALT activity and, much less frequently, AST activity (see Case 61). It is uncertain if the increases reflect a direct drug effect on altering membrane permeability or inducing aminotransferase production. The biochemical pattern mimics hepatobiliary disease, and occasionally a liver biopsy is required for the differential diagnosis. At this time, no other enzyme or function test (including bile acids) is conveniently available to assist in the differentiation of corticosteroid-induced abnormal hepatic tests.

Anticonvulsant medications (phenobarbital, phenytoin, primidone) are also potent inducers of ALP activity in the dog. No hyperbilirubinemia or marked hyperbilirubinemia develops, and there is minimal increase in the aminotransferase activities unless there is concurrent liver disease. This is important to realize since an anticonvulsant-associated hepatitis develops occasionally, and this differential should be entertained if hyperbilirubinemia or moderate to marked increases in serum ALT and, especially, AST (with no increase in CK) are detected.

γ-Glutamyltransferase is a membrane-associated enzyme that is located in a number of tissues but *not bone*. Increased serum activity reflects increased production and release from hepatobiliary tissue. The enzyme was used initially in the differential diagnosis of hepatobiliary disease from bone disease in human patients with increased serum ALP activity. *Cholestasis* causes increased serum activity in all species with better diagnostic utility than ALP in the cat, horse, and ruminants (Fig. 5–6) (see Cases 30 and 31). Although acute hepatic damage causes little to no increase in the serum GGT activity in the dog and cat, a mild to moderate increase does occur in the horse (Fig. 5–4) and ruminants (see Case 31) (Fig. 5–5). The increase may result from enzyme-rich membrane fragments released from damaged cells since these species appear to have relatively high hepatobiliary activity.

Increased hepatobiliary production of GGT is also stimulated by corticosteroids in the dog (Fig. 5–7). In contrast to ALP anticonvulsant drugs do not appear to cause increased serum GGT activity in the dog.

The renal tubules have a relatively high tissue GGT activity. Damage to these cells results in a rapid increase in urine (but not serum) GGT activity. Determination of urinary GGT activity has been used in the differential diagnosis of suspected renal toxicity, such as a marker of aminoglycoside toxicity, before an increase in serum creatinine concentration.

Colostrum/milk contains remarkably high GGT activity. Consequently nursing animals will have high serum GGT activities.

FUNCTION TESTS

Metabolized or Excreted

Bilirubin is formed from the metabolic degradation of hemoglobin from aged erythrocytes by the macrophage. The *unconjugated* (indirect reacting) bilirubin is released from the macrophage and carried by albumin to the liver. The hepatocyte removes the bilirubin from albumin and forms a diglucuronide (referred to as *conjugated* bilirubin) in preparation for secretion by the canalicular membrane into the bile. The measurement of total bilirubin includes both unconjugated and conjugated. In jaundice, an increase in total bilirubin imparts a yellow color to plasma when greater than 1 mg/dL (17.1 μmol/L) and to other tissues at concentrations greater than 2 to 3 mg/dL (34.2 to 51.3 μmol/L).

An increase in total bilirubin will occur when there is accelerated destruction of erythrocytes (see Case 5), primary hepatobiliary disease (see Case 33), or extrahepatic obstruction to bile flow (see Case 32), referred to as *prehepatic, intrahepatic* and *extrahepatic,* respectively. It used to be thought that the ratio of unconjugated and conjugated components of the total bilirubin was diagnostically useful in placing the cause of the icterus into one of these three classifications. Although conceptually attractive, neither the ratios nor the predominant component provides dependable information in the differentiation for icterus; *yellow is yellow.* An increased bilirubin directs one to measure the erythrocyte mass (packed cell volume), evaluate other liver tests, and examine the biliary system (ultrasonography and/or laparotomy).

In the *horse* a physiologic phenomenon with regard to bilirubin metabolism poses a fascinating diagnostic dilemma. Fasting (anorexia) for more than 24 hours can result in icterus caused, in part, by metabolites (such as fatty acids) competing with bilirubin for hepatocyte uptake (see Case 49). Resuming food consumption ameliorates the hyperbilirubinemia. The caveat needs to be integrated into the differential considerations for icterus in this species.

Bile acids are made by the liver, excreted in the bile, reabsorbed efficiently by the ileum into the portal circulation, and removed effectively by the hepatocytes, referred to as an *enterohepatic circulation* (Fig. 5–8). A very low concentration of bile acids appears in the peripheral blood. Any disturbance involving one or more structural components of the liver can cause the bile acids to escape into the peripheral circulation. Serum bile acids are a much more sensitive test of liver function than is bilirubin, and they will increase prior to the development of icterus. Determination of bile acids in an icteric patient will not be diagnostically useful *except* in the anorectic horse for the differential diagnosis of hyperbilirubinemia. Fasting does not affect bile acids as it does bilirubin; an abnormal bile acid value corroborates liver dysfunction in the jaundiced horse.

The measurement of the serum bile acid concentration following an overnight fast appears to be a diagnostically rewarding test in selected situations. It is critical to ensure that no stimulus for gallbladder contraction occurs prior to sampling since contraction will increase the serum bile acid concentration. Nor-

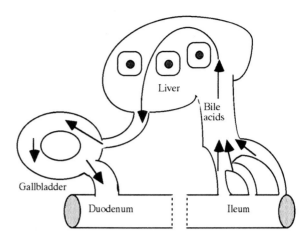

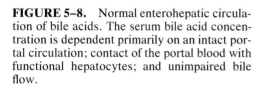

FIGURE 5–8. Normal enterohepatic circulation of bile acids. The serum bile acid concentration is dependent primarily on an intact portal circulation; contact of the portal blood with functional hepatocytes; and unimpaired bile flow.

mal fasting values are approximately less than 5 μmol/L for the cat, less than 10 μmol/L for the dog, and less than 15 μmol/L for the horse. Increased values suggest the presence of a pathologic process which will be evident histologically, or, if other clinicopathologic parameters are supportive, the presence of a congenital portosystemic vascular anomaly. It should be emphasized that, just as for the other hepatic tests, an increase in the serum bile acid concentration is not specific for a certain type of disease process and does not replace the histologic examination of tissue.

As alluded to earlier, contraction of the gallbladder temporarily challenges the bile acid clearing mechanisms (Fig. 5–9). The determination of the serum bile acid concentration 2 hours following meal-stimulated contraction of the gallbladder (except in the horse, of course) appears to increase test sensitivity but the diagnostic implications are premature. Postprandial values should not exceed 25 μmol/L for the dog and 15 μmol/L for the cat. The interpretation of the postprandial serum bile acid concentration should be made only by the experienced.

FIGURE 5–9. After a meal, contraction of the gallbladder bathes the gut with bile acids. The normal liver can remove most of the increased bile acids from the portal circulation by 2 hours postprandial. With liver disease a greater proportion of the bile acids escape into the peripheral circulation.

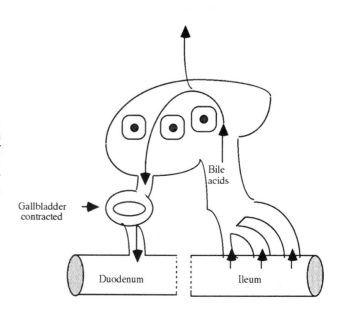

The determination of the serum bile acid concentration in the lactating cow does not appear to be diagnostically useful.

Serum bile acids are most diagnostically useful for detecting congenital porto-systemic shunts and for supporting liver dysfunction in the *nonicteric* patient when clinical signs are vague and other clinicopathologic parameters are suggestive of liver insufficiency (Figs. 5–10 and 5–11) (see Cases 9, 33, 34, and 35).

Ammonia is derived primarily from the catabolism of amino acid enteric bacteria, absorbed into the portal circulation, removed by the liver, and incorporated into the urea cycle with the resultant formation of urea and eventual excretion by the kidney (Fig. 5–12). By default, *urea* (urea nitrogen) can be considered a liver function test, that is, decreased secondary to hepatic insufficiency. Ammonia, along with other protein-derived metabolic products which escape liver detoxification, is toxic to the central nervous system and causes the neurologic syndrome referred to as *hepatic encephalopathy* (Fig. 5–13). Ammonia is the metabolite clinically used to reflect dysfunction of the central nervous system secondary to liver insufficiency because of its relative ease of measurement. Since a fasting plasma ammonia concentration will be normal in some cases, we adapted an ammonia tolerance test that can be used to challenge the liver. Ammonium chloride salt is administered, 100 mg/kg body weight (3 gm maximum), in 20 to 30 mL of water, either orally or rectally. A second blood sample is taken at approximately 30 minutes. Normally, there is less than a two-fold increase; more than a three-fold increase is indicative of liver insufficiency. *Caveat:* the ammonia tolerance test should only be used if the fasting ammonia concentration is normal. Since ammonia is volatile, the heparinized sample should be kept in crushed ice

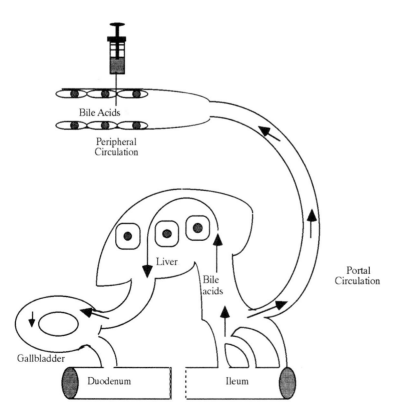

FIGURE 5–10. Congenital portal vascular anomaly: altered enterohepatic circulation of bile acids.

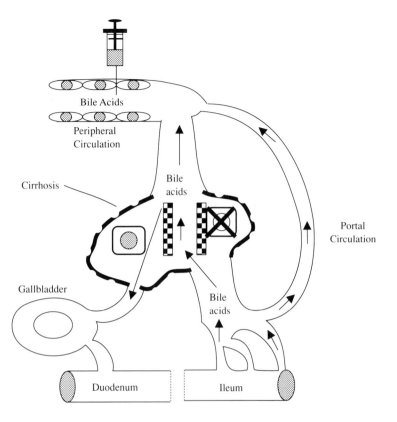

FIGURE 5–11. Chronic liver disease/cirrhosis; shunting of bile acids around (acquired extrahepatic shunts) and through the diseased liver (intrahepatic shunts) as a result of altered physioanatomy (loss of hepatocytes, abnormal blood flow, and cholestasis).

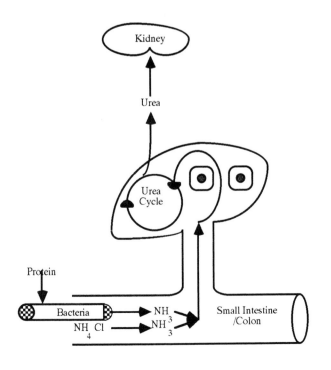

FIGURE 5–12. Ammonia is formed in the intestinal tract, absorbed, carried to the liver by the portal vascular system, and metabolized forming urea. (Modified from Meyer, D. J.: The liver. Part 1: Biochemical tests for the evaluation of the hepatobiliary system. Comp. Contin. Educ. Small Anim. Pract. 4:663, 1982.)

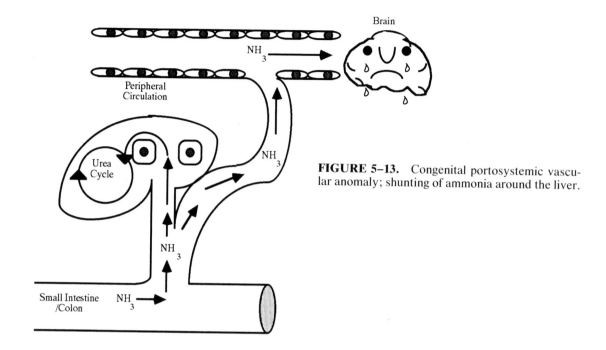

FIGURE 5–13. Congenital portosystemic vascular anomaly; shunting of ammonia around the liver.

and assayed within 2 or 3 hours. The dry chemistry-based reagent systems facilitate the clinical use of this liver function test.

Illustrated in Figures 5–13, 5–14, and 5–15 are the causes of hyperammonia: congenital malformation of the portal circulation (a differential for dysfunction of the central nervous system in all species), cirrhosis/chronic liver disease, and

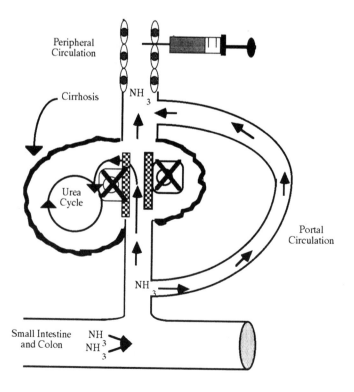

FIGURE 5–14. Ammonia metabolism in chronic liver disease/cirrhosis; intrahepatic and extrahepatic shunting of ammonia through and around the liver.

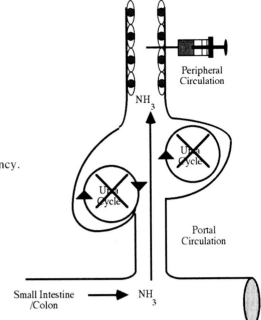

FIGURE 5–15. Congenital urea enzyme cycle deficiency.

congenital enzyme deficiency of the urea cycle. It is noteworthy that the serum bile acid concentration also will be abnormal in the first two disorders but *not* the last. In the ruminant, ammonia intoxication also may occur secondary to the ingestion of large amounts of urea in the diet.

Dyes such as *sulfobromophthalein* (BSP) and *indocyanine green* (ICG) are dyes which, after intravenous administration, are cleared by the liver similar to bilirubin. The dyes, like bile acids, are more sensitive to liver dysfunction than is bilirubin. The advent of bile acids has replaced the diagnostic use of dyes for the evaluation of liver function in most clinical settings with the exception of some academic institutions which have the dye and the methodology available for the procedure.

Cholesterol. While a number of disturbances in lipid metabolism have been documented to occur in association with liver disease, few are useful diagnostically. The liver is the focal point for the elimination of cholesterol from the body in the form of bile acids. *Hypercholesterolemia* may occur in patients with extrahepatic biliary obstruction (see Case 32) but icterus has already developed. *Hypocholesterolemia* may develop secondary to congenital portal vascular anomalies (see Case 35); the reason is unknown. One nonspecific reflection of aberrant lipid metabolism is the formation of poikilocytes and target cells in association with some liver disorders as a result of abnormal erythrocyte membrane lipid accumulation (causes of hypercholesterolemia and hypocholesterolemia are listed in Table 3–1).

Produced by the Hepatocyte

Albumin. The measurement of total protein reflects a combination of albumin and globulins. The plasma total protein value determined with a refractometer is greater than the value biochemically determined on serum, the difference repre-

TABLE 5–1. Causes of Changes in Serum Cholesterol

Increased
  Hypothyroidism
  Postprandial
  Diet high in fat
  Extrahepatic biliary obstruction
  Diabetes mellitus
  Nephrotic syndrome
  Hyperlipidemia syndrome (schnauzers and other breeds)
  Primary (idiopathic) associated with corneal lipodystrophy
  Primary hyperchylonmicronemia in cats
  Congenital lipoprotein lipase deficiency in cats

Decreased
  Maldigestion/malabsorption
  Exocrine pancreatic insufficiency
  Protein-losing enteropathy
  Congenital portosystemic shunts

senting the fibrinogen concentration utilized during clot formation. Albumin, which represents about half of the adult total protein, is produced solely in the liver; one differential consideration for *hypoalbuminemia* is liver insufficiency (see Cases 29, 34, and 35). Albumin is not a sensitive test of hepatic function, and its diagnostic sensitivity varies among species. Concomitantly, the globulin concentration is usually normal or slightly increased. Other differential considerations for hypoalbuminemia include increased urinary loss associated with glomerulonephropathy (globulins are usually normal); a protein-losing enteropathy (globulins are usually decreased); starvation (globulins are usually normal); and secondary to hyperglobulinemia. When there is a hyperglobulinemia, either polyclonal or monoclonal, the hyperviscosity signals the liver to down-regulate albumin production (causes of hypoalbuminemia are listed in Table 3–2).

Urea is produced by the liver, and measurement of serum levels is usually done to evaluate renal function but may be decreased in association with hepatic failure and congenital portosystemic venous anomalies (see Case 35).

Coagulation factors, for all practical purposes, are produced in the liver. In addition, some of the factors (V, VII, IX, and X) are dependent on vitamin K for

TABLE 5–2. Causes of Hypoproteinemia (Usually Hypoalbuminemia)

Decreased production
  Intestinal malabsorption (primary or secondary)
  Maldigestion (exocrine pancreatic insufficiency)
  Malnutrition (parasitic or dietary)
  Chronic liver disease (atrophy or fibrosis)

Increased loss
  Renal disease with chronic proteinuria
  Exudative skin lesions[a]
  External hemorrhage[a]
  Protein-losing enteropathy[a]

[a] Globulins may also be decreased.

formation. Vitamin K is a fat-soluble vitamin, and since bile acids are an integral component of intestinal fat absorption, diseases that impair the flow of bile to the gut may prolong clotting times. The subcutaneous administration of vitamin K_1 to a patient with a clotting disorder secondary to extrahepatic cholestasis will return the clotting time toward normal within 6 to 8 hours, a useful *presurgical* procedure in any jaundiced surgical patient. Although coagulation tests have limited diagnostic utility, the predisposition for a bleeding disorder in a patient with any type of liver disease should be kept in mind (see Case 33).

Glucose is stored in the liver in the form of glycogen, which provides for a readily available source. Although clinical *hypoglycemia* is not a common association with liver insufficiency, a slight decrease in the fasting glucose, more common in association with congenital portal vascular anomalies, should be pursued with a more sensitive liver test in the nonicteric patient (see Case 34). The diseased liver or the liver associated with a congenital portal vascular anomaly is unable to maintain adequate glycogen stores, predisposing the patient to stress/fasting hypoglycemia, an important *postoperative* consideration.

IMPACT OF DISEASE

While liver tests have been divided into (1) parameters that reflect hepatobiliary function including an intact portal circulation, and (2) serum enzyme tests that serve as markers of hepatocellular injury or increased enzyme production secondary to impaired bile flow or drug induction, they should not be interpreted as separate entities. Because of the intimate hepatic physioanatomic interdependence, a pathologic event affecting one structural component (and causing an attendant biochemical abnormality) often rapidly impacts on one or more of the other components (causing further biochemical abnormalities). This complex interrelationship results in *patterns* of functional and liver enzymes test abnormali-

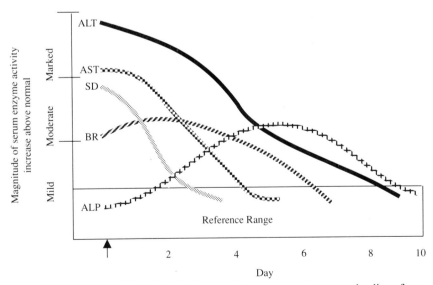

FIGURE 5–16. Relationship among liver enzyme tests and a liver function test (*BR*, total bilirubin) after acute hepatic injury. Increased ALT activity is appropriate in the dog and cat. The increased ALP activity is more dramatic in the dog. ↑ indicates the point of acute insult.

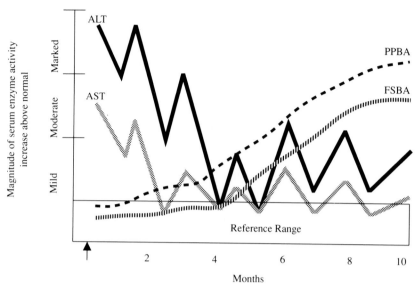

FIGURE 5–17. Relationship among liver leakage enzymes and a liver function test (*FSBA*-fasting bile acids), PPBA-2-hour postprandial bile acid in chronic active liver injury progressing to cirrhosis prior to the development of icterus. The time course is arbitrary; the pathologic process may be faster or slower; ↑ indicates first recognition of abnormal liver tests.

ties which are diagnostically more useful than attempting to interpret each test as a separate entity. For example, an icteric dog, historically sick for 2 days, with markedly increased serum ALT and AST activities and mild to moderate increased ALP activity most likely has severe liver insufficiency associated with acute diffuse hepatocellular injury (Fig. 5–16). A differential diagnosis of congenital portal vascular anomaly or cirrhosis (Fig. 5–17) should be considered in a nonjaundiced dog or cat showing nondescript central nervous system signs with hypoalbuminemia, a markedly increased fasting serum bile acid concentration, and normal or mild increases in serum ALT and ALP activities.

6

URINARY TRACT TEST ABNORMALITIES*

The functional unit of the kidney is the nephron, which consists of the glomerulus, containing a vascular bed that serves as a filtration unit, and the tubule which modifies the filtrate (Fig. 6–1). The end product is urine.

URINALYSIS

Urine can be collected by cystocentesis, catheterization, and free catch (voided). Midstream (voided) collections are adequate for examination if results are negative. Interpretation of cell counts, protein, and culture of these specimens may lead to misleading results. Abnormal findings should be reaffirmed by a second specimen collected by cystocentesis or catheterization.

Urinalysis should be completed on freshly collected urine; refrigerated specimens are acceptable for up to 6 hours.

Physical Properties

Appearance

The color and transparency of urine should be recorded. The normal yellow color of urine is a result of urochromes. Dark yellow urine usually indicates a concentrated specimen whereas dilute samples are often colorless. The presence of blood or hemoglobin produces a red urine that changes to brownish discoloration on standing.

Urine is transparent except in the horse, in which the thick and cloudy appearance is a result of mucus and calcium carbonate crystals. Cloudy urine may be observed if cells, bacteria, fat, crystals, or mucus is present in a large concentration. The cause of cloudy urine can be determined by microscopic examination of sediment.

Specific Gravity

Specific gravity is the ratio of the mass of a solution compared with the mass of an equal volume of water. It is not a direct measurement of the number of solute particles, as is osmolality. However, the two determinations are related, and the

---

* See Algorithms 10 and 11.

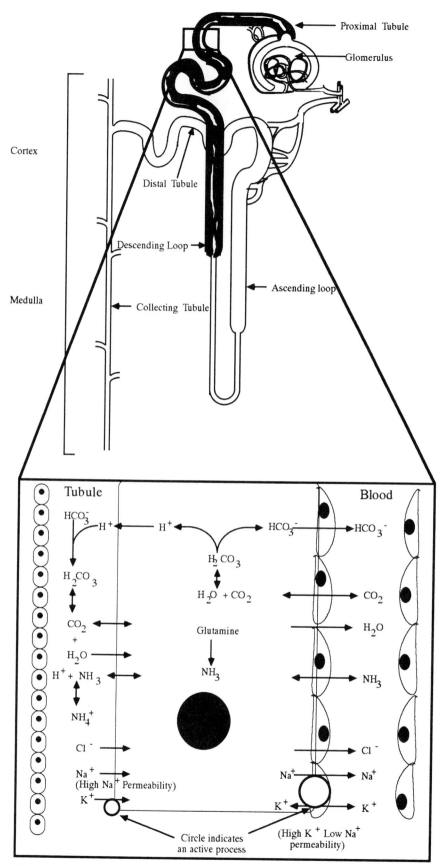

FIGURE 6–1. See legend on opposite page.

specific gravity is a clinically useful test since loss of concentrating ability is one of the first signs of renal tubule disease.

The specific gravity of the glomerular filtrate is between 1.008 and 1.012. A urine specific gravity above 1.012 or below 1.008 requires tubular cell function.

The specific gravity can range from 1.001 to 1.060 and reflects the hydration status of the animal (Fig. 6–2).

A specific gravity greater than 1.030 in the dog and 1.035 in the cat suggests adequate concentrating ability. Evaluation of the specific gravity should *always* be made with a *concurrent* serum urea nitrogen and/or creatinine value as outlined in Figure 6–3.

It is emphasized that these are only general guidelines, and the patient's history and other clinicopathologic parameters should be taken into consideration.

Although renal disease is one cause of low specific gravity (see Cases 39, 40, and 41), many other factors such as excessive fluid intake, diuretic therapy, and the administration of fluids must be considered.

Chemical Examination

Chemical examination of urine routinely includes assay for pH, protein, glucose, ketones, occult blood, and bilirubin.

FIGURE 6–1. The glomerulus filters creatinine and urea nitrogen from the blood but retains albumin. Decreased glomerular blood flow (prerenal) or disease involving the glomerulus (renal) can be recognized by azotemia (increased urea-nitrogen and/or creatinine). In addition, certain types of glomerular injury permit albumin to escape into the filtrate, resulting in proteinuria. Tubular function can be reflected crudely by determining the urine specific gravity. Consequently, determination of serum urea nitrogen/creatine plus the urine specific gravity can be used to screen nephron function. The renal tubular cell plays a pivotal role in maintaining acid/base and electrolyte homeostasis. Hydrogen ions (H^+) are secreted into the tubular fluid whereas bicarbonate ions (HCO_3^-) are transported to the blood; for every mol of acid secreted, 1 mol of bicarbonate appears in the blood. Chloride (CL^-) reciprocates with HCO_3^- as the major anion as needed. Similarly, when acid (H^+) is secreted a sodium (Na^+) ion is exchanged to maintain cationic electrical neutrality. In addition, the secretion of potassium (K^+) and H^+ are inversely related. Consequently metabolic alkalosis can develop (or be perpetuated) if there is a potassium deficiency since H^+ is secreted preferentially into the urine in order to conserve K^+. Aldosterone (secreted by the zona glomerulosa of the adrenal glands in response to the plasma potassium concentration, as well as angiotensin II) acts on the distal tubule and collecting ducts to increase K^+ secretion into the urine and conserve Na^+. Ammonia (NH_3), formed primarily from glutamine, diffuses into the tubular fluid where it combines with H^+, facilitating the conservation of Na^+. One can readily appreciate that with renal disease these complex interrelationships are disrupted and can result in metabolic acidosis, hyperkalemia, and accelerated loss of Na^+ in the urine. Interestingly hypokalemia appears to develop initially in cats during the early stages of chronic renal failure for unknown reasons. Aldosterone is mentioned in this discussion on renal physiology because a deficiency of the hormone (hypoadrenocorticism) results in a combination of hyperkalemia, hyponatremia, and prerenal azotemia secondary to vomiting, which can mimic renal failure clinicopathologically.

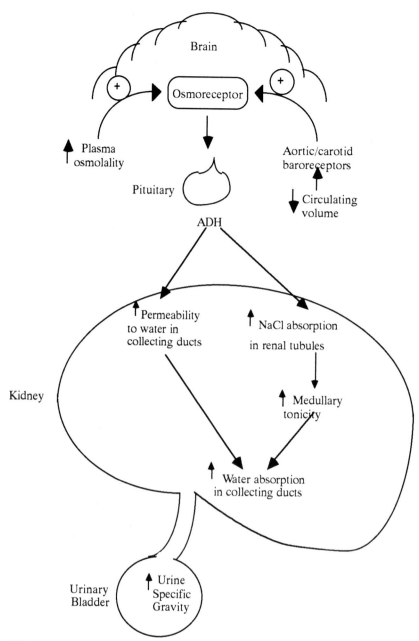

FIGURE 6–2. The urine specific gravity is a crude index of renal tubule function in response to fluid homeostasis. A decrease in circulating blood volume or an increase in plasma osmolality stimulates the release of *antidiuretic hormone* (ADH) which facilitates the absorption of water by the collecting ducts. The action of ADH is reflected by an increase in urine specific gravity. Lack of ADH secretion or resistance of the collecting ducts to the stimulus of ADH (*diabetes insipidus, central or nephrogenic*) is associated with an inappropriate specific gravity in relation to the hydration status; the resulting plasma hyperosmolality may be reflected by *hypernatremia* and the dehydration by *azotemia*. The azotemia and inappropriate (low) specific gravity, along with the signs of polydipsia/polyuria, mimic chronic renal insufficiency. With the judicious use of the water deprivation test (limiting dehydration to 5% of the body weight and frequent monitoring of the urea nitrogen) followed by ADH administration, the specific gravity will increase with central diabetes insipidus but will not change if nephrogenic. It is emphasized that diabetes insipidus is an *uncommon* cause of polydipsia/polyuria, and the other more common causes should be ruled out exhaustively.

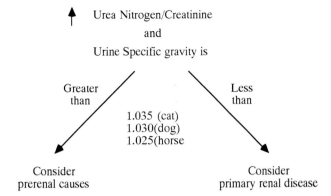

FIGURE 6–3. Relationship of urine specific gravity to serum urea nitrogen, and creatinine values.

pH

Urine pH is dependent upon the diet. Herbivorous animals have an alkaline pH, and carnivores and omnivores will vary from acid to alkaline depending upon the amount of animal protein in the diet.

Increased urine acidity may result from starvation, fever, metabolic or respiratory acidosis, prolonged muscular exercise, or the administration of acid salts such as ammonium chloride.

Increased urine alkalinity may accompany metabolic or respiratory alkalosis, bacterial cystitis (see Case 46), and may follow ingestion of sodium bicarbonate.

Protein

A small quantity of protein passes the glomerular filter but is reabsorbed by the renal tubules, consequently, normal urine is usually negative when tested for protein. In concentrated urine (specific gravity greater than 1.050) trace to 1+ reactions may be normal.

A slight transitory proteinuria may be associated with fever, muscular exercise, and seizures. A false positive may occur with an alkaline urine (pH greater than 8.5).

Proteinuria must be interpreted in association with urine specific gravity and urine sediment. A slight proteinuria in urine of low specific gravity is more significant than the same quantity of protein in concentrated urine. The significance of protein loss through the kidney can be determined by calculating the urine protein to urine creatinine ratio (UP/UCr) as follows:

$$\frac{\text{Urine protein (mg/dL), g/L} \div 10}{\text{Urine creatinine (mg/dL), } \mu\text{mol/L} \div 84 \div 100} = \frac{\text{UP}}{\text{UCr}} \text{ ratio}$$

A $\dfrac{\text{UP}}{\text{UCr}}$ ratio greater than 1.0 for the dog or greater than 0.7 for the cat indicates renal disease (see Case 41).

The detection of proteinuria should prompt several differential considerations. *Renal proteinuria* occurs as a result of abnormal glomerular permeability. Glomerulonephritis and renal amyloidosis are the most common causes of altered glomerular permeability. *Postrenal proteinuria* occurs when there is inflammation of the lower urinary tract. It is usually accompanied by hematuria or pyuria or both. The most common cause of postrenal proteinuria is cystitis. A midstream urine sample may also contain protein secondary to prostatitis, urethritis, and vaginal or preputial discharges.

A *nonrenal* source of proteinuria (*prerenal*) occurs when low molecular weight proteins (light chain immunoglobulins) pass through the glomerulus. A plasma cell tumor is the most common cause. One characteristic of finding these Bence Jones proteins is that the pad on the test tape remains negative, but the sulfosalicylic acid (Bumintest*) test is usually positive (see Case 13).

Both *hemoglobinuria* and *myoglobinuria* may cause a positive protein reaction.

Glucose

Glucose passes the glomerular filter and is completely reabsorbed by tubule cells, therefore glucose is not detected in normal urine.

The usual method of testing urine for glucose is the enzyme (glucose oxidase) dipstick. False negative reactions may occur in urine containing a large quantity of ascorbic acid. Because dogs synthesize variable amounts of ascorbic acid, an alternative method should be used to detect glucosuria. A commercial tablet (Clinitest*) that detects reducing substances can be used. Cats with cystitis may also give a false positive reaction with the dipstick method.

Renal Glucosuria

When the blood glucose is normal, renal glucosuria is a component of the Fanconi-like syndrome caused by an inability of tubules to reabsorb urine constituents. This syndrome, which often leads to severe renal pathology, has been reported in several breeds of dog including basenji, Norwegian elkhound, Shetland sheepdog, and miniature schnauzer. Affected patients also have an aminoaciduria. Primary renal glucosuria has been reported (as an isolated finding) in Scottish terriers, Norwegian elkhounds, and mixed breeds. It is not apparently associated with clinical disease and should not be confused with diabetes mellitus.

Ketones

Excessive ketone formation results from accelerated oxidation of fatty acids as an energy source. Slight ketonuria can be seen in malnourished dogs and cats. It frequently accompanies advanced cases of canine diabetes mellitus (see Case 53). If the predominant ketone is β-hydroxybutyrate, ketonuria will not be detected because the test tape is insensitive to this ketone.

Ketonuria in ruminants is also associated with abnormal carbohydrate metabolism. Acetoacetate and β-hydroxybutyrate predominate with a lesser amount of ketone.

Occult Blood

A positive reaction indicates erythrocytes, free hemoglobin, or myoglobin. A positive reaction must be interpreted in light of urine sediment findings. After centrifugation, a positive test in the supernatant suggests hemoglobinuria, RBC lysis in hypotonic urine, or myoglobinuria. Myoglobinuria and hemoglobinuria can be differentiated crudely using an ammonium sulfate precipitation test. (2.8

---

* Ames Company, Elkhart Indiana.

mg of ammonium sulfate should be added to 5 ml of urine, mixed well, and centrifuged. If the supernatant fluid remains dark, myoglobin is probable. Myoglobinuria may be supported by finding an increase in serum creatine kinase (CK) activity.

Hematuria reflects hemorrhage in the urinary tract, and hemoglobinuria suggests intravascular destruction of erythrocytes.

Bilirubin

Conjugated bilirubin appears in urine if there is an increase in the serum concentration (see Case 32). Dogs have a low renal threshold for bilirubin, and a trace or 1+ reaction in urine with a specific gravity greater than 1.020 is insignificant. However, a stronger (3+ or more) reaction suggests hepatic disease and the need for a more sensitive liver function test if the patient is not jaundiced since bilirubinuria precedes bilirubinemia in the dog. Bilirubinuria may be also detected in dogs with hemoglobinemia secondary to increased erythrocyte destruction (see Case 5).

Urobilinogen

Urobilinogen lacks diagnostic utility.

Microscopic Sediment

Urine collected by cystocentesis normally contains sparse numbers of cells and other formed elements from the urinary tract.

The method for examining urine sediment should be consistent. Five ml is sedimented to provide a uniform semiquantitation. We recommend the examination of unstained sediment since stain precipitate and bacteria and yeasts introduce erroneous findings. It is important to *rack* the condenser down when examining urine sediments. Altering the light in this fashion emphasizes urine particulate constituents.

Leukocytes

Zero to 3/hpf leukocytes are normally present in urine collected by cystocentesis. Increased numbers of leukocytes (pyuria) support the presence of an inflammatory process. The sample should be cultured even if bacteria are not seen.

Erythrocytes

Normal urine has a few erythrocytes (0 to 3/hpf). An increased number of RBCs in urine is an indication of inflammation or hemorrhage (see cases 44 and 46). If the RBCs are in a cast, renal hemorrhage is suggested. Hematuria may be associated with uroliths, neoplasia, bacterial infections, trauma, sterile cystitis, nephritis, nephrosis, urinary parasites, and thrombocytopenia. Leukocytes and/or erythrocytes in urine collected midstream may reflect hemorrhage/inflammation in the genital tract.

Epithelial Cells

Epithelial cells may appear in small numbers in urine, but the number may be increased in animals with cystitis, neoplasia, or other inflammation of the urinary tract. In a patient with persistent hematuria and stranguria, cytologic examination of the urine is a useful screening procedure for neoplasia. A small drop of sediment is spread on a glass slide, air dried, and stained similarly to a blood smear. Neoplastic cells can be more readily identified in this type of preparation.

Casts

Urine casts are formed within renal tubules.

Urine from normal animals contains only a few hyaline casts (2 or less/lpf) and/or granular (1 or less/lpf) casts. Hyaline, granular, and waxy casts represent a continuum regarding formation.

The causes and significance of urine casts are summarized in Table 6–1.

Bacteria

Bacteria are not present in normal urine collected by cystocentesis but may be present in varying numbers in catheterized or midstream collections. Bacteria in urine collected by cystocentesis indicate an infectious process.

Yeasts and Fungi

In the urine these are usually contaminants. Contamination usually occurs during collection. Urine sediment stains may become contaminated with yeasts as well as bacteria.

Crystals

Certain crystals are of diagnostic significance. Ammonium biurate suggests hepatic insufficiency; cystine crystals may be associated with cystine uroliths; calcium oxalate monohydrate (hippuric acid appearing crystals) occur with ethylene glycol (antifreeze) toxicity as well as with the more common Maltese cross variety.

Sperm

Sperm are found in about one fourth of urine samples taken by cystocentesis from intact males and in recently bred females.

TABLE 6–1. Urine Casts

Type of Cast	Associated with	Interpretation
Hyaline	Proteinuria	Insignificant
Epithelial	Tubular sloughing	Acute severe tubular damage
Granular	Tubular epithelial cell degeneration	Suggest tubular nephrosis
Leukocyte	Renal inflammation	Suggest pyelonephritis
Erythrocyte	Hemorrhage	Usually the result of trauma

RENAL FUNCTION TESTS-BLOOD CHEMISTRY

Renal function tests can be used as markers of renal function but do not provide a diagnosis. Sequential evaluation is useful for monitoring treatment and disease progression.

Urea Nitrogen

Urea is formed by the liver and represents the principal product of protein catabolism in carnivorous and omnivorous species. Urea passes through the glomerular filter, and 25 to 40% of filtered urea is reabsorbed as it passes through the tubules. Increased urine diminishes urea reabsorption while slow flow rates facilitate reabsorption.

Urea nitrogen levels may be increased (carnivores and omnivores) with a dietary increase in protein and catabolic breakdown of tissue and hemorrhage into the gastrointestinal tract (see Case 51) (Table 6–2). The creatinine concentration is unchanged.

Azotemia

Prerenal Azotemia

This condition is associated with decreased blood flow through the kidney secondary to dehydration and cardiovascular insufficiency. Prerenal azotemia should be accompanied by an increased urine specific gravity (1.030 or more in dog; 1.035 or more in cat) if there is no concurrent primary renal disease (see Cases 33 and 56).

Primary or Renal Azotemia

Primary azotemia occurs with glomerular damage; proteinuria may also be present (see Cases 39 through 44).

TABLE 6–2. **Causes of Azotemia (Increased Urea Nitrogen and/or Creatinine)**

Classification	Cause
Prerenal	Dehydration Cardiovascular disease Shock (septic or traumatic) High protein diet (urea-nitrogen increase only) Hemorrhage into gastrointestinal tract (urea-nitrogen increase only)
Renal	Renal diseases causing two thirds to three-fourths of nephrons to be destroyed
Postrenal	Obstruction of urinary tract Rupture of urinary tract

Postrenal Azotemia

Postrenal azotemia occurs with urethral obstruction or subsequent to rupture of the urinary bladder (see Case 45).

Creatinine

Creatinine is formed during skeletal muscle metabolism. As with urea nitrogen serum creatinine is a crude index of glomerular filtration. Serum creatinine is not markedly influenced by diet or intestinal hemorrhage. Severe muscle wasting will reduce the quantity of creatinine formed.

As with urea nitrogen a reduced glomerular filtration rate (GFR) increases the serum concentration of creatinine. The same prerenal, renal, and postrenal factors that influence urea nitrogen also affect serum creatinine.

Other Blood Chemistry Determinations

Because kidneys play an important role in the elimination and conservation of many chemical components of the blood, renal disease may alter their serum values. These are summarized in Table 6–3.

Electrolytes

A more detailed consideration of electrolytes will be found in Chapter 8. The following discussion will be directed toward alterations observed in renal disease and some mechanisms involved.

Potassium. Potassium is filtered and is actively excreted. The quantity of potassium handled by the kidneys reflects potassium intake. Patients with renal disease may retain potassium, and hyperkalemia will develop.

Sodium. The ability to retain sodium is frequently lost in chronic renal disease.

Chloride/Bicarbonate. The chloride composition of the body varies inversely with the bicarbonate concentration. Bicarbonate deficiencies may occur with advanced renal disease.

TABLE 6–3. Electrolyte and Nonelectrolyte Changes in Advanced Renal Disease

	Renal Alteration	Result
Electrolytes		
Sodium	↑ Fractional excretion	Hyponatremia
Postassium	↓ Fractional excretion	Hyperkalemia
Bicarbonate	↓ Conservation	Acidemia
Phosphate	↓ Excretion	Hyperphosphatemia (dog and cat)
Calcium	↑ Excretion as phosphate ↑	Hypocalcemia
Nonelectrolytes		
Blood pH	↓ Removal of H^+ and acid products	Acidemia
Lipids	↑ Synthesis of lipids	Hypercholesterolemia
Serum proteins	Persistent proteinuria	Hypoalbuminemia

Phosphate.   Hyperphosphatemia occurs with regularity in dogs and cats with a decreased GFR (see cases 39, 41, 43, and 44). Hyperphosphatemia is not constant in cattle or horses with decreased GFR (see Cases 40 and 42).

Calcium.   There are usually no changes in serum calcium in acute renal disease, but hypocalcemia may be observed with chronic renal disease. Hypercalcemia frequently occurs in *horses* with advanced renal disease (see Case 40) and has been reported in dogs occasionally.

Nonelectrolytes

Blood pH.   Metabolic acidosis is relatively consistent in patients with renal failure. Reduced renal function affects H^+ removal from the blood as well as the capacity to remove acid products of metabolism. This reduced ability is compounded by a deficiency to conserve bicarbonate.

Lipids.   Hyperlipidemia is a common association with the nephrotic syndrome (proteinuria, hypoalbuminemia, edema). Enhanced synthesis of cholesterol-containing lipoproteins by the liver is thought to be related to the hypoalbuminemia and/or decreased oncotic pressure.

Serum Proteins.   Generalized renal disease with a persistent proteinuria will result in hypoalbuminemia. Patients with primary glomerular disease usually have the most severe protein loss, especially if associated with amyloidosis (see Case 41).

PANCREATIC AND INTESTINAL TESTS

Endocrine and Exocrine Deficiencies; Intestinal Tests*

The pancreas has two types of functions: hormonal (endocrine) and digestive (exocrine). Hormonal functions include the interaction of insulin and glucagon, which is important in the regulation of glucose metabolism.

THE ENDOCRINE PANCREAS

Carbohydrate Metabolism

Insulin

The release of insulin by the pancreatic β-cells is regulated primarily by the feedback effect of blood glucose on the pancreas. When the blood glucose concentration is increased insulin secretion increases, and when the blood glucose concentration decreases so does insulin release. Studies suggest that the serum insulin concentration is near zero when the blood glucose approaches 30 mg/dL (1.65 mmol/L). This is the rationale for including the value of 30 mg/dL in the formula for the amended insulin to glucose ratio (AIGR) that is used to aid in the diagnosis of hyperinsulinism.

Fatty acids, selected amino acids, and ketones also have a stimulatory effect on insulin secretion. Glucagon, in small amounts, will stimulate insulin secretion. Growth hormone, glucocorticoids, estrogen, and progesterone increase peripheral resistance to insulin in increased pancreatic secretion of insulin (Fig. 7–1).

Glucagon

Glucagon is produced by pancreatic α-cells and cells in the wall of the duodenum and stomach.

Glucagon is also regulated by plasma glucose levels. A rise in glucose causes decreased secretion whereas fasting causes increased secretion. Glucagon increase the glucose concentration primarily through hepatic glycogenolysis and gluconeogenesis (Fig. 7–1).

---

* See Algorithms 12, 13, and 14.

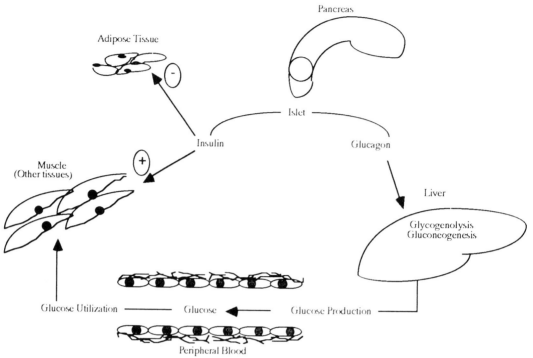

FIGURE 7–1. Regulation of the blood glucose concentration. Insulin promotes glucose utilization and inhibits lipolysis. Glucagon facilitates glucose production.

Diseases

Hypoinsulinism (Diabetes Mellitus; Hyperglycemia)

Glucose, in the absence of insulin, is utilized inefficiently by muscle, adipose tissue, or the liver. Insulin deficiency along with the continued activity of glucagon results in hyperglycemia and glycosuria (Fig. 7–2). Diabetic animals may also develop weight loss and polyphagia because, in spite of large quantities of blood glucose, body tissues are starved, resulting in the catabolism of fat and muscle. The longer hypoinsulinism exists the more likely ketoacidosis will develop. Diabetes mellitus may also occur in patients with hypersomatotropism (see Chapter 9 for discussion).

Diagnosis. Laboratory findings, in addition to hyperglycemia and glycosuria, include hypercholesterolemia (plasma is frequently lipemic), increased serum alkaline phosphatase, and alanine aminotransferase activities as a consequence of hepatic lipidosis, and ketonemia and ketonuria (see Case 53).

Other causes of hyperglycemia are summarized in Table 7–1.

Uremic animals often have a diabetic-like glucose tolerance curve. The fasting glucose may not be increased, but hyperglycemia may develop after parenteral or oral administration of glucose. This is thought to occur because of peripheral resistance to insulin. Since insulin is catabolized by the kidney, it is ironic that glucose intolerance develops despite peripheral insulin values in the high normal range, inappropriate for the blood glucose concentration.

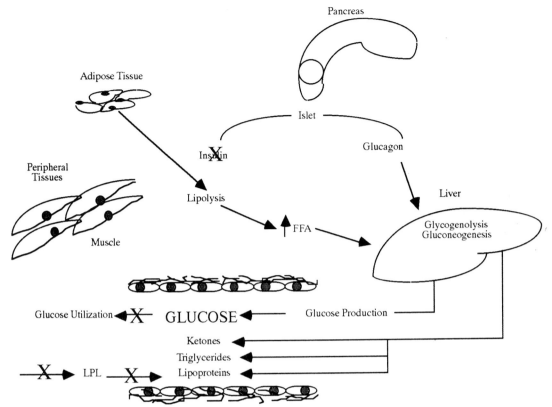

FIGURE 7–2. Diabetes mellitus. Because of insulin deficiency, hyperglycemia develops secondary to decreased utilization. Insulin deficiency permits lipolysis to generate free fatty acids (*FFA*), which are transported to the liver in which some are stored as triglycerides (fatty liver) and some are converted to lipoproteins (resulting in lipemia). Lipoprotein lipase (*LPL*) activity declines with insulin deficiency, contributing to the hyperlipoproteinemia. The altered glucagon to insulin ratio also activates fatty acid oxidation, resulting in ketone production.

The increase in plasma glucose associated with excess glucocorticoid activity is usually not marked (see Case 60). However, stressed cats frequently have a marked increase in plasma glucose as well as glycosuria, and this must be differentiated from diabetes (see Case 7).

Hyperglycemia occurs frequently in animals poisoned with ethylene glycol (see Case 43). The mechanism is not well understood, but it is thought that there may

TABLE 7–1. Causes of Hyperglycemia

Postprandial (monogastric animals)
Exertional epinephrine (very common in cats)
Increased glucocorticoids (stress, hyperadrenocorticism, administration of corticoids or ACTH)
Diabetes mellitus
Acute pancreatitis
Drug induced-thiazide diuretics, morphine, intravenous fluids with glucose, Ovaban in some cats, ethylene glycol
Glucagon-secreting pancreatic tumor (no ketonuria)

TABLE 7–2. Causes of Hypoglycemia

Delayed separation of serum from erythrocytes
Hepatic disease
Hyperinsulinism (islet cell neoplasm or insulin therapy)
Extrapancreatic tumors (rare)
Idiopathic in toy breeds and puppies
Septicemia/endotoxemia
Endocrine hypofunction (hypopituitarism,
   hypoadrenocorticism, hypothyroidism
Canine renal glycosuria (severe cases)
Drug induced (salicylates, sulfonyurea, exogenous
   insulin, ethanol)
Glycogen storage disease
Starvation

be (1) an inhibition of glycolysis and the Krebs cycle by aldehydes; (2) increases in glucocorticoid and epinepherine activity; and (3) inhibition of insulin release because of hypocalcemia.

Glucose Tolerance Tests. Glucose tolerance tests are indicated in patients that are mildly hyperglycemic (125 to 180 mg/dL) (6.875 to 9.9 mmol/L). Intravenous glucose tolerance is the most common test performed. There are several protocols for the glucose tolerance test and the clinician should contact the laboratory being used. Prediabetic animals have a prolonged hyperglycemia after glucose administration.

Hyperinsulinism

Hyperinsulinism is associated with neoplasia of the pancreatic β-cells (insulinoma).

Excessive production of insulin results in fasting hypoglycemia. Affected animals have a history of intermittent periods of episodic weakness and collapse.

A tentative diagnosis of hyperinsulinism can be made by demonstrating fasting hypoglycemia or marginally normal blood glucose associated with an inappropriate insulin concentration in a patient with a typical history (see Case 54). Other causes of hypoglycemia are summarized in Table 7–2.

AIGR. The amended insulin to glucose ratio has been used to assist in the diagnosis of hyperinsulinism using the following formula:

$$\frac{\text{Serum insulin } (\mu\text{U/mL}) \times 100}{\text{Serum glucose (mg/dL)} - 30} = \text{AIGR.}$$

AIGR values greater than 30 support the diagnosis of an insulin-producing neoplasm; however, the formula is not unique to insulinomas.

THE EXOCRINE PANCREAS

The function of the exocrine pancreas is to produce and secrete digestive enzymes. Most of these enzymes are stored in the pancreas as inactive precursors (zymogens). Amylase and lipase are notable exceptions. The secretions respond to both neural and hormonal stimuli (Fig. 7–3).

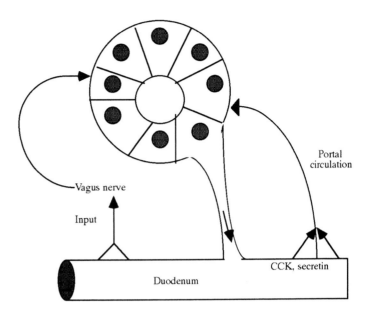

FIGURE 7–3. The exocrine pancreas is responsive to both neural and hormonal stimuli. Gastric acid and long-chain fatty acids cause secretin release into the portal circulation, which causes pancreatic water and bicarbonate secretion Cholecystokinin (*CCK*) is released secondary to the metabolic production of fat and protein digestion and stimulates the secretion of pancreatic enzymes.

Exocrine pancreatic disorders can be classified as inflammatory (pancreatitis, acute or chronic) or insufficiency (reduced production and secretion of digestive enzymes).

Inflammatory Disease

Amylase and *lipase* are the two enzymes that are measured most frequently as markers of acute pancreatitis. Although the majority of normal plasma activity of amylase and lipase is not of pancreatic origin, marked increases of both occur subsequent to experimental pancreatitis in the dog. In naturally occurring disease, the association is less consistent for unknown reasons. Additionally, controversy continues to surround which enzyme is the better marker of acute pancreatitis. It appears prudent to determine both in the differential diagnosis, with a greater than two-fold increase in serum activity considered supportive of acute pancreatitis (see Case 48). Recurrence of the disease (chronic pancreatitis) results in a scarred organ with limited capacity for the production of digestive enzymes. Neither amylase nor lipase would be expected to increase (or decrease) in the plasma at this stage of the disease process.

There are numerous causes of acute pancreatitis, but in most cases the underlying etiology is not known (idiopathic). Some associated causes include diets rich in fat, drugs (glucocorticoids, azathioprine, sulfa antibacterials, organophosphates), trauma, and ischemia. The underlying pathophysiologic events appear to occur within the pancreatic acinar cells and involve impaired secretion of the inactive digestion enzymes. Eventually, intracellular lysosomal hydrolases, normally shielded from the zymogens, activate the enzymes, which initiates autodigestion of the organ (Fig. 7–4). It remains unclear how extrapancreatic events (inflammation, spasm, or obstruction of the pancreatic duct) are related to the intracellular activation of the digestive enzymes.

The kinetics of both amylase and lipase is affected by kidney function in the dog. *Chronic renal insufficiency* can cause an increase in one or both enzymes.

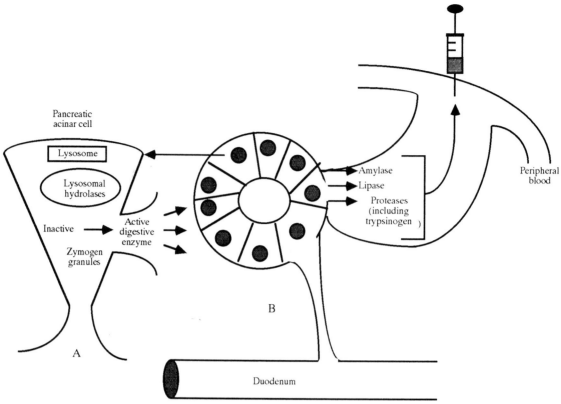

FIGURE 7–4. *A*. Impaired cellular secretion of zymogen granules results in the fusion of the zymogen granules and lysosome. Subsequent activation of the digestive enzymes by the lysosomal hydrolases causes autodigestion, allowing release of the enzymes into the peripheral circulation. *B*. The degree of tissue pathology may limit the exposure of the enzymes to the peripheral blood affecting the magnitude of the increase.

Since acute pancreatitis can be associated with acute renal decompensation and the clinical signs can appear similar, values for amylase greater than three- to four-fold are supportive of acute pancreatitis when there is concurrent renal insufficiency.

Although pancreatitis occurs in the cat, very little is known regarding the clinical disease process or its diagnosis. Experimental pancreatitis in the cat was shown to cause a minimal increase (two-fold) in lipase and a decrease in amylase. Based on that study and on clinical experience, the biochemical diagnosis of pancreatitis differs from the dog. The normal range for amylase and lipase is lower for the cat than the dog. A lipase or, based on our clinical experience, an amylase value greater than two-fold increase supports the differential consideration of pancreatitis. It should be noted that feline pancreatitis differs from that in the dog in that vomiting is not a prominent feature. Loss of appetite, lethargy, nondescript abdominal discomfort, and a painful mass in the anterior abdomen on palpation are the more common findings.

The administration of glucocorticoids can cause a mild increase in plasma lipase activity and a decrease in plasma amylase activity without causing clinical or histologic evidence of pancreatitis in the dog, a dichotomy since glucocorticoids have been incriminated as a cause of acute pancreatitis. An exploratory laparotomy can also result in a mild increase in plasma lipase activity without evidence of pancreatitis. Other associations with hyperlipasemia and/or hyperamylasemia are listed in Table 7–3.

Liver Enzyme Tests

Abnormal liver enzyme tests and liver function reflected as hyperbilirubinemia can occur in association with acute pancreatitis (see Case 48). Although mechanical obstruction of the common bile duct may occur secondary to the closely associated inflamed peripancreatic/pancreatic tissue, direct dumping of proteases into the portal circulation with alteration of intrahepatic cellular structure and function probably occurs with greater frequency (Fig. 7–5). The observation of abnormal liver tests in a dog with acute, repetitive vomiting should prompt the determination of serum lipase and amylase activities. The abnormal liver tests will return toward normal within 7 to 10 days as the pancreatitis resolves. Persistence of hyperbilirubinemia beyond 10 days in a dog diagnosed as having acute pancreatitis implies an extrahepatic obstructive process that should be pursued diagnostically with ultrasonography and with surgery as a consideration.

The continued search for more reliable diagnostic tests for acute pancreatitis in humans and veterinary medicine implies the diagnostic liabilities associated with amylase and lipase. Electrophoresis of serum amylase results in several isoamylases. Although abnormal isoamylase patterns develop subsequent to acute pancreatitis, an overlap with other diseases occurs. Perhaps with improved methodology for separation and clinical utility the procedure will find future application.

Exocrine Pancreatic Insufficiency (EPI)

Trypsinogen (measured as trypsin-like immunoreactivity, TLI) is pancreas specific, and increased plasma activity is associated with acute pancreatitis. Chronic renal insufficiency will cause increased plasma TLI. The primary limitation for its diagnostic use is limited access to laboratories for quick differential diagnostic use. The radioimmunoassay for TLI measurement in humans does not cross-react with canine TLI. A canine immunoassay kit for TLI became available recently. If the commercial product proves satisfactory, the differential diagnosis of pancreatitis in the dog may be enhanced. As discussed next, serum TLI has become the cornerstone in the differential diagnosis of exocrine pancreatic insufficiency (see Case 47).

**TABLE 7–3. Causes of Increased
Serum Amylase or Lipase**

Pancreatic inflammation, necrosis, and neoplasia
Obstruction of pancreatic ducts
Chronic renal insufficiency
Slight increase with glucocorticoids (lipase only)
Intestinal perforations

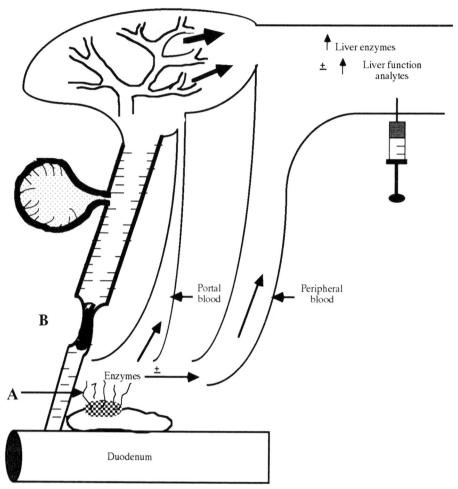

FIGURE 7–5. Acute pancreatitis may be associated with abnormal liver tests by *A,* release of active digestive enzymes into the portal circulation with subsequent intrahepatic injury or *B,* obstruction (temporary or permanent) of the common bile duct due to the impingement of the inflamed pancreatic/peripancreatic tissue. (Modified from Meyer, D. J. and Burrows, C.B.: The liver. Part 2: Biochemical diagnosis of the hepatobiliary disorders in the dog. Comp. Contin. Educ. Small Anim. Pract. 5:706, 1982.)

Maldigestion and Malabsorption

The *exocrine pancreas and small intestine* are integral in facilitating digestion and absorption of ingested nutrients. Dysfunction of one or both organs results in chronic diarrhea and weight loss. Numerous serum and fecal tests have been developed for diagnostic use, indicative of the difficulty in evaluating the function of these organs. Because of the pragmatic limitations in adapting many of these tests for clinical use or because of unreliable results the following tests are not recommended: Sudan staining for fecal fat (before and after addition of acetic acid), iodine staining for fecal starch, assessment for fecal muscle fibers, fecal trypsin-gel tube or radiographic film digestion, plasma turbidity test, oral glucose tolerance test, and xylose absorption. The *most reliable* approach to the differential diagnosis of canine maldigestion/malabsorption is by concurrently assessing the function of the exocrine pancreas and small intestine combined with endoscopic/surgical biopsy of the small intestine when indicated. Exocrine pancreatic insufficiency should always be ruled out in all cases of *chronic diarrhea/weight loss* so that the diagnostic focus can be shifted to the assessment of small intestinal function.

Trypsinogen and Bentiromide Test

Both serum TLI and the bentiromide test can be used for the diagnosis of EPI (Fig. 7–6). Serum TLI is determined on one fasted sample, thus offering simplicity and accuracy. A decreased value is supportive of EPI. The bentiromide test is technically more difficult. Oral bentiromide is administered, and chymotrypsin, normally secreted by the pancreas, cleaves off the P-aminobenzoic acid (PABA) which can be measured at four 30-minute time points. In EPI the PABA concentration curve is blunted. The limited diagnostic advantages of the bentiromide test over determination of TLI include EPI secondary to obstruction of the pancreatic duct and in cases of EPI with concurrent acute pancreatitis. Replacement pancreatic enzyme supplements and antibiotics should not be given 1 week prior to assessing pancreatic function.

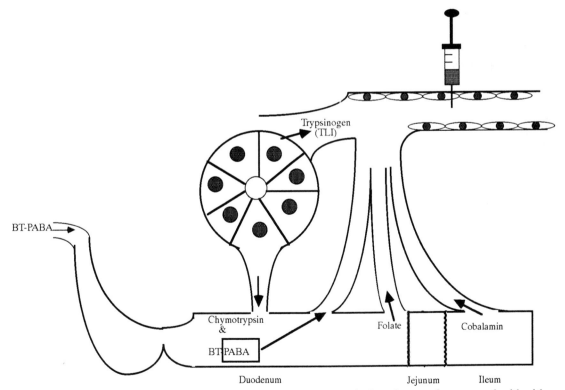

FIGURE 7–6. Exocrine pancreatic function can be assessed with either serum TLI or measurement of the serum PABA concentration after oral administration of bentiromide. The absorptive function of the proximal part of the small intestine can be assessed by measurement of serum folate concentration and distal small intestine function by the serum cobalamin concentration.

Neither the determination of TLI nor the bentiromide test is diagnostically useful in the cat. A radial enzyme diffusion test to assess fecal proteolytic enzyme using an azocasein substrate has been found to be diagnostically useful. Three fecal samples, not necessarily sequential, should be measured. Fresh feces or samples stored at $-20°$ C can be used. Commercial availability is the primary limitation.

Folate and Cobalamin

Although the accurate biochemical diagnosis of EPI has been enhanced greatly, functional assessment of the small intestine is hampered by the tremendous surface area of the affected organ and by varying degrees of pathology. Folate is absorbed primarily in the proximal small intestine, and cobalamin (vitamin B_{12}) is absorbed predominantly by the ileum (Fig. 7–6). Pathology sufficient to result in chronic diarrhea can cause decreased serum values depending on the diseased site. Bacterial overgrowth, which appears to complicate both pancreatic and intestinal diseases secondarily, can cause increased serum folate values because of increased bacterial production (see Case 47). Occasionally bacterial consumption of cobalamin is sufficient to cause a concurrent decrease. Marked increases in both folate and cobalamin suggest B-vitamin supplementation.

Biochemical assessment of pancreatic and intestinal disorders in the equine remain problematic and restricted to institutions with research interests.

8

ELECTROLYTE, ACID-BASE HOMEOSTASIS AND DISTURBANCES

The subject of water and electrolyte balance has been obscured by a long series of efforts to establish short cuts. Attempts to simplify it usually has led to faulty thinking and, as a result, to inadequate care of those patients who need it most— Carl Moyer in *Surgery,* 4th ed., Lippincott.

Approximately 60% of an adult's body weight is water; 40% is intracellular, and 20% is extracellular (5% plasma plus 15% interstitial). The young animal has a higher per cent of body weight in water. Vomiting, diarrhea, and polyuria are the most frequent causes of altered water and electrolyte balance.

The major factors that determine the plasma solute concentration and water content are shown in Figure 8–1. The input and output are normally maintained in a steady state. An abnormality will develop if the homeostatic mechanisms balancing input and output are altered. For example, the plasma sodium concentration is most commonly altered as a result of a primary change in the input rate or an altered mechanism for water balance. An abnormal plasma potassium is commonly a reflection of accelerated renal tubular loss or impaired renal tubular secretion. Since a number of physiologic mechanisms are involved in plasma solute homeostasis, function tests and hormone measurements are often necessary to define the nature of the disturbance.

Sodium is the principal cation in the *extracellular* fluid, and potassium is the principal *intracellular* cation. The osmotic pressure of extracellular fluid is determined largely by the sodium concentration. It also determines the extracellular fluid volume as water tends to flow in or out in response to changes in the sodium concentration. Intracellular osmolality is determined predominantly by potassium. Large potassium losses associated with chronic vomiting, diarrhea, or hy-

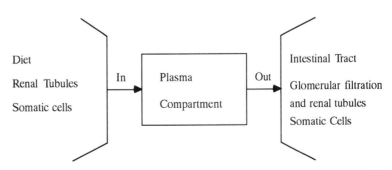

FIGURE 8–1. Factors that determine plasma solute concentration and water content.

Diet
Renal Tubules
Somatic cells

In → Plasma Compartment → Out

Intestinal Tract
Glomerular filtration and renal tubules
Somatic Cells

persecretion of aldosterone, cause cells to shrink as intracellular water is lost. The principal anion within the cells is phosphate whereas chloride and bicarbonate predominate in the extracellular fluid. Active transport mechanisms located in the cell membrane are responsible for maintaining these large solute gradient differences.

The maintenance of plasma volume is illustrated in Figure 8–2. Albumin is the principal protein that contributes to oncotic (osmotic) pressure because of its low molecular weight and high concentration. Despite the influence of albumin, sodium is the main determinant of plasma volume. As a consequence, the albumin concentration has to fall by at least 50% before effecting a change in plasma oncotic pressure (manifested clinically as edema). Disturbances in osmolality are adjusted by the water intake or excretion. Dehydration stimulates thirst and stimulates the posterior pituitary to secrete *antidiuretic hormone (ADH)*, which promotes renal tubular reabsorption. Overhydration inhibits thirst and the release of ADH (Fig. 6–2).

ELECTROLYTES

Sodium Disturbances

Plasma sodium is filtered by the glomerulus, and the majority is reabsorbed by the proximal and distal renal tubules. The distal tubular exchange of sodium and potassium is accelerated by *aldosterone,* promoting sodium retention and potassium excretion.

Hyponatremia (less than 140 mEq/L (mmol/L) in dogs; less than 147 in cats; less than 137 in horses; and less than 132 in cattle) occurs with gastrointestinal loss (vomiting and diarrhea) (see Case 48). If severe enough, a metabolic acidosis can develop which contributes to electrolyte shifts that mimic those associated with hypoadrenocorticism. However, the ACTH stimulation will not be abnormal. Other causes of hyponatremia include uroperitoneum ("third space" loss) (see discussion of Case 48), congestive heart failure, diuretic administration, and diabetes mellitus (see Case 53). Some dogs with adrenal insufficiency have only a glucocorticoid deficiency and may have a hyponatremia with a normokalemia.

Facetious hyponatremia (pseudohyponatremia) may result when a lipemic sample is measured by flame photometry or indirect potentiometry (see Case 30). This may also occur with severe hyperglobulinemia. The falsely decreased sodium value does not occur if an ion-selective electrode is used for the electrolyte determination. A more detailed list of disorders associated with hyponatremia is presented in Table 8–1.

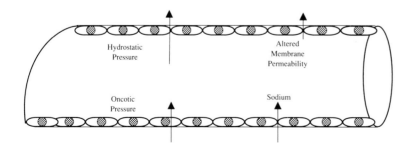

FIGURE 8–2. Maintenance of plasma volume.

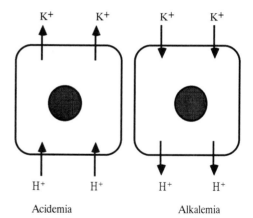

FIGURE 8–3. Cellular movement of H^+ and K^+ with acidemia and alkalemia.

Hypernatremia (more than 155 mEq/L (mmol/L) in dogs; more than 161 in cats; more than 148 in horses; and more than 152 in cattle) is associated with dehydration secondary to inadequate water intake or excessive pure water loss. This is especially prominent in diabetes insipidus if the patient is not allowed free access to water. An increased sodium value may occur with cirrhosis and be exaggerated by the osmotic catharsis used in the management of hepatic encephalopathy. Hypernatremic hypovolemia may develop in patients with chronic renal failure and inadequate water intake. A more detailed list of the causes of hypernatremia is presented in Table 8–2.

Potassium Disturbances

Hypokalemia (K^+ less than 4.2 mEq/L (mmol/L) in dogs; less than 4.0 in cats; less than 2.8 in horses; and less than 3.8 in cattle) results from decreased intake, excessive loss, extracellular to intracellular shift, and dilution. The use of potassium-poor intravenous fluids may enhance the renal loss plus dilute further the marginal plasma potassium in an anorectic animal, resulting in hypokalemia. Gastrointestinal loss (vomiting and diarrhea) is a common cause of hypokalemia, often exacerbated by inadequate dietary intake. Excess loss will also occur with

TABLE 8–1. Disorders Associated with Hyponatremia

Gastrointestinal loss (vomiting, diarrhea)
Congestive heart failure (edema)
Hypoadrenocorticism (glucocorticoid deficiency)
Diuretic treatment
Administration of hypotonic fluid (e.g., 5% dextrose in water)
Third space loss (pancreatitis, peritonitis, uroperitoneum)
Diabetes mellitus
Renal disease (polyuric acute renal failure, horse)
Factitious
Ptyalism (horse)
Cellulitis (horse)
White muscle disease (horse)

TABLE 8–2. Disorders Associated with Hypernatremia

Diabetes insipidus
Increased insensible water loss (fever, high environmental temperature)
Gastrointestinal loss (vomiting, diarrhea)
Inadequate intake
Renal failure (acute and chronic)
Diabetes mellitus (following insulin treatment)
Diuretic treatment
Increased salt intake or intravenous administration
Hyperaldosteronism
Artifact caused by improper sample handling (allowing evaporation of serum)

hyperaldosteronism (hypernatremia is also present) and renal tubular acidosis (hyperchloremic acidosis is present). Diuretics also enhance renal loss of potassium. The use of insulin in the management of the ketoacidotic diabetic patient will carry potassium into the cell (along with glucose). Table 8–3 contains a more detailed list of disorders associated with hypokalemia.

Hyperkalemia (K^+ more than 5.7 mEq/L (mmol/L) in dogs; more than 4.7 in cats; more than 5.1 in horses; and less than 6.0 in cattle) develops secondary to increased intake, decreased secretion (kidney dependent), or a shift from the rich intracellular store to the extracellular fluid. Life-threatening hyperkalemia most frequently occurs secondary to adrenal insufficiency or renal failure (both represent decreased excretion). A sodium to potassium ratio of less than 27:1 with an abnormal ACTH stimulation test (decreased response) confirms the diagnosis of hypoadrenocorticism. There are anectodal cases of pure aldosterone deficiency (ratio of less than 27:1) with a normal ACTH stimulation test. One should be aware of this uncommon possibility.

Since cells are rich in potassium there is a potential for its shift to the extracellular fluid to cause hyperkalemia. With acidosis the cell helps maintain acid-base balance by exchanging intracellular potassium for the extracellular hydrogen ion. The kidney can usually increase potassium excretion blunting this effect unless there is concomitant organ dysfunction that facilitates the development of hyperkalemia. Diffuse cell necrosis or altered membrane permeability allowing potassium leakage may accompany shock, circulatory failure, crush-type injury, and rhabdomyolysis.

TABLE 8–3. Disorders Associated with Hypokalemia

Gastrointestinal loss (vomiting, diarrhea)
Intravenous administration of potassium poor fluids
Bicarbonate therapy
Diuretic treatment
Hyperaldosteronism
Renal tubular acidosis
Chronic renal failure (especially cats)
Insulin treatment of ketoacidotic diabetic
Alkalosis (translocation)
Prolonged anorexia (horse)
Excessive sweating (horse)
Factitious (hyperlipidemia, improper sample handling)
Reduced dietary intake (rarely the sole cause)

TABLE 8–4. Disorders Associated with Hyperkalemia

Hypoadrenocorticism
Renal failure (including urethral obstruction)
Diffuse cell death secondary to shock, circulatory stasis
Acidosis
Rhabdomyolysis (horse)
Periodic paralysis (horse)
Uroperitoneum
Factitious
  Hemolysis
  Delayed separation of clotted blood (Akita breed, herbivores, excessive
    leukocytosis or thrombocytosis)
  Collection in potassium heparin
  Collection from intravenous tube when potassium administered

Factitious hyperkalemia (pseudohyperkalemia) may occur secondary to a delay in separating serum from blood with extreme leukocytosis or thrombocytosis, cellular elements rich in potassium. A breed peculiarity has been noted in the Akita dog wherein delayed separation of the clotted specimen can result in an increased potassium value. The Akita's erythrocyte apparently has more potassium than that of other breeds (see Case 50). Hemolysis may also result in an abnormal potassium determination in horses and cattle. A more detailed list of disorders with hyperkalemia is presented in Table 8–4.

Chloride Disturbances

Chloride is the extracellular anion in highest concentration. Since it cannot accept the hydrogen ion at physiologic pH, it cannot act as a buffer. Because of electrochemical neutrality, chloride does not vary inversely with bicarbonate. Its measurement provides the least clinical information of the electrolytes. It is helpful for determining the anionic gap. Hyperchloremia is associated with dehydration and renal tubular acidosis. Decreased concentrations occur in metabolic acidosis and prolonged vomiting (hypokalemic, hypochloremic metabolic alkalosis).

Fractional Urine Creatinine/Electrolyte Clearance in the Horse

Fractional clearance (Fc) of electrolytes can be estimated by comparing the urine and serum concentration of creatinine with that of the electrolyte. The formula used is

$$\% \text{ CrCl(Fc)(E)} = \frac{\text{Cr serum}}{\text{Cr urine}} \times \frac{\text{E urine}}{\text{E serum}} \times 100.$$

Normal per cents CrCl(Fc)(E) for the horse are: sodium, 0.02 to 1; potassium, 15 to 65; chloride, 0.04 to 1.6; and phosphate, 0 to 0.2. Dietary intake has a substantial effect on clearance; particularly with respect to potassium. The normal values given above were established in the presence of an oats and prairie hay ration. Consumption of brome or alfalfa hay or green grass may raise normal potassium values to as high as 150%.

If furosemide is given the fractional clearance percentages are: sodium, 12; potassium 200; clorides 9.5; and phosphate, 0. Thus, a diuretic cannot be used to collect urine for determining electrolyte Fc.

Only an increased sodium Fc is of diagnostic significance. Increases occur with excessive sodium intake, hypoadrenocorticism, dehydration, and with renal tubular insufficiency. Increased sodium Fc must be evaluated in association with urinalysis results. If the sodium Fc is increased with normal but dilute urine and a normal phosphate Fc the finding is highly suggestive of hypoadrenocorticism. If the increased sodium Fc is found in association with high urine specific gravity it suggests dehydration. If the high sodium Fc is a result of tubular insufficiency the Fc for potassium, chloride, and phosphate will also be elevated, and there is usually a low urine specific gravity. These changes are summarized in Table 8–5.

Potassium Fc increases occur with high dietary levels of potassium if the urine is normal or with renal disease if the Fc for sodium chloride and phosphate is also increased.

Potassium Fc decreases are of importance as they indicate depletion of body potassium. Fc of potassium and pH of blood and urine should be assessed together because blood pH has a significant effect on hydrogen excretion and therefore urine pH. If body potassium is depleted, more hydrogen is excreted by the distal renal tubules in exchange for sodium resulting in acid urine. Acidic urine with low potassium Fc is consistent with metabolic alkalosis (inappropriate aciduria) because potassium is depleted and hydrogen is excreted in its stead. Potassium Fc is also reduced in chronic laminitis and recurrent myositis.

Phosphate Fc is increased with primary hyperparathyroidism, hypercalcemia of neoplasia (pseudohyperparathyroidism), with renal failure, with phosphate wast-

TABLE 8–5. Disorders Associated with Abnormal Electrolyte Fractional Clearances in the Horse

Electrolyte Fc Alteration	Other Laboratory Findings	Interpretation
Sodium increase	Normal dilute urine Normal PO$_4$ Fc	Hypoadrenocorticism
	High urine specific gravity	Dehydration
	High PO$_4$ Fc, Cl Fc, and K Fc with dilute urine	Renal tubular insufficiency
Potassium Increase	Normal urine	High dietary level of K
	High Cl Fc, Na Fc and PO$_4$ Fc	Renal disease
Potassium decrease	Acid urine, acidemia	Metabolic acidosis
	Alkaline urine	Low level dietary K Lack of K absorption Body depletion of K
Phosphate Increase	Increased serum Ca and normal urine[a]	Primary hyperparathyroidism Hypercalcemia of neoplasia
	Normal Ca and Urine	Secondary to nutritional hyperparathyroidism
	Dilute urine, abnormal urinalysis, high Na Fc, Cl Fc, and K Fc	Renal failure[b]

[a] If there is secondary renal calcinosis urinalysis findings may be abnormal.
[b] Horses with renal failure often have a high serum calcium.

ing nephropathy associated with multifocal recurrent lameness, and is secondary to nutritional hyperparathyroidism.

Use of Fractional Excretion of K$^+$ as a Diagnostic Aid for Hypokalemic Polymyopathy Syndrome in Cats

The Fc of K$^+$ has been used to study this condition. The ratio is calculated as follows:

$$\% \ CrCl(Fc)(K^+) = \frac{Cr_s}{Cr_u} \times \frac{K_u^+}{K_s^+} \times 100$$

where Cr_s = serum creatinine; Cr_u = urine creatinine; K_u^+ = urine potassium; and K_s^+ = serum potassium.

The normal per cent Fc of K$^+$ in healthy cats ranges from 11.99 to 14.26. The mean value for cats with hypokalemic polymyopathy is 26.71% with a range of 5 to 40%.

The normal fractional excretion percentages for domestic animals are presented in Table 8–6.

ACID-BASE BALANCE

The metabolism of fats, carbohydrates, and proteins for energy results in the formation of large quantities of CO_2. Although CO_2 forms a weak acid HCO_3 in plasma, the process is reversed in the lung, and CO_2 is eliminated rapidly. Incomplete oxidation of metabolites results in the formation of nonvolatile acids which rely on the kidney for excretion. When tissues are subjected to oxygen deficiency (anoxia, inadequate perfusion) the H$^+$ is incompletely transferred to O_2 to form water, and acidosis develops.

Normal blood pH is maintained between 7.35 and 7.45; intracellular pH is 6.8 to 7.0. Several buffer systems are utilized in the regulation of blood pH. The bicarbonate/carbonic acid buffer system is the most important one because of the rapidity with which CO_2 can be eliminated by the lung after the conversion from H_2CO_3. The rate of CO_2 elimination depends upon the rate and depth of respiration. The hemoglobin buffer system and phosphate buffer system also contribute to maintenance of normal blood pH but are not used clinically in assessing acid-base disturbances.

TABLE 8–6. Normal Per Cent Fractional Urine Creatinine/Electrolyte Clearance of Domestic Animals[a]

	Dog	Cat	Horse	Cow	Sheep
Sodium	0–0.7	0.24–0.1	0.02–1.0	0.2–1.43	0–0.071
Potassium[b]	0–20	6.7–23.9	15–65	15–63	80–180
Chloride	0–0.8	0.41–1.3	0.04–1.6	0.4–2.3	0–4.7
Phosphate	3–39	17–73	0–0.2		0–0.53

[a] Calculated using formula: $\% \ CrCl(Fc)(E) = \frac{Cr \ serum}{Cr \ urine} \times \frac{E \ urine}{E \ serum} \times 100.$

[b] The Fc for potassium in herbivorous animals is largely dependent upon the diet.

TABLE 8–7. Disorders Resulting in Metabolic Acidosis and Abnormal Anion Gap

Increased anion gap (chloride normal)
  Diabetic ketoacidosis
  Uremia
  Shock, anoxia, exercise (overproduction of acid, e.g., lactate)
  Grain overload in cattle (>lactic acid)
  Ethylene glycol toxicity
  Salicylate toxicity
Normal gap (increased chloride)
  Severe diarrhea
  Chronic vomiting
  Renal tubular acidosis
  Diuretics (carbonic anhydrase inhibitors)
  Oral acidifying agents

An abnormal blood pH occurs when the HCO_3^- (metabolic)/P_{CO_2} (respiratory) ratio deviates from 20:1 (based on the Henderson-Hasselbalch equation). As we mentioned, the lung can respond rapidly (hours) to changes by blowing off CO_2 whereas the kidney takes 12 to 24 hours to respond and days for complete metabolic compensation. Base excess is a measurement used to assess metabolic changes. A positive base excess (increased HCO_3^-) indicates an excess of base (metabolic alkalosis), and a negative value (decreased HCO_3^-) indicates a base deficiency (metabolic acidosis). Conversely an increase in P_{CO_2} (which actually causes the $[H_2CO_3^-]$ to increase) is referred to as a *respiratory acidosis,* and a decrease is called *respiratory alkalosis.* Since the body is well endowed with buffering systems, compensation (an attempt to correct the acid-base disturbance) is seen clinically. Thus a pure metabolic/respiratory acidosis/alkalosis is uncommon. The primary acid-base disturbance is usually indicated by determining blood pH (acidemia or alkalemia) and the respiratory (P_{CO_2}) and metabolic (HCO_3^-) components. The one that deviates greater from normal suggests the primary disturbance. For example, if the blood pH is below the normal range; the HCO_3^- is decreased (base deficit) and shows a greater deviation from normal than the decreased P_{CO_2}, a metabolic acidosis would be suggested.

Some of the most common causes acidosis and alkalosis are summarized in Tables 8–7 through 8–10.

The biochemical profile often contains a measurement referred to as total CO_2 (CO_2 content). Since most of the total CO_2 is comprised of bicarbonate, it gives a crude indication of the acid (decreased total CO_2)-base (increased CO_2) status. Its limitation is that both metabolic and respiratory factors affect the value.

TABLE 8–8. Disorders Resulting in a Metabolic Alkalosis

Vomiting (acute, gastric contents only)
Gastric (abomasal) sequestration
Small intestine obstruction
Cecal volvulus (cattle)
Excess use of potassium-depleting diuretics
Excess administration of sodium bicarbonate
Endurance competition (horse)
Excessive sweating (horse)
Ptyalism (horse, cow)

**TABLE 8–9. Disorders Resulting
in Respiratory Acidosis
(Depressed Respiration)**

Central (respiratory center)
   Drugs (anesthetics, narcotics)
   Trauma
   Tumor, inflammation
Impaired pulmonary function
   Pneumonia
   Pneumothorax
   Airway obstruction
   Pulmonary edema
   Hydrothorax
   Deficient diaphragm (muscle/chest wall movement)

**TABLE 8–10. Disorders Causing
Respiratory Alkalosis**

Central (stimulation of respiratory center)
   Anxiety
   Pain
   Pathologic lesions
Hypoxemia
   Severe anemia (with hyperventilation)
   Congestive heart failure
Excessive mechanical ventilation

Anion Gap.

The term *anion gap* refers to difference between the measured cations and measured anions: anion gap = $(Na^+ + K^+) - (Cl^- + HCO_3^-)$. The normal range is 12 to 18 mEq/L (mmol/L) and represents the gap or unmeasured anions. These include phosphate, sulfate, and lactate. Ketones, ethylene glycol metabolites, and salicylate are examples of unmeasured anions not normally present in the blood. The anion gap can facilitate the classification of metabolic acidosis. If the total $[HCO_3^-]$ is not available, the total CO_2 value can be substituted (see Cases 43, 53, and 58).

There is a relationship between acid-base status and potassium transcellular flux (see Fig. 8–3). This concept is of particular importance when therapeutically approaching the management of metabolic acidosis. The acidemia shifts the potassium extracellularly and is then excreted by the kidney, thus depleting the total body potassium. The more chronic the disorder, the greater the potassium depletion. When managing the disorder (thereby correcting the acidemia), the extracellular potassium returns into the cell, precipitating abrupt hypokalemia. The serum potassium concentration (which is a poor reflection of the total body stores) should be monitored frequently when managing disorders listed in Tables 8–7 and 8–9.

9

EVALUATION OF ENDOCRINE FUNCTION AND DISORDERS*

PARATHYROID AND MINERAL BALANCE

The minerals calcium, phosphorus, and magnesium are of importance in the normal physiologic activities of the body. Alterations in the serum concentration of these chemicals occur in several endocrine/metabolic disorders.

Calcium and Phosphorus Metabolism

Control of calcium metabolism and in particular the extracellular level of ionized calcium is mediated through the actions of parathormone, calcitonin (thyrocalcitonin), and vitamin D (Fig. 9–1). Other hormones such as estrogens, corticosteroids, somatotropin, glucagon, and thyroxine may influence calcium homeostasis.

Parathormone impacts on three target organs: bone, kidney, and intestinal mucosa. The principal function of parathormone is maintenance of a normal serum calcium level by action on target cells. Most action occurs as mobilization of calcium from bone but also includes enhancement of calcium reabsorption and action on intestinal mucosa to promote calcium absorption. Parathormone enhances phosphorus excretion by kidney tubules, which assists in maintaining the serum calcium to phosphorus ratio.

Parathormone is produced by the secretory cells of the parathyroid and is stored in small quantity in these cells providing a parathormone reserve. Release of stored parathormone and the production of additional hormone is controlled by the serum concentration of ionic calcium. When the plasma concentration decreases parathormone is released and the parathyroid gland is stimulated.

Calcitonin (thyrocalcitonin) is produced by parafollicular (C) cells of the thyroid gland. Its action is the opposite of that of parathormone. As the plasma concentration of calcium increases, calcitonin is released to inhibit bone resorption of calcium. Calcitonin has no appreciable effect on intestinal absorption of calcium or renal metabolism of calcium.

Vitamin D control of serum calcium and phosphorus levels is similar to that of parathormone although its major target organ is intestinal mucosa where it stimulates calcium absorption. Vitamin D stimulates bone resorption by dissolution of mineral salts and destruction of collagen fibers.

---

* See Algorithms 15, 16, 17, and 18.

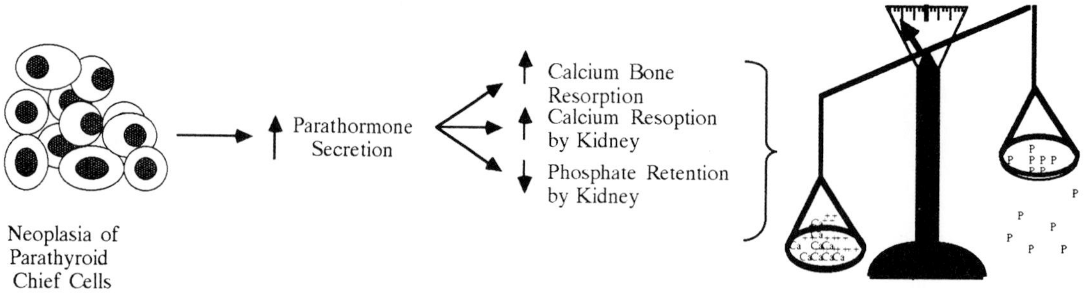

Neoplasia of
Parathyroid
Chief Cells

FIGURE 9–1. Endocrine control of mineral balance depends on the interaction of parathormone from the parathyroid glands, calcitonin from the parafollicular cells of the thyroid gland, and vitamin D after activation to 1,25-dihydroxycholecalciferol by the kidney.

Abnormalities in Serum Calcium and Phosphorus Concentration

Effect of Serum Albumin and Acid-Base Balance

Serum calcium values are affected by the serum albumin concentration. Approximately 40% of total serum calcium is bound to albumin, and 10% is associated with anions as phosphorus and citrate. The remaining 50% is ionized. Only ionized calcium is biologically active. The proportion of serum calcium which is bound varies with the total albumin concentration; ionized calcium is not affected. Total serum calcium decreases in animals that have hypoalbuminemia and increases when albumin increases. Hypercalcemia can be masked if the total serum calcium is not corrected for hypoalbuminemia (see Case 39).

In *dogs* the total serum calcium can be adjusted by one of two methods.

1. Using serum albumin:

$$\text{Adjusted serum calcium} = \text{Ca(mg/dL)} - \text{albumin(g/dL)} + 3.5.$$

$$\text{SI} = \left[\text{Ca(mmol/L)} \times \left[4 - \frac{\text{albumin (g/L)}}{10} \right] + 3.5 \right] \times 0.25$$

2. Using total serum protein:

$$\text{Adjusted serum calcium} = \text{Ca(mg/dL)} - (0.4 \times \text{total protein [g/dL]}) + 3.3.$$

$$\text{SI} = \left[\text{Ca(mmol/L)} \times 4 - \left[0.4 \times \frac{\text{total protein (g/L)}}{10} \right] + 3.3 \right] \times 0.25$$

The proportion of ionized calcium decreases with metabolic alkalosis, increases with metabolic acidosis, and is almost always increased in animals that have hypercalcemia.

The causes of hypercalcemia and hypocalcemia are summarized in Tables 9–1 and 9–2, respectively.

Serum phosphorus is regulated primarily by the kidneys but is also influenced by age. Parathormone stimulates phosphorus excretion by the kidney. Growing animals have a higher serum phosphorus than adults.

The causes of hyperphosphatemia and hypophosphatemia are summarized in Tables 9–3 and 9–4, respectively.

TABLE 9–1. Disorders Causing Hypercalcemia

Hyperalbuminemia (dehydration)
Hypercalcemia of neoplasia (pseudohyperparathyroidism)
Primary hyperparathyroidism
Hypoadrenocorticism
Hypervitaminosis D
Renal disease (horse and cow, uncommonly in dog)
Osteolytic bone lesions (*e.g.,* septic osteomyelitis)
Plant toxicity (jasmine in dogs and cats, *Cestrum* sp. and
    Solanum sp. [nightshade] in herbivores)
Calciferol-containing rodenticides
Certain granulomatous diseases (*e.g.,* caning blastomy-
    cosis)

TABLE 9–2. Disorders Causing Hypocalcemia

Hypoalbuminemia
Alkalosis (especially in ruminants)
Hypoparathyroidism
Secondary renal hyperparathyroidism
Ethylene glycol toxicity (dogs and cats)
Necrotizing pancreatitis
Dietary imbalance (hypovitaminosis D, excess phos-
phorus)
Eclampsia (bitch, mare, ewe) or parturient paresis (cow)
Hypomagnesemic tetany in ruminants (three fourths of
    cases)
Intestinal malabsorption (dog)
Blister beetle poisoning in horses
Hypercalcitonism
Transport tetany (sheep)
Factitious (sample run on EDTA plasma)
Iatrogenic, after thyroidectomy (bilateral)

TABLE 9–3. Disorders Causing Hyperphosphatemia

Reduced glomerular filtration rate (renal, prerenal, or post-
    renal azotemia from any cause)
Factitious; sample held too long before analysis (phosphorus
    released from erythrocytes)
Growing animals
Dietary phosphorus excess
Phosphorus enema or administration of phosphorus-containing
    fluids
Hypervitaminosis D
Osteolytic bone disease (neoplasia)
Jasmine toxicity
Tissue trauma
Hypoparathyroidism with normal glomerular filtration
Hypercalcemia of malignancy with normal gomerular filtration
Hyperthyroidism in cats without renal insufficiency
Slight increases occasionally from drug treatment (anabolic ste-
    roids, furosemide, minocycline, hydrochlorothiazide)

TABLE 9–4. Disorders Causing Hypophosphatemia

Primary hyperparathyroidism (early stages before renal calcinosis)
Hypercalcemia of neoplasia (early stages before renal calcinosis)
Lack of dietary calcium
Hypovitaminosis D
Dogs and cats with diabetes mellitus and ketoacidosis
Respiratory alkalosis due to hyperventilation
Hyperadrenocorticism (about one third of dogs with disorder)
Eclampsia
Hypomagnesemic tetany of ruminants
Parturient paresis in cattle
Malabsorption or starvation
Canine Fanconi-like syndrome
Chronic renal failure in horse
Vitamin D intoxication
After insulin administration in diabetics

Conditions with Hypercalcemia (Table 9–1)

Primary Hyperparathyroidism. This condition is caused by a functional neoplasm or idiopathic hyperplasia of the parathyroid gland. In the early stages there is a significant hypercalcemia accompanied by hypophosphatemia (Fig. 9–2). If renal calcinosis develops secondary to hypercalcemia, the serum phosphorus will increase as renal function deteriorates and is accompanied by azotemia and other laboratory changes associated with renal failure. If bone lesions develop the increased metabolic activity in the bone may result in an increase in serum alkaline phosphatase. The condition can be confirmed biochemically by demonstration of an increase in the serum parathormone concentration (see Case 52).

Idiopathic parathyroid hyperplasia has been reported in German shepherd puppies.

Humoral Hypercalcemia of Malignancy (Pseudohyperparathyroidism). Laboratory findings associated with the paraneoplastic syndrome are similar to those seen in primary hyperparathyroidism with hypercalcemia and hypophosphatemia in the early stages followed by hyperphosphatemia and azotemia if renal calcinosis develops. In contrast, the serum parathormone level is normal to decreased. Neoplasms that have been associated with hypercalcemia include lymphosarcoma, mammary gland adenocarcinoma, squamous cell carcinoma, pancreatic carcinoma, and nasal adenocarcinoma. Some of these neoplasms produce a parathormone-related protein that affects calcium and phosphorus metabolism. The paraneoplastic syndrome is the most common cause of hypercalcemia (see Case 57).

Vitamin D Intoxication. Overzealous owners who supplement a diet with excess quantities of vitamin D may induce hypercalcemia accompanied by hyperphosphatemia. Hyperphosphatemia often occurs prior to renal damage from calcinosis.

Renal Disease. The horse is biochemically unusual with regard to renal disease as hypercalcemia develops secondary to decreased urinary excretion (see Case 40). Serum phosphorus is low or low normal (Fig. 9–3). Hypercalcemia occurs in dogs occasionally in the late stages of renal disease. The mechanism is not well established.

Hypoadrenocorticism in the Dog. An increase in serum calcium occurs in some dogs with adrenal insufficiency. Increased renal tubular resorption of calcium is thought to be involved.

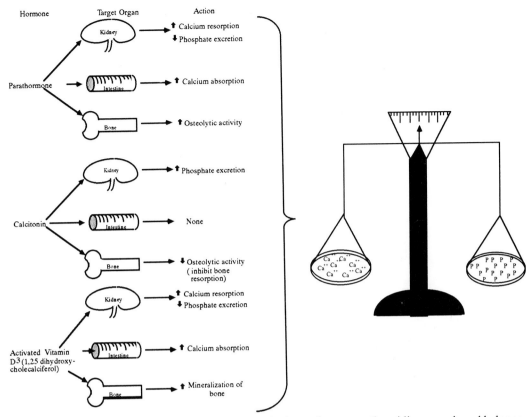

FIGURE 9–2. Effect of primary hyperparathyroidism on mineral balance. Increased production of parathormone increases calcium resorption from bone and calcium reabsorption by the kidney. It also causes increased phosphate loss (reduced retention). The net result is hypercalcemia and hypophosphatemia. Note: If the condition exists for some time renal calcinosis may develop, and when this occurs hyperphosphatemia may replace hypophosphatemia.

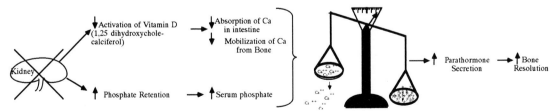

FIGURE 9–3. Effect of renal failure on mineral balance. Renal failure causes an increase in phosphate retention. This results in an increase in total mineral mass, and calcium excretion is increased. Vitamin D activation is also dependent upon renal function, and when renal failure intercedes vitamin D activation is reduced, causing decreased intestinal absorption of calcium and decreased bone mobilization. The cumulative effect is a decrease in serum calcium which in turn stimulates parathormone secretion by the parathyroid gland and an increase in bone mobilization of calcium and bone resolution.

Osteolytic Bone Lesions. Hypercalcemia may occur after marked bone resorption. Neoplasia of the bone in which hypercalcemia has been reported include carcinoma, osteosarcoma, myeloma, and lymphosarcoma. Hypercalcemia may occur with severe osteomyelitis, particularly blastomycosis. It has been suggested that humans infected with blastomycosis have a hyperreactivity to vitamin D.

Plant Intoxication. The ingestion of jasmine (*Cestrum* sp.) by dogs and cats and *Solanum* and *Cestrum* sp. by herbivores will produce hypercalcemia and soft tissue mineralization. As the disease progresses the serum calcium will fall. The mechanism for this alteration is not known.

Cholecalciferol-containing Rodenticides. Some rodenticides contain cholecalciferol (vitamin D_3) and will cause hypercalcemia. Such occurrences have been reported in both cats and dogs. One should consider the possible ingestion of either rodenticide or poisoned rodent in a dog and cat with unexplained hypercalcemia. The development of clinical signs is dose dependent and can be divided into neurologic, gastrointestinal, cardiovascular, and renal signs. The parathormone concentration will be low normal to low.

Conditions with Hypocalcemia (Table 9–2)

Hypoalbuminemia and Alkalosis. When the serum albumin is low or an animal is alkalotic (especially ruminants) the serum calcium will be below the normal range. In an animal with metabolic alkalosis (increased total CO_2 or bicarbonate) there will be a decrease in the ionized calcium level and if sufficient may produce neuromuscular signs. These factors should be considered prior to attempting differentiation of the cause of the hypocalcemia.

Hypoparathyroidism. This condition is characterized by hypocalcemia and a normal or slightly increased serum phosphorus; serum parathormone concentration is low. Hypoparathyroidism may appear after parathyroidectomy for removal of parathyroid neoplasms, in association with lymphocytic parathyroiditis, secondary to infection with canine distemper virus, or, most commonly is idiopathic.

Renal Disease. Hypocalcemia may occur in renal failure even though there is increased parathyroid activity. This occurs because there is a decreased conversion of vitamin D to its active form (1,25-dihydroxycholecalciferol), the reduction in calcium in response to hyperphosphatemia and decreased responsiveness to parathormone.

These mineral changes are seen in both acute and chronic renal failure, and with postrenal urinary obstruction in the cat. If there is systemic acidosis clinical signs associated with the hypocalcemia may be masked as there is an increase in ionized calcium. However, rapid correcting of the altered acid-base state may cause a reduction of ionized calcium and precipitate clinical signs.

Dietary Imbalances. Hypocalcemia as a result of excess dietary phosphorus, lack of vitamin D, or a dietary calcium deficiency is rare. Secondary hyperparathyroidism will occur with any of those conditions. If there is a dietary lack of calcium, serum phosphorus is normal and decreased. It is increased or normal if there is excess dietary phosphorus.

Parturient Paresis and Hypomagnesemic Tetany (Cattle) and Eclampsia (Horse, Dog, Sheep). Hypocalcemia is a consistent finding in parturient paresis and hypomagnesemic tetany (cattle) and eclampsia (horse, dog, sheep) and is secondary to lactation and the consequent depletion of calcium. It most commonly occurs in cattle that have been fed a prepartum diet of high calcium, which has a tendency to depress parathormone secretion. Prolonged suppression prevents rapid mobilization of bone calcium which is needed when a negative calcium balance occurs with the beginning of lactation.

In hypomagnesemic tetany the majority of affected cows also have hypocalcemia. Hypomagnesemic tetany can be differentiated from parturient paresis by measuring urine magnesium. Magnesium is markedly decreased in urine of cattle with hypomagnesemic tetany (normal = about 50 mg/dL (25 mmol/L) urine).

Acute Pancreatitis. In dogs this condition occasionally may be accompanied by hypocalcemia (see Case 48). The mechanism is probably multifactorial. If fat necrosis accompanies pancreatitis, calcium is bound to free fatty acids in the area. It has also been suggested that increased glucagon release associated with pancreatitis produces a decrease in ionized calcium or an increase in calcitonin.

Ethylene Glycol Toxicity (Dogs and Cats). This may be accompanied by hypocalcemia as calcium oxalate crystals are formed in excess (see Case 43).

Other Causes of Hypocalcemia. Hypocalcemia may also be caused by blister beetle poisoning in horses, intestinal malabsorption in dogs, hypercalcitonism secondary to neoplasia of thyroid parafollicular (C) cells in cattle, transport tetany in sheep, and idiopathic acute hypocalcemic tetany in horses. Hypocalcemia produced by these mechanisms is poorly understood.

Conditions with Hyperphosphatemia (Table 9–3)

Young Animals. Serum phosphorus levels are above adult normals in growing animals as a consequence of rapid bone turnover (see Case 46).

Renal Disease. Hyperphosphatemia associated with renal disease in the dog and cat is a result of a reduction in glomerular filtration and is preceded by azotemia. Hyperphosphatemia (as well as azotemia) is not consistent in herbivorous animals with renal failure since phosphorus can also be eliminated via the digestive tract (see Cases 40 and 42).

Exogenous Phosphorus. Administration of phosphorus-containing fluids and phosphorus (Fleet) enemas will result in hyperphosphatemia if given in excessive volume (see Case 56).

Other Causes of Hyperphosphatemia. Hypervitaminosis D (preceding renal calcinosis), osteolytic bone disease, jasmine (*Cestrum* sp.) toxicity (dog and cat), excess dietary intake of phosphorus, and hypoparathyroidism are accompanied by hyperphosphatemia in addition to the serum calcium changes described earlier.

Improper Specimen Handling. Serum held too long on RBCs will often have a high serum phosphorus concentration. This is because of the release of the mineral from erythrocytes. Excessive hemolysis will also produce a falsely increased serum phosphorus. Factitious hyperphosphatemia appears to be common.

Causes of Hypophosphatemia (Table 9–4)

In the early stages of primary hyperparathyroidism and hypercalcemia of neoplasia (pseudohyperparathyroidism) hypophosphatemia may be present.

Patients with secondary nutritional hyperparathyroidism resulting from avitaminosis D or the lack of dietary calcium have a normal or decreased serum phosphorus.

Patients with diabetes mellitus compounded by ketoacidosis and hypokalemia may have hypophosphatemia. In the ketoacidotic diabetic patient, phosphorylation is depressed which causes decomposition of intracellular phosphate compounds. Inorganic phosphate moves into extracelluar fluid and is excreted in urine. Hyperglycemia, polyuria, and ketonuria produce an osmotic diuresis, which enhances phosphate elimination in urine.

Respiratory alkalosis from hyperventilation causes phosphate to move into intracellular space, resulting in hypophosphatemia.

About one third of the dogs with hyperadrenocorticism have hypophosphatemia.

Hypophasphatemia also accompanies eclampsia, hypomagnesemic tetany in ruminants, parturient paresis in cattle, malabsorption, starvation, canine Fanconi-like syndrome, and insulin administration.

In the horse, hypophosphatemia may occur in association with chronic renal failure (see Case 40) as well as vitamin D intoxication, pseudohyperparathyroidism, and after insulin administration.

THYROID GLAND

Function Tests

Evaluation of the functional status of the thyroid gland depends upon the measurement of the serum concentration of the thyroid hormones thyroxine (T_4), triiodothyronine (T_3), unbound thyroxine, and triiodothyronine (free T_4 and free T_3) (Fig. 9–4).

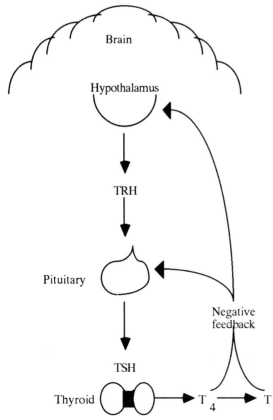

FIGURE 9–4. A simplified regulatory mechanism is illustrated for the hypothalamic-pituitary-thyroid axis. Thyrotropin-releasing hormone stimulates the pituitary gland to release thyroid-stimulating hormone which initiates thyroid hormone release. Both T_3 and T_4 inhibit the pituitary gland and hypothalamus.

Most (more than 90%) of the secreted hormone is T_4, and the remainder is T_3. T_3 is more biologically active than T_4 at the cellular level. Almost all thyroid hormone in serum (99%+) is bound to the thyroid binding proteins TBPA (thyroid-binding prealbumin) and TBG (thyroid-binding globulin). Unbound (free) thyroxine accounts for approximately 0.1% of the serum thyroid hormone.

Secretion of thyroid hormone is controlled by the release of thyrotropin (TSH), which is controlled by the action of thyrotropin-releasing hormone (TRH) from the posterior pituitary gland. The feedback mechanism that controls the production of thyroxine is related to the concentration of free thyroxine in plasma. Any reduction in the level of free (unbound) thyroid hormone stimulates the pituitary gland to release TRH whereas an excess of hormone reduces TRH secretion.

Hypothyroidism

Hypothyroidism typically causes symmetric hair loss, lethargy, and obesity. Myxedema, stupor, and coma are an extreme clinical expression of hypothyroidism. Prompt recognition and treatment are essential to prevent death. Biochemically, an increased cholesterol, increased triglycerides, and a decreased T_4 (or lack of response to TSH) support the diagnosis.

Laboratory Findings

Hematology. Nonregenerative anemias (usually mild) are seen frequently with hypothyroidism. Thyroid imbalance has also been incriminated as a factor in the development of immune-mediated diseases (see Case 3).

Hypothyroidism seems to increase the clinical manifestation and severity of hemorrhage in canine von Willebrand's disease (VWD). The common occurrence of hypothyroidism and VWD in some dog breeds (Doberman pinscher, golden retriever, Pembroke Welsh corgi, basset hound, Scottish terrier, standard poodle, Manchester terrier) suggests a relationship between the synthesis and metabolic regulation of thyroid hormones and the von Willebrand factor (VFW), which is deficient or abnormal in VWD (see Case 28).

Thyroid Hormone Concentrations. Hypothyroidism causes low serum T_3 and T_4 values in dogs and horses. Recent studies that applied linear analysis to available thyroid profile tests suggested that the best test combination for the diagnosis of hypothyroidism in dogs is free (unbound) T_4 and cholesterol. Using this information a K value is calculated. The formula is

$$K = [9.0 \times \text{free } T_4 \text{ (ng/dL)}] - [0.026 \times \text{cholesterol (mg/dL)}]$$

$$K = 9 \times \left(\frac{\text{free } T_4 \text{ (pmol/L)}}{4} \right) - \text{cholesterol (mmol/L)}$$

If the K value is lower than −4, the dog is suspected of having primary hypothyroidism, K values greater than +1 mean that the dog is normal or has a nonthyroidal illness. K values between +1 and −4 should usually be interpreted as meaning primary hypothyroidism or a nonthyroidal illness.

Care should be taken in interpreting the K value especially when other laboratory data or clinical signs support hypothyroidism. About 30 to 40% of dogs with hypothyroidism do not have hypercholesterolemia. In these patients the K value may be within the normal range even though the T_3 and T_4 as well as the free T_4

are low. Conversely, dogs with a serum cholesterol over 500 mg/dL (13 mmol/L) but with normal thyroid hormone levels often have a low K value. The hypercholesterolemia is usually a result of other diseases.

Serum concentrations of T_4 can also be altered by *nonthyroidal illness* in dogs and cats. Conditions known to produce decreases in the amount of circulating thyroid hormones include diabetes mellitus, hypoadrenocorticism, hyperadrenocorticism, renal failure, liver disease, and systemic neoplasia. Drugs that may cause a decreased serum concentration of thyroid hormones include glucocorticoids, particularly if given over a long time; antithyroid drugs such as propylthiouracil and radiocontrast dyes; antiepileptics such as diphenylhydantoin and phenobarbital; and a few other drugs such as phenylbutazone and furosamide have also been incriminated.

Measurement of free (unbound) thyroxine concentrations may be useful in assessing patients with decreased T_3/T_4 without primary thyroid disease, as this reduction is often the result of decreased thyroxine binding. Such a decrease does not reduce free T_3 and T_4 levels in serum. Free T_3 and T_4 levels are usually normal to slightly increased in the euthyroid sick patient and those on drugs. Assays for free T_4 and T_3 are now available from some commercial laboratories serving the veterinary profession.

TSH Test. Confirmatory diagnosis of thyroid insufficiency rests with completion of a TSH stimulation test. This test is conducted by measuring T_3 and T_4 just prior to and 8 hours after the administration of TSH intramuscularly at the rate of 5 units/20 lb (2.3 units/9.1 kg) of body weight (maximum of 10 units) or prior to and 4 hours after intravenous injection of 0.1 units TSH/lb (0.22 units/kg) (maximum of 5 units). Serum thyroxine levels should at least double after TSH stimulation. Failure to do so suggests primary hypothyroidism. If the patient has been on thyroid therapy, it may be necessary to discontinue therapy for 10 days to 2 weeks prior to conducting the test. Therapeutic administration to patient with a functioning thyroid will depress the gland, and it will not react to TSH.

Occasional patients with all of the clinical signs of hypothyroidism will have increased T_3 or T_4 values or both. This occurs in patients with an immune mediated thyroiditis in which antibodies to thyroxine have developed. These antibodies interfere with the radioimmunoassay and result in false high values. In such patients a test for antithyroid antibodies can be used for confirmation of the condition. Serum titers of antithyroglobulin antibodies can be determined in some veterinary laboratories. Positive titers are observed in about half of the canine patients with hypothyroidism as they have an immune mediated thyroiditis.

Specialized Tests. Increased serum canine thyrotropin, measured with a verified immunoassay, would be valuable in the diagnosis of hypothyroidism. Such assays are used for evaluating thyroid function in man but are not suitable for measuring TSH in domestic animals.

Radioiodine uptake can be used to rule out hypothyroidism in cases of drug-induced lowering of total serum thyroxine. This test is not available to most general practitioners and is subject to variation with dietary intake of iodine.

Hyperthyroidism

Hyperthyroidism in dogs and cats is usually accompanied by an increase in the serum levels of T_4.

Cats

The most common cause of hyperthyroidism in cats is functional adenomatous hyperplasia. It is a multisystemic disease occurring because of the circulation of excessive quantities of thyroid hormones.

Cats with hyperthyroidism generally have an increase in T_4. If the cat has a severe concurrent nonthyroidal illness high normal or only slightly increased total T_4 may be seen on initial examination. A few cats will have an increased T_4 with a normal T_3. It is likely that conversion of T_4 to T_3 may be inhibited in these cats while the total T_4 is reduced because of decreased protein binding associated with the nonthyroidal illness. T_4 may be increased artificially in cats with autoantibodies to thyroxine depending upon the type of radioimmunoassay used.

TSH Stimulation. At 1.0 units/kg body weight TSH stimulation is not followed by a T_4 increase in cats with hyperthyroidism.

T_3 Suppression Test. This test may also be used as an aid in the diagnosis of feline hyperthyroidism. A resting T_4 is completed, T_3 at a dose of 25 mg is given every 8 hours for 2 days. One more dose is given, and the T_4 posttreatment sample is collected 2 to 4 hours later. In normal animals there will be a decrease of at least 50% whereas in hyperthyroid cats or those with autoantibodies there is little or no decrease in serum T_4.

Diagnosis of hyperthyroidism should be based on clinical findings of hyperthyroidism and laboratory data. Cats with increased T_4 levels which are asymptomatic or do not have typical signs and cats that appear to be euthyroid but have typical signs should be retested for serum T_4 in 3 or 4 weeks or alternative testing should be completed.

Additional laboratory findings may include elevations in serum alkaline phosphatase (SAP), alanine aminotransferase (ALT), aspartate aminotransferase (AST), lactic dehydrogenase (LD), and hyperphosphatemia (see Case 63). Hematologically there may be a mild polycythemia or, conversely, a mild nonregenerative anemia.

Thyroid imaging is also a useful technique for confirming a diagnosis of hyperthyroidism, particularly if there is no clinical enlargement of the gland.

Dogs

Hyperthyroidism in the dog is uncommon and commonly the result of thyroid neoplasia. It is usually accompanied by increased concentrations of circulating T_3 and T_4. A dog with thyroid neoplasia may show clinical signs of hypothyroidism.

ADRENAL CORTEX

Adrenal cortical function is controlled by the serum level of cortisol (Fig. 9–5).

The primary syndromes affecting the adrenal cortex are hypoadrenocorticism (Addison's disease) and hyperadrenocorticism (Cushing's syndrome).

Primary hypoadrenocorticism most often results from atrophy of the adrenal cortex. This results in decreased production of glucocorticoids and mineralocorticoids. The cause of atrophy remains undetermined, but there is increasing evidence that immune mediated destruction of the gland is important. Addison's disease may also occur as a result of any destructive lesion of the adrenals, such as those seen with metastatic tumors, infarction of the adrenals, amyloidosis, or

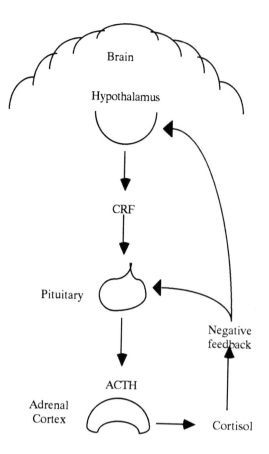

FIGURE 9–5. A simplified regulatory mechanism for the hypothalamic-pituitary-adrenal axis. Corticotropin-releasing hormone (CRF) stimulates the pituitary to release ACTH, which stimulates cortisol release. Glucocorticoids inhibit both the pituitary and the hypothalamus.

by infections involving both adrenal glands. Secondary hypoadrenocorticism develops if there is lack of ACTH production associated with an underlying hypothalamic-pituitary disorder or can result from drugs that suppress pituitary production of ACTH.

Hyperadrenocorticism occurs by two mechanisms: (1) as a result of a functioning pituitary neoplasm that autonomously secretes ACTH causing bilateral hyperplasia of the adrenal cortex (pituitary-dependent hyperadrenocorticism[PDH]); and (2) resulting from a functional adrenal neoplasm. Clinical signs of hyperadrenocorticism may appear in patients that have been on long-term glucocorticoid therapy (iatrogenic Cushing's) (see Case 61).

Hyperadrenocorticism (See Case 60)

Hyperadrenocorticism is accompanied by clinical signs that reflect the actions of glucocorticoids. One of the earliest manifestations and the most frequent owner complaint involves polyuria and polydipsia. As the condition progresses symmetric alopecia develops, and in severely affected dogs hair loss may extend over most of the body except for the head and lower limbs. The abdomen may become pendulous if the condition has persisted for some time.

Hematology

There may be a leukocytosis that includes lymphopenia, eosinopenia, and mature neutrophilia. Monocytosis is frequent in dogs but is variable in cats and seldom occurs in other species. Neutrophilic hypersegmentation may occur as the excess glucocorticoids retard normal neutrophil migration into tissues. These findings are subject to variability depending on the presence of concurrent disease.

Plasma Cortisol

Some animals with hyperadrenocorticism have an increase in plasma cortisol concentration. However, the majority of the patients have normal to only slightly increased baseline values. These findings seem to prevail whether the cause is primary adrenal neoplasia or the consequence of increased ACTH activity resulting from a pituitary lesion. Thus, single baseline cortisol determinations are of little value in arriving at a diagnosis of hyperadrenocorticism.

ACTH Stimulation

An ACTH stimulation test is the most commonly used diagnostic device for hyperadrenocorticism. A number of different protocols have been employed. The protocol selected should be that recommended by the laboratory that will complete the tests. Porcine aqueous gelatin ACTH can be used at a dose of 1.0 IU/lb (2.2 units/kg) of body weight. Plasma samples for cortisol assay are obtained prior to and 2 hours after an intramuscular injection of ACTH. Synthetic ACTH at a dose of 0.25 mg/dog (entire vial) or ½ vial for a cat can also be used. If the synthetic product is used a 1-hour post-ACTH sample is used for the dog and a ½ hour post-ACTH sample for the cat. In the horse of 1 IU/kg is given if the porcine product is used or 100 IU of synthetic ACTH is administered intravenously. A post-ACTH sample is obtained in 2 to 8 hours in the horse.

Normal values must be established by each laboratory. Abnormal responses, those with postvalues greater than normal, are supportive of hyperadrenocorticism but do not aid in differentiating between pituitary dependent hyperadrenocorticism and adrenal neoplasia (adrenal neoplasia hyperadrenocorticism [ANH]). Patients with iatrogenic Cushing's syndrome will have little if any increase in baseline cortisol in response to ACTH stimulation; in fact, the post-ACTH value may be decreased.

If there is normal to increased pre-ACTH cortisol and normal post-ACTH cortisol it does not rule out hyperadrenocorticism. If the patient is showing clinical signs of the disorder, the ACTH stimulation test should be repeated in weeks or months or a dexamethasone suppression test completed.

If there is normal to increased pre-ACTH cortisol and abnormally high post-ACTH cortisol it confirms hyperadrenocorticism and the presence of an adrenal gland capable of responding to ACTH. It does not, however, differentiate PDH from ANH.

If there is a markedly increased pre-ACTH cortisol and little to no increase post-ACTH, it suggests an autonomous cortisol-secreting adrenal tumor.

Patients that are chronically stressed may have a slightly high baseline cortisol and demonstrate an abnormal response to ACTH stimulation. If the history and clinical signs do not strongly suggest a final diagnosis, a dexamethasone suppression test should be completed.

PD test
ACTH test
Routine Dex) Test
Suppression

Dexamethasone Suppression Screening (Low-dose) Test

This test is helpful in confirming hyperadrenocorticism in patients in whom the ACTH test results were equivocal. The test is conducted by obtaining a fasting plasma sample, administering 0.01 mg/kg dexamethasone IV, and intravenously collecting a second sample for cortisol assay 6 and 8 hours later.

Normal dogs will have an 8-hour post-dexamethasone cortisol value that is usually less than 1 μg/dL (0.0276 μmol/L). (Some laboratories use 1.4 μg/dL) (0.0386 μmol/L) because this dose of dexamethasone will consistently suppress serum cortisol levels for 8 hours. If the postdexamethasone value is greater than 1.0 μg/dL (1.4 μg/dL) (0.0386 μmol/L) one has confirmed the presence of hyper-adrenocorticism.

High-dose Dexamethasone Suppression

The test is conducted in the same fashion as the low dose except that dexamethasone is given at the rate of 0.1 mg/kg. Some practitioners use a megadose of 1.0 mg/kg. Such high doses of dexamethasone should completely suppress ACTH secretion from abnormal pituitary cells. Normal suppression is considered to be a cortisol that is less than 50% of base line. If the second value is more than 50% of the baseline, it suggests adrenal tumor or a large pituitary chromophobe adenoma. Some dogs with PDH do not suppress, even with a megadose of dexamethasone.

ACTH Assay

Differentiation between PDH and ANH is best accomplished with an assay for plasma ACTH. Because ACTH secretion appears to have a diurnal pattern in the dog, it is best to hospitalize the patient overnight and collect the plasma sample between 8 and 9 AM. The sample should be collected in cold heparin-treated syringes and the syringe placed on ice or the blood transferred to a cold plastic tube. The plasma is harvested, preferably in a cold centrifuge, and the separated plasma is frozen until analyzed. The laboratory should be contacted prior to obtaining the sample to confirm the handling procedure and to find out how frequently the assay is performed.

Normal plasma ACTH is from 20 to 100 pg/mL (4.4 to 22 pmol/L). In the dog or cat endogenous ACTH values that are less than 20 pg/mL (4.4 pmol/L) are highly indicative of adrenal neoplasm whereas ACTH values greater than 100 pg/ml (22 pmol/L) support PDH.

Serum Chemistry

Chemistry findings, other than cortisol and ACTH levels, are variable and may include any, all, or none of the following:

1. Fasting hyperglycemia (often low grade with no glucosuria); glucosuria common in horse
2. Hypercholesterolemia and lipemia
3. A marked increase in serum alkaline phosphatase activity (dogs)
4. An increase in ALT activity (usually a small increase) with a normal AST value
5. A low urine specific gravity less than 1.015, often 1.003 to 1.005

6. Hypophosphatemia in dogs (about one third of those affected)
7. A mild increase in sodium with a mild decrease in potassium in about half of affected dogs; values usually within the normal range
8. Low T_3, T_4 concentrations with normal TSH response

Hypoadrenocorticism (See Case 59)

Hypoadrenocorticism may be a result of a primary adrenocortical failure or secondary adrenocortical failure caused by the administration of exogenous corticosteroids (see Case 61) or, less commonly, as a consequence of spontaneous pituitary insufficiency. Patients with hypoadrenocorticism often have a vague history of depression, weakness, dehydration, weak pulse, bradycardia, and intermittent vomiting and diarrhea. Hemoconcentration, hypotension, and circulatory collapse may develop acutely. A chronic disease course is highlighted by recurrent episodes of vague clinical signs that respond to symptomatic treatment.

Hematology

Leukocyte counts are variable but may include normal lymphocyte and eosinophil counts in a patient that one would expect to have a stress leukogram (lymphopenia and eosinopenia). There is a normocytic, normochromic, nonregenerative anemia that is often masked by dehydration.

Serum Chemistry

Increases in urea nitrogen and creatinine frequently occur in patients with hypoadrenocorticism. The azotemia is prerenal and is accompanied by increases in other analytes affected by hemoconcentration: hyperphosphatemia, hyperproteinemia, and hyperalbuminemia. It occurs because of reduced glomerular filtration that accompanies dehydration. The azotemia is sometimes erroneously interpreted as an indication of primary renal disease. Differentiation can be made by determining urine specific gravity. In most patients urine specific gravity will be greater than 1.030 to 1.035 if the azotemia is prerenal. The urine specific gravity may not be as high as one would expect in a severely dehydrated patient due, in part, to the reduced concentrating ability of kidneys devoid of mineralocorticoid activity and renal sodium loss.

Serum electrolyte changes classically include decreased sodium and chloride with an increased potassium and a decreased sodium to potassium ratio (less than 27:1).

Hypercalcemia occurs in about one fourth of the dogs with hypoadrenocorticism and especially in those that are severely ill.

Plasma Cortisol

Patients with hypoadrenocorticism generally have a decreased plasma cortisol. Because normal plasma cortisol levels may be low, finding a single low value is not adequate to confirm decreased adrenal cortical function. In order to evaluate the adrenal properly the adrenal reserve must be tested.

ACTH Stimulation

The test is conducted as described above. A post-ACTH cortisol less than two standard deviations below the mean for the laboratory will confirm hypoadreno-corticism. If adrenal hypofunction is a result of reduced secretion of ACTH by the pituitary, the adrenals will not respond to a single dose of ACTH but may respond after repeated doses.

ACTH Assay

Because a patient with a primary hypoadrenocortical failure has a low endogenous cortisol, there is little negative feedback to the pituitary, and the plasma ACTH level is high. With secondary adrenocortical failure plasma ACTH levels will be low. If the secondary insufficiency results from a primary pituitary insufficiency there may be a response to ACTH stimulation if it is repeated several times.

GROWTH HORMONE (GH) (FIG. 9–6)

Hyposomatotropism

Decreased GH can be congenital, especially in German shepherd dogs, or it may be acquired in the adult animal.

Hypopituitarism (dwarfism) in German shepherds is characterized by short stature, hair abnormalities including retention of puppy-hair coat, deficiency of guard hairs, and partial or complete alopecia. The condition appears to be inherited through an autosomal recessive trait. Growth rate is retarded a few weeks after birth, but affected puppies remain alert.

Adult onset GH deficiency is rare and is sometimes, but not always, accompanied by deficiencies in other pituitary hormones. The condition occurs primarily in Pomeranians, chow chows, poodles, American water spaniels, keeshonden, and Samoyeds but can occur in any breed. Affected dogs are usually presented for a skin condition characterized by truncal alopecia and hyperpigmentation. Skin changes seldom occur over the head and neck. Causes of adult onset GH deficiencies are not completely understood.

Diagnosis of hyposomatotropism may be difficult because the measurement of resting concentration of GH is not adequate for the diagnosis of deficiencies. Many normal dogs have a low resting GH concentration. A GH-responsive test using clonidine hydrochloride (10 mg/kg) or its structural analog xylazine hydrochloride (100 μg/kg) should be completed. These agents induce production of growth hormone-releasing factor which stimulates GH release. Human growth hormone-releasing factor (1 to 5 mg/kg) can also be used. The usual procedure is to measure GH prior to and 15, 30, 45, 60, and 120 minutes after intravenous administration of clonidine hydrochloride, xylazine hydrochloride, or human growth hormone-releasing factor. A normal animal will have an increase in GH which peaks 15 to 30 minutes after injection and returns to the base line within 90 minutes. The absence of any increase in the concentration of GH is indicative of a deficiency.

Animals treated with GH should be monitored routinely as GH is diabetogenic, and patients may develop transient or permanent diabetes mellitus.

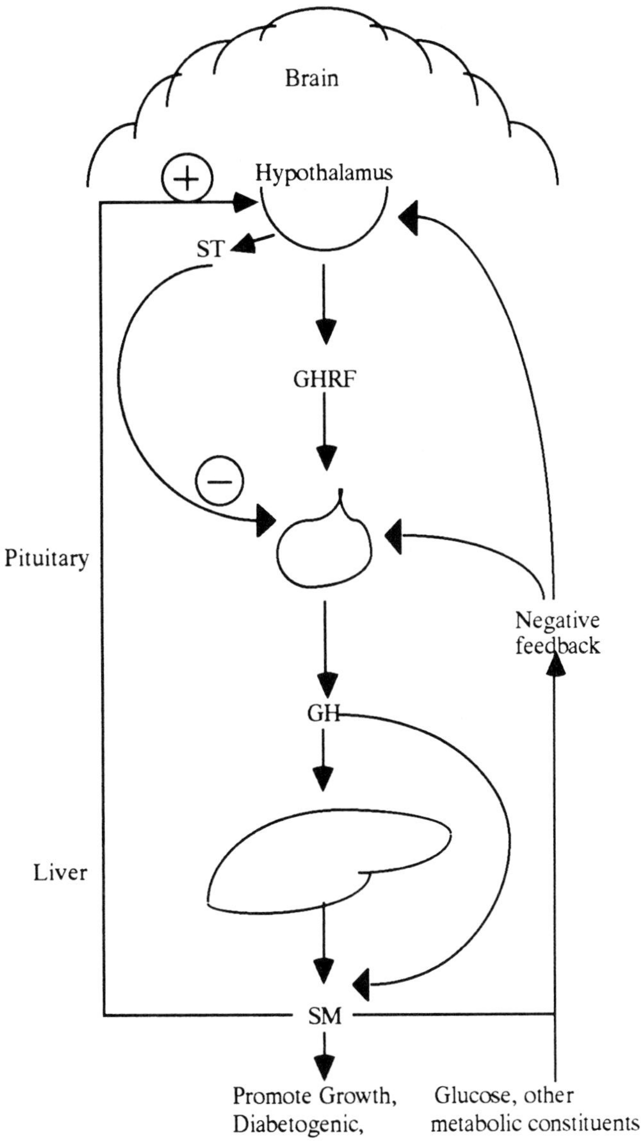

FIGURE 9–6. A simplified regulatory mechanism is illustrated for growth hormone. Growth hormone-releasing factor (GHRF) stimulates the pituitary gland to release growth hormone which interacts with the liver and possibly other organs to produce somatomedins (SM). GH appears to facilitate SM activity directly for some metabolic functions. The negative feedback axis for GH is complex and involves multiple peripheral metabolic substances (SM, glucocorticoids, increased glucose, increased fatty acids) and, centrally by stomatostatin (ST). Somatomedins may have a positive effect on stomatostatin release.

Hypersomatotropism (Diabetes Mellitus-Acromegaly)

Diabetes mellitus occurs in association with oversecretion of GH because GH is an insulin antagonist or because of an increased concentration of insulin-like growth factor.

Acromegaly in dogs appears to be confined to females and has been associated with treatment with progestagens or occurs during diestrus when progesterone levels are naturally high. Clinically, acromegaly in dogs is characterized by polyuria/polydipsia, inspiratory stridor, fatigue, prominent skin folds (particularly in the head and neck region) that are a consequence of soft tissue proliferation, enlargement of intradental spaces, and increased abdominal size.

Progestagens apparently do not stimulate GH secretion in cats. Acromegaly has been reported in cats with insulin-resistant diabetes. Cats with a persistent hyperglycemia in spite of insulin treatments in excess of 25 units should be suspected of acromegaly especially if other signs such as cardiopathy or arthropathy are present.

Affected cats have many of the same clinical signs as dogs, but the condition is seen mostly in males.

Diagnosis of hypersomatotropism is confirmed by the demonstration of increased levels of circulating GH.

Because some patients without acromegaly have increased GH levels, a suppression test such as glucose tolerance must be done to verify a diagnosis. GH concentrations remain elevated after glucose administration. Few veterinary laboratories have the capacity to measure GH in animals, and tests designed for use in humans are not acceptable for dogs and cats. Measurement of insulin-like growth factors (somatomedins) may be helpful in the diagnosis of acromegaly in dogs because these peptides are GH dependent and are increased in patients with acromegaly.

10

EVALUATION OF CEREBROSPINAL FLUID

Cerebrospinal fluid (CSF) is a clear, colorless ultrafiltrate of the plasma which bathes the exterior of the brain and spinal cord. Pathology of the outer surfaces of these structures may cause changes in the CSF whereas pathologic changes deeper in the nervous tissue usually do not. Evaluation of the CSF minimally should include a nucleated cell count, cytologic examination, and protein determination. Other biochemical measurements which can be performed include glucose, creatine kinase, lactic dehydrogenase, protein electrophoresis, and specific immunoglobulin quantification. These measurements are usually restricted to use by clinical investigators at this time.

There are certain visually recognizable changes in the CSF. Turbidity implies abnormal numbers of nucleated cells (pleocytosis). A pink to red color indicates the presence of erythrocytes, and a yellow discoloration (xanthochromia) suggests the prior (days to weeks) presence of erythrocytes (hemorrhage) in the nonicteric patient.

ENUMERATION AND DIFFERENTIAL OF NUCLEATED CELLS

The normal CSF is devoid of erythrocytes and contains less than five to eight nucleated cells per microliter. Because of the low cell numbers, counts cannot be done on an automated counter but must be performed by directly loading a hemacytometer. The condenser of the microscope should be lowered to enhance the silhouette of the cells and aid in differentiating erythrocytes (anuclear with irregular, crenated surface) and nucleated cells. The cells in the nine large squares of the Neubauer-ruled chamber are counted and the nucleated and erythrocyte counts each multiplied by 10/9 to yield the cell number per microliter.

The microscopic examination of the cellular component must be performed soon after collection (preferably within 1 hour) to avoid the artifact of cell deterioration. Refrigeration (4° C) of the specimen will delay cell deterioration by several hours. All CSF specimens should be examined cytologically even if the total nucleated cell number is normal. A concentration procedure is necessary so that sufficient nucleated cells are present for cytologic examination. The use of a cytocentrifuge provides a cell preparation of uniform quality with good preservation of cell morphology. Although the expense of the equipment (about $5500) limits its widespread availability in veterinary practices, most medical facilities and commercial laboratories have a unit. Simplified sedimentation chambers have been adapted for use with CSF for economic reasons. These concentration methods can provide adequate cell preparations for those experienced with the procedure. Membrane filtration techniques also yield acceptable cytologic preparations, but special training or prior experience is again recommended.

Cell Types

Small to medium mononuclear (mature lymphocytes and monocytoid cells) monopolize the normal CSF microscopically. A lymphoplasmacytic pleocytosis is associated with certain viral infections and granulomatous meningoencephalitis (see Case 65). Macrophages may also be prominent in the latter pathologic process. A neutrophilic pleocytosis is most frequently associated with septic and certain sterile inflammatory processes (see Cases 64 and 67). Suppurative, nonseptic disorders include immune mediated disease, rickettsial infection, feline infectious peritonitis, cryptococcosis, trauma and myelographic procedures, and neoplasia (which have not exfoliated cells into the CSF). Lymphoma is the most commonly diagnosed neoplasm of the central nervous system cytologically. Much less frequently other types of neoplastic cells, often associated with metastatic lesions, are detected. Occasionally small clumps of epithelial-like cells will exfoliate from the choroid plexus and ependymal lining. These uniform cell clusters should not be confused with neoplastic cells.

BIOCHEMICAL DETERMINATIONS

Protein

Quantification of the total protein requires a dye-binding or turbidimetric procedure because of the small, milligram concentrations normally present. The reference range for normal values varies depending on the procedure used, usually it is more than 20 mg/dL (200 mg/L) or less than 40 mg/dL (400 mg/L). It is essential to know the normal range for the laboratory used. A urine dipstick may be used to get a rapid estimate of the protein concentration. A 1+ to 3+ relates to a mild to marked protein increase, respectively. A simple precipitation procedure, the Pandy test, which is selective for globulins, may also be used in a practice setting. Three to four drops of CSF are mixed with 1.0 mL of Pandy reagent (1.0 gr of carbolic acid crystals (phenol) in 10 mL of distilled water) and the degree of precipitation (cloudiness) graded from slight to marked. Increased protein concentrations are associated with a variety of pathologic processes, with or without pleocytosis (see Cases 65 and 67).

Glucose

The glucose concentration of CSF is 60 to 80% of plasma and may be measured by the same methodology. Hypoglycorrhacia, low CSF glucose, may be associated with hypoglycemia or bacterial meningitis (see Case 67).

Suppurative *Versus* Nonsuppurative Disease

Examination of the CSF is an adjunct to the neurologic examination and should minimally include a nucleated cell count, cytologic evaluation, and determination of the protein concentration. A positive finding may assist in the differential diagnostic considerations, especially between nonsuppurative and suppurative conditions. The latter often show fever, cervical rigidity, and vertebral pain.

A sterile, suppurative, corticosteroid-responsive meningitis appears to be a relatively common disease in large, young adult dogs (see Case 64). Certainly the observation of bacteria dictates a septic meningitis and the need for antibiotic treatment.

Neutrophils predominate (with occasional eosinophils) in the CSF infected with *Cryptococcus neoformans*. The organisms are recognized readily.

Granulomatous Meningoencephalitis

In granulomatous meningoencephalitis (see Case 65) the protein is increased, and lymphocytes, monocytes, and macrophages predominate with lesser numbers of neutrophils and plasma cells. Affected dogs are commonly young adult small breeds with an acute onset in the disseminated form and a more insidious onset in the focal form. Clinical signs reflect the form present, head signs that progress to signs reflecting involvement of the caudal fossa as well as changes in mental status.

Canine Distemper

Young, unvaccinated dogs are common candidates for distemper. The disease is usually multisystemic with progressive multifocal central nervous system involvement. Older dogs may develop a more insidious form with gradual loss of mentation and progressive posterior paresis. Changes in the CSF, when present, include an increase in protein and slight lymphocytic pleocytosis.

Rickettsial Infections

Rickettsial infections may also involve the central nervous system. The dogs usually show systemic signs of illness, a nonregenerative anemia and thrombocytopenia, and a neutropenia (ehrlichiosis) or neutrophilia (Rocky Mountain spotted fever whereas a lymphocytic pleocytosis appears more common in ehrlichiosis. Serologic titers are required to confirm the diagnosis.

Feline Infectious Peritonitis

In this disease the protein is markedly increased, and neutrophils and monocytes/macrophages predominate.

Neoplasia

Dogs with brain tumors may show an increased protein with normal to mild pleocytosis with variable cell types.

Disc Disease

Dogs with intervertebral disc disease usually have normal CSF and radiographic findings supportive of the diagnosis.

Many animals with clinical signs of a central nervous system disturbance, particularly those that have seizures, have unrewarding CSF findings.

EVALUATION OF EFFUSIONS

Pleural, Peritoneal, Pericardial*

Evaluation of body cavity fluids is usually diagnostically rewarding. It may provide an etiologic diagnosis or, more often, a general classification of the underlying disorder.

CELLULAR EVALUATION

Collection of fluid is usually done using a 20- to 22-gauge needle and a 10- to 12-ml syringe. After surgical preparation of the skin the needle with syringe attached is placed into the subcutaneous tissue and slight negative pressure applied as the needle is advanced at an angle. Fluid will appear in the syringe as soon as the needle penetrates the lining of the cavity. Angling the needle helps prevent fluid from potentially leaking from the cavity into surrounding tissue. A small drop of fluid is layered thinly on a glass slide. About three fourths of the way down the slide any excess fluid is *left on* the slide and allowed to *flow back* and dried with a hair blower. Such a two-part slide provides for an estimate of the cell count from the thin area, and the concentrated area can be searched for cell clumps or organisms. The remaining fluid should be placed in an EDTA tube (purple top) to prevent any potential clotting and the fluid used for cell counts and other biochemical parameters that may need to be determined at a later date.

TRANSUDATES AND EXUDATES

Analysis of fluid in the pericardial, pleural, and peritoneal cavities includes the measurement of certain physiochemical properties and a description of cells present on stained smears. Evaluation of the cell component includes an absolute and differential nucleated cell count. Fluids with very low cell counts are concentrated by routine centrifugation or with a cytocentrifuge. Fluids are generally classified as a transudate, modified transudate, or an exudate. Special classifications will be noted (Table 11–1).

Effusions form when there is an increase in hydrostatic pressure and/or a decrease in oncotic pressure in capillaries (Fig. 11–1).

---

* See Algorithm 19.

TABLE 11–1. Guidelines for Characterizing Effusions Other Than Hemorrhagic

	Transudate	Modified Transudate	Exudate
Total protein (g/dL)	<2.5	>2.5	>2.5
Nucleated cell count/μL			
Horse	<1000 <5000	<5000 <10,000	>5000 >10,000
Predominant nucleated cell type			
Horse	Mesothelial/ macrophage Up to 60% may be neutrophils	Mesothelial/ macrophage Up to 60% may be neutrophils	Neutrophil/ macrophage >60% are neutrophils
More common causes			
	Portal hypertension secondary to liver insufficiency	Ascites secondary to right-sided cardiac insufficiency	Inflammatory Septic Nonseptic
	Severe hypoalbuminemia	Intestinal disorder (equine)	Intestinal disorder (equine)

Transudates

Transudates are characterized by a protein concentration that is *less than 2.5 g/dL,* and *modified transudates* are characterized by a protein concentration *greater than 2.5 g/dL;* (25 g/L) that biochemical parameter is an important determination to make on an effusion. The transudate and modified transudate have low nucleated cell counts, the predominant cell type is the large mononuclear cell (mesothelial cells). The mesothelial cell may be either the reactive form or the macrophage type.

The pathophysiologic event leading to the formation of a transudate or modified transudate *ascitic fluid* can be related to the protein concentration in the lymphatic vessels. It is critical to understand that hepatic lymph, that is the lymph vessels within the hepatic parenchyma, is a relatively *high protein lymph.* The lymphatic vessels associated with the intestinal tract have a relatively *low protein lymph* (Fig. 11–2). A disease process that involves area 1 (in Fig. 11–2) will cause hepatic congestion and ultimately leaking of the high protein lymph from the hepatic parenchyma into the abdominal cavity. This will result in a *modified transudate.* The most common cause is right-sided heart failure, but less common causes include lesions that constrict the caudal vena cava. The important point to remember is that when an ascites is classified as a modified transudate one should direct

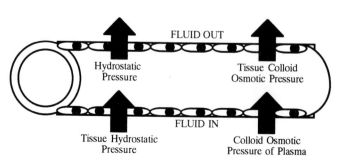

FLUID OUT

Hydrostatic Pressure

Tissue Colloid Osmotic Pressure

FLUID IN

Tissue Hydrostatic Pressure

Colloid Osmotic Pressure of Plasma

FIGURE 11–1. Diagram of a capillary.

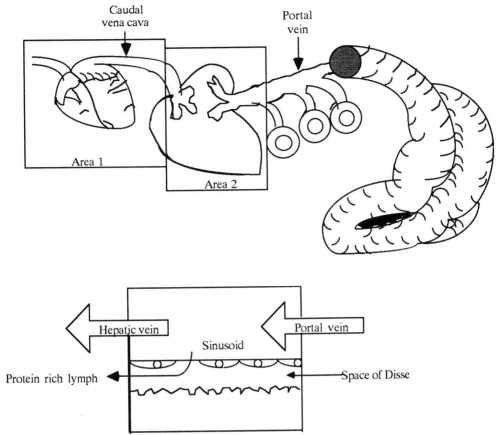

FIGURE 11–2. Normal vascular and lymphatic drainage of the abdominal cavity. *Bottom section* shows microscopic view of sinusoidal blood flow and lymph formation. (Modified from Greene, C.E.: Diagnostic and therapeutic considerations. Comp. Contin. Educ. Small Anim. Pract. 1:712–719, 1979.)

diagnostic efforts toward area 1. Modified transudates may also occur in association with a sterile inflammation (see Case 45).

The portal circulation drains the entire gastrointestinal tract and delivers the blood to the liver by the porta hepatis. A disease process that interferes with the blood flow through or to the liver will cause *portal hypertension,* resulting in the leakage of low protein lymph into the abdominal cavity, yielding a *transudate* (see Cases 33 and 34). The most common pathology involving area 2 (in Fig. 11–2) which results in portal hypertension is hepatic cirrhosis. A less common cause for the formation of portal hypertension resulting in an ascites classified as a transudate would be a constrictive lesion at the porta hepatis where the portal vessels enter the liver. Once again the important point to remember is that when an ascites is classified as a transudate the differential diagnostic focus should be toward area 2. Severe hypoalbuminemia (less than 1.0 g/dL) (10 g/L) can also predispose to the formation of an ascitic transudate without the presence of portal hypertension.

Exudates

An exudate is characterized by a protein concentration of greater than 3.0 g/dL (30 g/L) and an increased nucleated cell count composed primarily of *neutrophils* with lesser numbers of macrophages and lymphocytes (see Case 1). Infectious and noninfectious inflammatory causes of an exudate may be distinguished usually by the microscopic examination and biochemical determinations. *Septic exudates* are defined by the identification of bacteria in the fluid (see Case 17). Some bacteria contain potent toxins which cause neutrophils to undergo nuclear karyolysis giving the nuclei a mushy appearance. When these neutrophils are identified in an exudate, an extensive search for bacteria should be made using the oil objective. It is important to remember that the neutrophil and not the macrophage is the primary cell involved in phagocytosis of bacteria. Consequently, microscopic examination of neutrophils is the preferential cell when looking for bacteria.

One example of a noninfectious exudate (pleural or peritoneal cavities) is feline infectious peritonitis (FIP). Immune complex deposition within vessels causes two pathophysiologic events to occur: (1) altered vascular permeability, allowing protein to leak into the fluid; and (2) neutrophil chemotaxis. This results in an exudate with a particularly high protein concentration, sometimes becoming close to that of the plasma, and numerous numbers of "happy" neutrophils with lesser numbers of macrophages present. *Electrophoresis* of effusions resulting from FIP virus infection reveals that globulins predominate (see Case 38). An A : G ratio of less than 0.81 in an *effusion* from a cat is highly suggestive of FIP virus infection and may be used to supplement the cytologic examination.

Irritant substances may also cause a *nonseptic exudate*. Examples include bile from a ruptured gallbladder and urine from a ruptured urinary bladder (See Case 45). An irritant process may initially cause an effusion with a protein that is less than 2.5 g/dL (25 g/L) but with increased cell numbers comprised predominantly of neutrophils. This type of *modified transudate* is uncommon but should direct one's thinking toward an irritant process as discussed previously. We have also seen this type of effusion in association with *neoplasia* within the cavity.

EQUINE ABDOMINAL FLUID

The normal equine abdominal fluid is different from that of the dog and cat with regard to the normal total nucleated cell counts and the differential cell types. This takes on diagnostic importance when evaluating the equine patient for abdominal disorders. The nucleated cell count is approximately 5000/μL although some report up to 9000 nucleated cells/μL as normal. The most important difference from a diagnostic standpoint is that the *neutrophil* may comprise up to *60%* of the nucleated cells. This physiologic phenomenon creates increased diagnostic frustration when examining equine abdominal fluid. Total cell numbers as well as neutrophil morphology take on greater importance when evaluating equine abdominal fluid (see Table 11–1).

OPAQUE EFFUSIONS

White opaque fluid initially conjures a differential diagnosis of a chylous effusion. However, other types of effusion may have a similar physical appearance, emphasizing the importance of appropriately examining the fluid.

A *chylous effusion* (peritoneal or pleural) is associated with a ruptured thoracic duct and reflects its components, that is, triglyceride-rich chylomicrons and small to medium lymphocytes. This type of fluid is very irritating to the serosal surface, and within days to weeks increased exfoliation of mesothelial cells and an influx of neutrophils may even give the effusion an exudative appearance. The reader should also remember that lipid will cause the total protein on the refractometer to appear *factitiously* increased, and one could be misled into suspecting an inflammatory exudate. Therefore in the differential approach to a fluid that is suspected of being a chylous effusion the determination of the triglyceride concentration becomes critical. A specimen of the fluid and of the serum from the patient can be sent to a commercial laboratory for a quantitative triglyceride determination. A fluid value that is greater than the serum triglyceride concentration is supportive of a diagnosis of a chylous effusion. Any fluid for which an etiology cannot be determined or, in case of pleural effusions, recurs after symptomatic management should be examined for triglyceride concentration. It should be emphasized that in a patient who is not eating, the amount of chylomicrons being generated will be decreased and will result in a lower triglyceride value in the effusion. Consequently it is best to obtain a specimen after an animal has had a meal if the value obtained in the fluid is very close to that in the serum.

Lymphosarcoma involving the body cavity may also have an opaque fluid associated with it. Microscopic examination will reveal that the predominant cell type is a medium to large, sometimes blastic appearing lymphocyte characteristic of a lymphoid neoplasm. Since the neoplastic process may involve the lymphatic system it is not surprising that occasionally a chylous effusion may develop coincidentally.

Lastly, an opaque pleural effusion has been described in cats with *congestive cardiomyopathy*. The cell types include macrophages, small lymphocytes, and occasionally neutrophils; however, the triglyceride concentration of these fluids is less than serum, indicating a nonchylous effusion. In these patients the next diagnostic approach would be the echocardiographic examination of the heart.

Tests such as fat stains (Sudan) and ether clearance of effusions have not been discussed because of their variable results.

NEOPLASTIC EFFUSIONS

Occasionally the microscopic examination of an effusion will reveal cell types that are not normally present in an effusion. The neoplastic cell types most commonly associated with effusion are lymphosarcoma and carcinomas because of their ease of exfoliation. Exfoliation of reactive mesothelial cells in response to an irritation may be dramatic enough to cause confusion with neoplastic carcinoma cells. There are no simple guidelines for separating these confusing cell types, and the clinician is encouraged to submit these slides to a clinical pathologist for examination.

PERICARDIAL EFFUSIONS

Pericardial effusions are evaluated in the same way as are pleural or peritoneal fluids. Most pericardial effusions are bloody and contain a relatively small number of nucleated cells. It has been our limited experience that the evaluation of these hemorrhagic effusions does not help distinguish between the two more commonly caused in the dog: neoplastic (hemangiosarcoma, heart-base tumor) and the idiopathic disorder.

CELLS COMMONLY SEEN IN EFFUSIONS

Mesothelial cells comprise the serous lining of the pericardial, pleural, and peritoneal cavities. Their size is variable, but their morphology is similar. They are
observed singly or in hyperplastic clumps. The cell is usually oval to round; the
diameter is 10 to 30 μm. The cytoplasm is basophilic without vacuoles or phagocytized material. The centrally located nucleus is round, has a prominent nuclear
membrane, fine dark purple chromatin pattern, and one or two blue nucleoli.
Classically the reactive mesothelial has an eosinophilic villous-like cytoplasmic
membrane border, a sun burst effect. Binucleated and multinucleated forms are
normally observed. Occasional mitotic figures are seen.

At the slightest irritation the mesothelial cells undergo hyperplasia and exfoliate
readily. The cells enlarge and, pseudogranular structures or rosettes can be observed. These reactive or basophilic mesothelial cells subsequently undergo morphologic changes reflected as vacuolization in gray-blue cytoplasm. The cytoplasm may contain numerous pink staining granules. The nuclei stain pale, and the
chromatin is more coarse.

The *pale mesothelial cells* derived from basophilic mesothelial cells have lightly
basophilic abundant cytoplasm with varying degrees of vacuolization. The cytoplasm may contain pink staining granules which at times may be very prominent.
These cells are usually observed as singles or in small clusters. Similar cell types
may be observed with ingested neutrophils and amorphous debris and are referred
to as *macrophages*.

12

EVALUATION OF SYNOVIAL FLUID*

The cytologic examination of synovial fluid can provide clinically useful information for the identification of a number of joint disorders. Indications for obtaining synovial fluid include: (1) the patient with a swollen hot joint suggestive of an infective process; (2) the patient in which there are radiographic findings suggestive of a degenerative joint process and a synovial fluid analysis is obtained to rule out a concomitant inflammatory process; and (3) a broad group of disorders referred to as *polyarthritis* in which the patient has a history of nondescript pain, short choppy gait, or rotating leg lameness. In this last group of disorders multiple joints are frequently involved, and synovial fluid from the carpal joint will usually reflect the inflammatory process in the other joints.

SAMPLE COLLECTION AND EVALUATION

Synovial fluid is obtained using a 23- to 25-gauge needle attached to a 3-ml syringe. The procedure is not painful. The area over the joint is clipped and surgically prepared, and the leg is alternatively flexed and extended as the joint surface is palpated until a soft spot is located. The soft part is entered with the needle, and a few drops of synovial fluid are gently aspirated. In a patient with an inflammatory process it may be possible to remove as much as 0.5 to 1.0 ml of fluid. The suction is released, the needle removed, and the specimen is used to prepare at least two slides for cytologic examination. Cytology preparations are made in the same fashion as blood films for differential counts except that the spreader slide is drawn *slowly* into the drop of fluid on the slide, the fluid is allowed to spread, and the spreader slide is moved *slowly* away from the drop. The fluid should not go off the end of the slide. The slide is air dried and, if to be analyzed in the practice, it is stained using a polychromic stain. If the slide is to be forwarded to an outside laboratory it should be dried but not stained.

Care should be taken to make sure that the cytologic preparation is not too thick. Cells are difficult to evaluate on thick specimens as the nuclei are rounded up, making a differential count difficult.

After the slides have been prepared any remaining synovial fluid can be added to a *purple* top tube and submitted to the laboratory for cell counts or, since material remaining in the syringe is sterile, submitted to the laboratory for microbiology if the cytologic examination suggests an infectious process. Even if bacteria are seen, the fluid culture may be negative. If the neutrophils have been

---

* See Algorithm 20.

131

effective, ingested bacteria may be dead. Cytologic examination takes precedence over culture, and culture takes precedence over a cell count (an optional request).

The evaluation of synovial fluid lends itself to an algorithmic approach (see Algorithm 22).

The first decision to be made is whether the synovial fluid is normal or abnormal. Synovial fluid is low in cellularity (less than 3000 cells/μL) and usually has a lightly granular slightly eosinophilic background with small to medium mononuclear cells. These cells have a round to oval nucleus and a rim of pale blue cytoplasm. The presence of other cell types is abnormal.

Having identified an abnormal synovial fluid, the next procedure is to decide whether the fluid is inflammatory or noninflammatory. Noninflammatory disorders include hemarthrosis (hemorrhage into the joint) and degenerative joint disease.

NONINFLAMMATORY DISORDERS

Hemarthrosis is associated with trauma (which should be in the history) or coagulation deficiencies (usually found in young animals) and in patients with warfarin intoxication. Finding blood in a joint should prompt a reevaluation of the history, and a coagulation panel is indicated.

Blood can be aspirated as a contaminant during the procedure. This is suggested when clear fluid is obtained initially and then blood appears in the specimen. In such cases erythrocytes and neutrophils are present in approximately the same proportion as in peripheral blood.

Degenerative joint diseases have synovial fluid that contains macrophages with none to very few neutrophils. Macrophages are larger than the normal mononuclear cells and have a vacuolated cytoplasm and a coarse appearing nucleus. Eosinophilic granules may be noted in the cytoplasm.

INFLAMMATORY DISORDERS

Inflammatory joint diseases are characterized by the presence of many neutrophils.

Septic arthritis is suspected if neutrophils are identified. In this case they should be examined with the oil immersion objective to look for bacteria. Some neutrophils may have a mushy chromatin. These are "unhappy" neutrophils, highly suggestive of a bacterial etiology. If such cells are identified it is prudent to submit any remaining fluid for microbiologic examination.

Nonseptic arthritis (immune mediated) is characterized by an increased number of "happy" neutrophils with a clumped chromatin, a clear cytoplasm, and no evidence of bacteria. If the inflammation has been present for some time, days to weeks, macrophages and erythrocytes may be present. When blood is present, evidence of inflammation is suggested by comparing the number of neutrophils per number of erythrocytes. If the RBCs are a contaminant caused by hemorrhage during collection and the patient has a normal peripheral blood leukocyte count, the neutrophils present in the synovial fluid will be in a ratio of 1 WBC for every 750 RBC. If the patient has a leukocytosis then we allow about 1 WBC for every 250 RBC. If the WBC number exceeds this ratio it indicates an increase in the WBC count in synovial fluid in addition to the presence of blood.

Nonseptic (poly)arthritis is often *idiopathic;* however, other known associated causes should be ruled out. Drugs such as trimethoprim-sulfa will produce a nonspecific arthritis. It is thought that the sulfa component stimulates an immune-mediated process. Nonseptic arthritis is a common clinical sign of the uncommon immune-mediated disease lupus erythematosus. Patients suspected of lupus can be screened by use of an antinuclear antibody assay (ANA) (see Chapter 13). A strongly positive ANA titer is supportive of lupus. It must be remembered that lupus is a multiorgan disorder, and other organs should be evaluated for disease. For example, a marked proteinuria suggests glomerulonephritis, and hematologic aberrations such as hemolytic anemia and immune-mediated thrombocytopenia may also complicate the disease. Lupus erythematosus (LE) cells may be found in the synovial fluid of patients with systemic lupus erythematosus. These are neutrophils that contain an amorphous lump of protein. Although these cells are present in only a few affected animals, if present they are diagnostic for lupus.

Erosive polyarthritis synovial fluid contains numerous "happy" neutrophils, and when the joints are examined radiologically there are erosive, and proliferative lesions present. This immune-mediated disease is uncommon and can be verified by biopsy of the synovial membrane.

Patients with rickettsial or *Borellia* infections can be included under both noninfectious and infectious categories because cytologically when these organisms induce a polyarthritis the neutrophils are "happy". It is virtually impossible to identify any organisms in the specimen. If these infectious agents are endemic in one's geographic area, serologic tests can be used to aid in identifying the infection in the differential diagnosis of suppurative polyarthritis.

Bacterial arthritides have synovial fluid that contains few to many mushy neutrophils, and occasionally bacteria can be seen in the cytoplasm of such neutrophils.

13

TESTS FOR IMMUNE-MEDIATED DISEASE

The immune system is an integrated network comprised of several cell types and numerous soluble peptide hormones which work in synergy to eliminate infectious agents, parasites, and noxious antigens.

SPECIFIC IMMUNITY

Lymphocytes are the immunocompetent cells that respond to specific antigens. B-lymphocytes produce antibodies (humoral response) after interacting with antigen-specific T-lymphocytes. T-lymphocytes regulate the immune response by secreting soluble peptide hormones that activate receptors on B-lymphocytes, additional T-lymphocytes, and other cells (*e.g.,* macrophages) involved in nonspecific immune responses. Helper T-lymphocytes promote lymphocyte responses, suppressor T-lymphocytes down-regulate antibody production, and cytotoxic T-lymphocytes play pivotal roles in cell-mediated immunity directed at fungi, protozoan organisms and neoplastic cells. Genetics also influence the lymphocyte response to antigens.

An inappropriate or exaggerated immune response will cause *immune-mediated* tissue injury. The four classifications of immune-mediated processes are illustrated in Figure 13–1.

NONSPECIFIC IMMUNITY

Nonspecific immunity involves macrophages, mast cells, eosinophils, basophils, and platelets along with the complement system. The mucosal surfaces along with the secretions are another component of the nonspecific defense network. We now know that macrophages play a pivotal part in the processing and presentation of antigens to T-lymphocytes in addition to their traditional role in phagocytosis.

IMMUNODEFICIENCY

Primary immunodeficiencies, congenital or inherited, are probably uncommon but difficult to assess since neonates succumb soon after maternal protection (passive immunity) wanes. Acquired immunodeficiency can be associated with certain viruses (canine distemper, feline leukemia, feline immunosuppression), chronic stress (causing lymphoid depletion), neoplasia, and malnutrition.

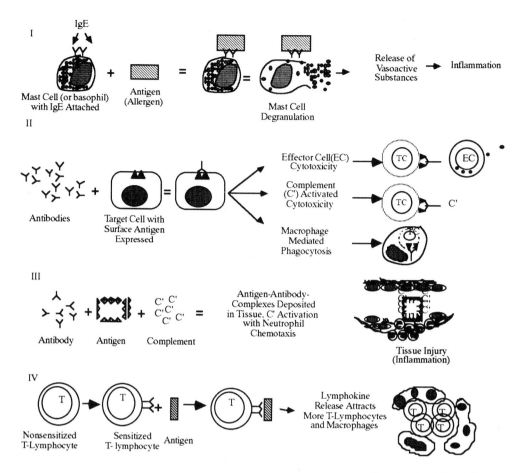

Granulomatous Inflammation

FIGURE 13–1. The four classical pathways of immune-mediated inflammation. *Type I,* when mast cells with IgE on the cell surface are exposed to an antigen (allergen) degranulation occurs, releasing eosinophil and neutrophil chemoattractants, platelet-activating factor, and vasoactive substances such as histamine culminating in inflammation. *Type II,* antibody-mediated cytotoxicity can occur via several mechanisms. When the target cell (*TC*) comes in contact with the appropriate antibody, an effector cell (*EC*), usually a mononuclear cell such as a large granular lymphocyte (NK cell), is stimulated to destroy the target cell. If complement is fixed, an antibody-complement-mediated destruction of the target cell occurs. Finally, macrophages with the appropriate receptors can phagocytize the target cell-antibody complex. *Type III,* when circulating antigens combine with immunoglobulins, circulating immune complexes form which may become trapped in small vessels in tissues, especially the glomeruli and synovial membranes. The immune complex fixes complement (*C'*) of which components C3a and C5a are chemoattractants for neutrophils which release lysosomal enzymes causing tissue injury/inflammation. *Type IV,* the delayed response occurs when a sensitized T-lymphocyte comes in contact with the appropriate antigen. This sensitized T-lymphocyte secretes lymphokines, which causes cell division or attracts additional T-lymphocytes and macrophages; the resultant inflammatory response is referred to as a granuloma.

Electrophoresis of the serum proteins is a crude screening test that can be used initially to identify immunodeficiency (Fig. 13–2). Measurement of specific immunoglobulins is a more sensitive method for assessing for adequacy of immunoglobulins. Patients with a disruption of the cell-mediated response will not be identified by this or any other readily available screening test.

AUTOIMMUNE DISEASE

The development of autoantibodies directed against a wide variety of normal cellular components is associated with immune-mediated diseases and may be the cause or the result of the pathologic process. The detection of these antibodies serve as diagnostic markers of these disorders. The common tests employed for the diagnosis of immune-mediated disorders include Coombs', the antinuclear antibody (ANA), and the rheumatoid factor (RF).

Coombs' Test

The Coombs' test detects antibody directed at the erythrocyte membrane causing immune-mediated hemolytic anemia. Underlying disorders that may give a positive Coombs' test should be ruled out. These include hemobartonellosis, drugs such as trimethoprim-sulfa antibacterials, and neoplasia such as lymphosarcoma.

There are a direct and an indirect Coombs' test. Since there is limited knowledge (diagnostic experience) in domestic animals with the latter, only the direct test is discussed here. This test is used primarily for the differential diagnosis of *regenerative* (reticulocytosis present) anemia. The Coombs' reagent, *species specific* antisera against IgG, IgM, and the third component of complement (C_3), detects the presence of one or more of these immunologic factors on the surface of the erythrocyte in the majority of immune-mediated hemolytic cases (Fig. 13–3). There is an immune mediated *nonregenerative* (no reticulocytosis) anemia which may be Coombs' positive. A bone marrow examination is required for diagnosis, that is, finding a low M : E ratio and evidence of erythrophagocytosis (see Case 4).

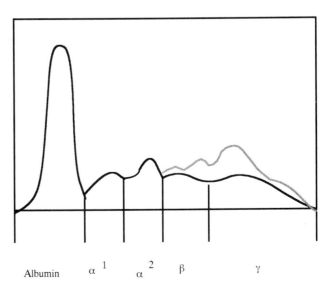

FIGURE 13–2. Serum protein electrophoresis from an immunodeficient patient. The β and γ peaks are markedly attenuated (flat) supporting a humoral deficiency. The broken line represents a normal tracing.

Albumin α^1 α^2 β γ

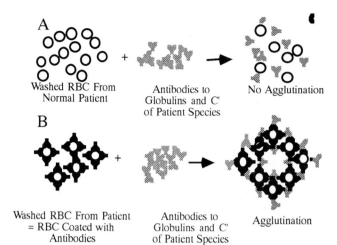

A

Washed RBC From
Normal Patient

Antibodies to
Globulins and C'
of Patient Species

No Agglutination

B

Washed RBC From Patient
= RBC Coated with
Antibodies

Antibodies to
Globulins and C'
of Patient Species

Agglutination

FIGURE 13–3. Direct Coombs' test for the presence of globulins or complement on the surface of erythrocytes. *A,* negative test; *B,* positive test.

The patient for which the Coombs' test is evaluated should be selected carefully since the test can be positive secondary to chronic infections, neoplasia, parasitic infections (*e.g.,* heartworms in dogs and hemobartenellosis in cats), viral infections (feline leukemia [FeLV] and equine infectious anemia [EIA], drugs (*e.g.,* sulfa antibacterials), and after transfusions. In fact, a primary (no underlying etiology apparent) Coombs'-positive hemolytic anemia is uncommon in the cat, and an underlying cause especially hemobartonellosis, should be suspected.

The test can be negative if there are insufficient immunologic components on the erythrocyte surface. Conversely, when there is an excess of antibody, agglutination is inhibited causing a negative test, referred to as a *prozone phenomenon.* Routinely using serial dilutions of the Coombs' reagent will unmask this type of false negative. Cold agglutinins elute from the erythrocyte surface during preparation of standard Coombs' test (37° C), resulting in a negative Coombs' test. If the history indicates a possible relationship to cold ambient temperatures, the Coombs' test should be determined at 4° C.

When blood is drawn from the anemic patient into an EDTA tube, the glass surface should be examined for agglutination (evidence of warm agglutinins) as the tube is slowly tilted while holding it up against fluorescent lighting. If agglutination is suspected, a drop of EDTA blood is thoroughly mixed with physiologic saline on a glass slide and examined with low power on a microscope. The observation of grape-like clustering of erythrocytes is equated to a positive Coombs' test. Again, if the history relates the disease to cold temperatures, the EDTA tube should be refrigerated for 10 minutes before looking for erythrocyte clumping (suggesting the presence of cold agglutinins).

A practical application of the Coombs' test principle is in cross-matching blood prior to transfusion. The *major cross-match,* donor erythrocytes plus recipient serum, is similar to the indirect Coombs' test (donor/control erythrocytes plus patient's serum), and the *minor cross-match,* donor serum plus recipient erythrocytes, is similar to the direct Coombs' test (Coombs' reagent plus the patient's erythrocytes). The end point is also similar; an incompatible blood is indicated by observing microscopically grape-like clustering of the erythrocytes or pink/red discoloration in the supernatant, indicative of hemolysis. The steps in cross-matching are illustrated in Figure 13–4.

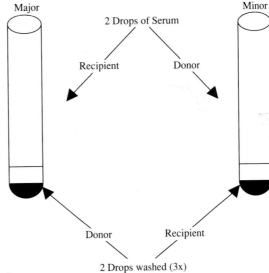

FIGURE 13–4. Method for cross-matching blood.

1. Mix by "flicking" tubes several times with finger
2. Allow tubes to sit at room temperature 30 minutes
3. Centrifuge (3000 rpm) for 15 minutes
4. Observe supernatant for pink/red discoloration indicative of incompatibility
5. Gently "flick" tube with finger once or twice and look for erythrocyte clumping suggestive of incompatibility
6. Place 1 drop on a glass slide, coverslip, and look for clustering of erythrocytes microscopically with low power, the more common indicator of incompatibility

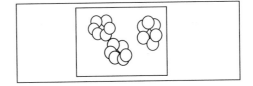

Enzyme-linked immunosorbent assay (ELISA)-based methods for Coombs' testing, not currently available commercially, are technically easier and appear to be more sensitive.

Antinuclear Antibody (ANA) Test

The development of autoantibodies directed against a wide variety of normal cellular components is associated with certain immune-mediated diseases, most notably, systemic lupus erythematosus (SLE). The detection of antinuclear antibodies directed to nucleic acids is the most clinically useful marker of SLE. Serum from the patient is layered on a tissue-covered slide, incubated, washed off, and is followed by incubation with a fluorescein-labeled, species-specific antiserum (Fig. 13–5). Nuclear fluorescence indicates a positive ANA reaction.

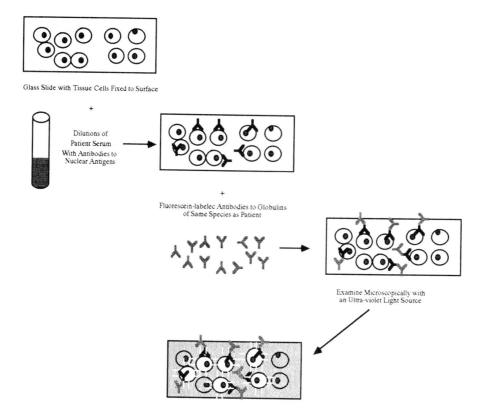

Glass Slide with Tissue Cells Fixed to Surface

+

Dilutions of
Patient Serum
With Antibodies to
Nuclear Antigens

+

Fluorescein-labelec Antibodies to Globulins
of Same Species as Patient

Examine Microscopically with
an Ultra-violet Light Source

Positive ANA Antibody Test with
Fluoresence of Cells with Anti-nuclear
Antibodies Attatched.

FIGURE 13–5. Principals of ANA test.

Systemic lupus erythematosus is a polyorgan immune-mediated disease. The more common manifestations include nonerosive polyarthritis, glomerulonephropathy, hemolytic anemia (often Coombs' positive), thrombocytopenia, neutropenia, polymyositis, persistent/recurring fever, and facial/mucocutaneous dermatitis. When two or more of these inflammatory processes are recognized, an attendant positive ANA supports the diagnosis of SLE. Various nuclear "patterns," which are recognized in humans and used for differential diagnosis and prognostic purposes, do not appear to have additional meaning in domestic animals. Serum from the patient, along with *species-specific* antisera, are used in the test system. It is advisable to *communicate* with the laboratory relative to the need for species-specific antisera for both the Coombs' and ANA tests. Chronic bacterial infections (*e.g.,* bacterial endocarditis), parasites (*e.g.,* heartworm), rickettsial infections, viral infections (*e.g.,* FeLV and feline infectious peritonitis), and neoplasia can give positive results (usually low titers). A test for double-stranded DNA which gives greater specificity in humans is not valid in domestic animals.

The lupus erythematous (LE) cell, as the name implies, is associated with SLE. It is a neutrophil that has ingested nuclear material freed from a damaged cell and altered by the antinuclear antibody. These cells may be cytologically observed, on rare occasion, in tissue specimens such as synovial fluid, bone marrow aspirates, and pleural fluid. *In vitro,* the potentiation for the formation of the LE cell can be performed with either EDTA blood or clotted blood (red top tube) depending on the procedure used; one should communicate with the laboratory. Although the LE cell test is not as sensitive as the ANA test, it is more specific and does not require the use of species-specific antisera.

Rheumatoid Factor (RF)

Antibodies directed against autologous IgG (possibly altered structurally) are referred to as rheumatoid factors. These antibodies are usually IgG in the dog but may be IgM, and their detection is used in the differential diagnosis of erosive arthritis. The use of the RF test to support the diagnosis of immune-mediated erosive arthritis is controversial in part because of the nature of the test system. Use of the Rose-Waaler method requires meticulous attention to detail and should only be performed, and interpreted, by a laboratory familiar with its use in veterinary medicine.

Platelet Factor 3 Test

The platelet factor 3 test was developed to detect antibodies against platelets, that is, immune-mediated thrombocytopenia. Unfortunately, the test system that is currently used lacks consistent diagnostic sensitivity and specificity. An ELISA method, not currently available commercially, appears to offer meaningful diagnostic utility. Consequently, the diagnosis of immune-mediated thrombocytopenia is often supported by ruling out underlying causes of thrombocytopenia such as drugs (*e.g.*, sulfa antibacterials), rickettsial infections (including *Ehrlichia platys*, which specifically infects canine platelets), disseminated intravascular coagulation, and myelophthistic disorders along with the response to immunosuppressive treatment.

Tissue Immunofluorescence

The presence of antibody and/or complement fixed to tissue can be detected by the use of fluorescein-conjugated antisera and fluorescent microscopy. Skin, kidney (glomenruli), and blood vessels are the more common specimens examined in the differential diagnosis of immune-mediated skin disease, glomerulonephritis, and vasculitis, respectively. Biopsy specimens are usually submitted in special fixatives, such as Michel's; the laboratory should be contacted prior to obtaining the tissue specimen.

Part II

Case Histories

Patient: Cat, domestic shorthair, male, 3 years old.

Presenting Signs and Complaints: Gone for 10 days, returned showing labored breathing.

Physical Examination: Shallow rapid respirations; no lung sounds auscultated; dull chest on percussion.

Radiographs: Bilateral fluid in chest.

Problem List: 1. Fluid in chest. 2. Dyspnea.

Hematology		Thoracic Fluid Analysis	
↓ RBC × 10⁶/μL	4.3 (4.3 × 10¹²/L)	↑ RBC/μL	630,000 (0.63 × 10¹²/L)
↓ Hemoglobin (g/dl)	2.1 (1.3 mmol/L)	↑ Nucleated cells/μL	99,100 (99 × 10⁹/L)
↓ PCV (%)	7.1 (0.71 volume fraction)	↑ Total protein (g/dL)	4.8 (48.0 g/L)
MCV (fL)	50		
Plasma Protein (g/dL)	6.0 (60 g/L)	**Differential**	
MCHC (g/dL)	32 (19.8 mmol/L)	85% neutrophils, karyolytic and karyorrhectic	
NRBC/100 WBC	0	forms present, some containing bacteria; 15%	
RBC morphology	Normal	macrophages, some containing nuclear debris.	
↓ WBC × 10³/μL	0.8 (0.8 × 10⁹/L)	*Opinion:* **septic exudate**	
Myelocytes/μL	0		
Metamyelocytes/μL	0		
Band neutrophils/μL	96 (0.096 × 10⁹/L)		
↓ Segmented neutrophils/μL	400 (0.4 × 10⁹/L)		
↓ Lymphocytes/μL	144 (0.144 × 10⁹/L)		
Monocytes/μL	160 (0.16 × 10⁹/L)		
↓ Eosinophils/μL	0 (0 × 10⁹/L)		
Basophils/μL	0 (0 × 10⁹/L)		
↑ Toxic neutrophils	3+		
↓ Platelets × 10³/μL	62 (0.062 × 10¹²/L)		
Platelet estimate	Decreased		
Blood parasites	None		
↑ Fibrinogen (mg/dL)	500 (5.00 gm/L)		
↑ FeLV (ELISA)	Positive		

THORACIC FLUID ANALYSIS

There is a septic exudate characterized by a marked increase in neutrophils and the presence of bacteria.

HEMOGRAM

There is a normocytic normochromic nonregenerative anemia. In this case anemia may be associated with the feline leukemia virus (FeLV) infection or the anemia of chronic disease.

On first appearance leukopenia and mature neutropenia suggest a peracute inflammatory response, perhaps related to the pyothorax. However, the absence of either a degenerative a regenerative left shift or a mature neutrophilia in relation to the pyothorax leads one to suspect an underlying bone marrow problem affecting myelopoiesis. The FeLV infection would be the most likely candidate to cause such a bone marrow disturbance. The toxic morphology of the neutrophils is compatible with a bacterial infection. These morphologic changes occur in the bone marrow, and, although FeLV can cause morphologic aberrations, these findings are most suggestive of an underlying bacterial infection.

There is a thrombocytopenia that may be associated with the bone marrow abnormalities although an endotoxin-induced thrombocytopenia cannot be ruled out.

Hyperfibrinogenemia is compatible with the inflammatory process.

BONE MARROW EXAMINATION

Prior to the initiation of medical management of the pyothorax a bone marrow examination was completed. The specimen was 80% cellular, the M : E ratio was 2.7 : 1.0, megakaryocytes were sparse and had abnormal morphology. The erythroid series was present and complete through the metarubricyte stage with few polychromatophils. The myeloid series was present and complete to the myelocyte stage, but band and segmented neutrophils were rare.

Opinion

Dysmyelopoiesis with ineffective granulopoiesis, erythropoiesis, and abnormal megakaryocytosis compatible with FeLV-induced bone marrow disturbance.

DIAGNOSIS

FeLV infection producing bone marrow dysplasia. Pyrothorax.

COMMENT

It is probable that the FeLV-induced bone marrow dysplasia predisposed to the pyothorax. Further considerations for the medical management of the pyothorax should be weighed against the dysmyelopoiesis in this patient.

Patient: Cat, domestic shorthair, neutered male, 5 years old.

Presenting Signs and Complaints: Lethargy and not eating for 3 days.

Physical Examination: Cat is depressed; normal temperature, pulse, and respiration; abdomen palpated doughy, suggestive of some fluid. Cat was hospitalized.

Problem List: 1. Depression. 2. Anorexia. 3. Possible ascites.

Hematology	
RBC × 10⁶/µL	5.6 (5.6 × 10^{12}/L)
Hemoglobin (g/dL)	11 (6.82 mmol/L)
PCV (%)	32 (0.32 volume fraction)
MCV (fL)	47
MCHC (g/dL)	32 (19.8 mmol/L)
NRBC/100WBC	1
RBC morphology	Normal
↓ WBC × 10³/µL	1.2 (1.2 ×
↑ Metamyelocytes/µL	168
↑ Band neutrophils/µL	
↓ Segmented neutrophil	
↓ Lymphocytes/	
Monocyt	
Eo	
Bas	
↑ Toxi	
↓ Platel	
Plasma	
Fibrino	
FeLV (E	
FIV (ELI	

[Handwritten note overlapping table: "In my opinion this is a lymphosarcoma — probably histiocytic type MJCE 5:00 AM KRP 1=800-343-5244 Call Warrin"]

Abdominal radiographs were ... noted throughout the abdomen, sugg ... performed, and only a few drops of thick ... Direct smears were made. Numerous neutrophils w ... phages were present. The neutrophils showed both normal n ... and various stages of karyolysis. A small percent of neutrophils contai ... rod-shaped bacteria.

Opinion

Septic exudate.

HEMOGRAM

The neutropenia with a marked left shift and toxic neutrophils is compatible with a degenerative left shift and is probably associated with the septic exudate in the abdomen which, because of the excessive demand, results in depletion of the marrow storage and maturation pools. This is in contrast to Case 1 in which there was also a septic condition, but the neutropenia was caused by bone marrow dysplasia resulting from FeLV infection. The presence of a degenerative left shift aids in differentiating between neutropenia caused by excessive tissue demand and ineffective myelopoiesis.

The slight thrombocytopenia is probably a result of an endotoxemia causing increased vascular margination.

Hyperfibrinogenemia is compatible with the inflammatory process.

DIAGNOSIS

The patient was taken to surgery for a laparotomy, and a small *rupture in the duodenum* was found leaking intestinal contents into the abdomen. A reason for the rupture of the viscus was not apparent. The defect was repaired, and the cat made an uneventful recovery.

Patient: Dog, mixed breed, spayed female, 11 years old.

Presenting Signs and Complaints: Nosebleed for the last 6 to 7 weeks; hemorrhage is bilateral; incessant itching and chewing at backside.

Physical Examination: Hemorrhage from nostril; thin hair coat, particularly over back and on legs; moderately enlarged lymph nodes; small hemorrhages on pale mucous membranes.

Problem List: 1. Epistaxis. 2. Bilateral alopecia over dorsum. 3. Patchy alopecia involving all four limbs. 4. Generalized peripheral lymphadenopathy. 5. Petechia on mucous membranes of mouth. 6. Pale mucous membranes.

Hematology[a]		Serum Chemistry	
↓ RBC × 10⁶/μL	2.27 (2.27 × 10¹²/L)	AST (SGOT) IU/L)	37 (37 U/L)
↓ Hemoglobin (g/dL)	8.1 (5.03 mmol/L)	ALT (SGPT) (IU/L)	75 (75 U/L)
↓ PCV (%)	18 (0.18 volume fraction)	ALP (IU/L)	50 (50 U/L)
↑ MCV (fL)	82	Total protein (g/dL)	6.7 (67 g/L)
↑ Plasma protein (g/dL)	9.8 (98 g/L)	Albumin (g/dL)	2.7 (27 g/L)
↑ MCHC (g/dL)	45 (27.9 mmol/L)	Globulin (g/dL)	4.0 (40 g/L)
↑ Reticulocytes (%)	25 (0.25 number fraction)	Glucose (mg/dL)	107 (5.9 mmol/L)
↑ Corrected reticulocytes (%)	10 (0.10 number fraction)	Urea nitrogen (mg/dL)	18 (6.4 mmol/L)
↑ Absolute reticulocytes/μL	567,500 (567.5 × 10⁹/L)	Creatinine (mg/dL)	0.9 (79.6 μmol/L)
↑ NRBC/100 WBC	13	Calcium (mg/dL)	10.0 (2.5 mmol/L)
RBC morphology		Phosphorus (mg/dL)	10.8 (3.5 mmol/L)
↑ Polychromasia	3+		
Spherocytes	None seen	↓ Total T₃ (ng/dL)	35 (0.54 nmol/L)
↑ Anisocytosis	+	↓ Total T₄ (μg/dL)	0.8 (10.3 nmol/L)
↑ Poikilocytosis	+		
↑ WBC × 10³/μL	30.3 (corrected) (30.3 × 10⁹/L)		
Differential			
↑ Band neutrophils/μL	1,515 (1.52 × 10⁹/L)		
↑ Neutrophils/μL	21,210 (21.2 × 10⁹/L)		
↓ Lymphocytes/μL	1,818 (1.8 × 10⁹/L)		
↑ Monocytes/μL	2,717 (2.7 × 10⁹/L)		
↑ Eosinophils/μL	3,030 (3.0 × 10⁹/L)		
Basophils/μL	0 (0 × 10⁹/L)		
Toxic neutrophils	None seen		
↓ Platelets × 10³/μl	10[a] (0.01 × 10¹²/L)		
Fibrinogen (mg/dL)	300 (3 g/L)		
PT (sec)	9/9		
APTT (sec)	11/12		
↑ Sample lipemic			
E. canis titer	Negative		
↑ Coombs' test	Positive		
ANA	Negative		
Antiplatelet factor 3	Negative		

[a] Platelets showed moderate to marked variation in size.

Urinalysis (Cystocentesis)	
Appearance	
Specific gravity	1.027
pH	6.5
Protein	Negative
Glucose	Negative
Ketones	Negative
Blood	Negative
Bilirubin	Negative
Sediment	
WBC/hpf	Rare
RBC/hpf	Negative
Casts/lpf	2–4 hyaline
Crystals	Negative
Bacteria	Negative

HEMOGRAM

Evaluation of the hemogram indicates a macrocytic anemia. The MCHC is increased. This is not physiologically possible and indicates the presence of hemolysis or lipemia or both. Lipemia is confirmed by cloudiness of the plasma; therefore this erythrocyte parameter is not used to characterize the type of anemia in this patient. The increase in plasma proteins, determined by refractometry, is caused by the presence of lipemic serum.

A macrocytic anemia suggests regeneration, and this is supported by the increased reticulocyte count (normal = $60,000/\mu L$ or less). There is nearly a 10-fold increase, which indicates a moderate to strongly regenerative anemia. Although there is an increase in nucleated RBCs they are not used to characterize an anemia as regenerative because they can be increased in several other conditions. The reticulocyte response should always be used to differentiate a regenerative from a nonregenerative anemia.

There is a decrease in platelet numbers, and the size variation is indicative of increased turnover.

There is a neutrophilia with a left shift, indicative of an acute inflammatory process in this patient, which is suspicious of an immune-mediated process; cytokines may be nonspecifically released from activated macrophages and cause release of granulocytes from the bone marrow (see Fig. 3–2).

An immune-mediated process is supported by the positive Coombs' test. The Coombs' test is positive in approximately two thirds to three fourths of the immune-mediated hemolytic anemias. The negative antinuclear antibody suggests that a multiple organ immune mediated process such as lupus erythematosus is not involved in this patient.

The test for antiplatelet factor 3 is of questionable value with current methodologies as an aid in the differential diagnosis of thrombocytopenia. Better indicators for increased platelet turnover are the variation in platelet size along with a bone marrow, which shows megakaryocytic hyperplasia.

BONE MARROW

Very cellular aspirate and large numbers of megakaryocytes of all stages of development were present. The myeloid series and the erythroid series were completed; with normal morphology. Stainable iron was present.

Opinion

Megakaryocytic and erythropoietic hyperplasia. Marrow is compatible with increased platelet and erythrocyte production. This supports increased platelet utilization or destruction as well as increased erythrocyte destruction or loss.

BIOCHEMICAL PROFILE

The T_3 and T_4 are both decreased, supportive of hypothyroidism. There has been an association between decreased function of the thyroid and immune-mediated hemolytic anemia. Both immunosuppressive therapy for the immune-mediated process as well as thyroid replacement medication should be used for the complete management in this patient.

DIAGNOSIS

Immune-mediated hemolytic anemia.

COMMENT

A bone marrow aspirate was not essential in this patient. One could treat and watch for the expected response. However, knowing that the bone marrow was capable of responding allowed one to pursue immunotherapy with greater confidence.

Patient: Dog, schnauzer, spayed female, 9 years old.

Presenting Signs and Complaints: Inappetence, lethargy, excessive panting for 2 or 3 weeks.

Physical Examination: 3/6 systolic murmur over mitral area; large spleen palpated; pale mucous membranes.

Problem List: 1. Heart disease. 2. Splenomegaly. 3. Anemia. 4. Anorexia.

Hematology	September 30	October 5	Serum Chemistry	September 30
↓RBC × 10⁶/µL	3.4 (3.4 × 10¹²/L)	2.9 (2.9 × 10¹²/L)	AST (SGOT) (IU/L)	17 (17 U/L)
↓Hemoglobin (g/dL)	8.3 (5.15 mmol/L)	6.9 (4.28 mmol/L)	ALT (SGPT) (IU/L)	48 (48 U/L)
↓PCV (%)	24 (0.24 volume fraction)	20 (20 volume fraction)	ALP (IU/L)	50 (50 U/L)
MCV (fL)	70.5 (70.5 fl)	69 (69 fl)	Total bilirubin (mg/dL)	0.5 (8.6 µmol/L)
Plasma protein (g/dL)	8.2 (82 g/L)		Total protein (g/dL)	7.9 (79 g/L)
MCHC (g/dL)	35 (21.7 mmol/L)	34 (21.1 mmol/L)	Albumin (g/dL)	2.5 (25 g/L)
↓Reticulocytes (%)	0.2 (0.002 number fraction)	0.2 (0.002% fraction)	↑Globulin (g/dL)	5.5 (55 g/L)
NRBC/100 WBC	3	0	Glucose (mg/dL)	88 (4.8 mmol/L)
RBC morphology	Normal	Normal	Urea nitrogen (mg/dL)	15 (5.4 mmol/L)
↓WBC × 10³/µL	2.5 (2.5 × 10⁹/L)	15.0 (15 × 10⁹/L)	Creatinine (mg/dL)	0.6 (53 µmol/L)
Myelocytes/µL	0	0	Carbon dioxide (mEq/L)	22 (22 mmol/L)
Metamyelocytes/µL	0	0	Chloride (mEq/L)	103 (103 mmol/L)
↑Band neutrophils/µL	75 (0.075 × 10⁹/L)	900 (0.9 × 10⁹/L)	Sodium (mEq/L)	141 (141 mmol/L)
↓Segmented neutrophils/µL	1050 (1.05 × 10⁹/L)	↑12,450 (12.5 × 10⁹/L)	Potassium (mEq/L)	4 (×4 mmol/L)
↓Lymphocytes/µL[a]	830 (0.83 × 10⁹/L)	900 (0.9 × 10⁹/L)	Na : K ratio	35.3
Monocytes/µL	490 (0.49 × 10⁹/L)	1200 (1.2 × 10⁹/L)	Calcium (mg/dL)	9.9 (2.5 mmol/L)
Eosinophils/µL	75 (0.75 × 10⁹/L)	150 (15 × 10⁹/L)	Phosphorus (mg/dL)	3.3 (1.1 mmol/L)
Basophils/µL	0	0		
Toxic neutrophils	None	None		
↓Platelet × 10³/µL	5.0[a] (0.05 × 10¹²/L)	91 (0.91 × 10¹²/L)		
Fibrinogen (mg/dL)	300 (3.0 gm/L)			

[a] Mild to moderate variation in platelet size.

HEMOGRAM

There is a nonregenerative anemia, neutropenia, and thrombocytopenia. The constellation of deficiencies in all three cell lines mandates an examination of the bone marrow. The lack of an appreciable reticulocyte count in light of anemia of this severity suggests that the marrow is either not producing them or they are being retained or destroyed in the marrow.

The thrombocytopenia resolved by October 12, and a RBC regenerative response occurred after 3 weeks of immunosuppressive therapy.

BIOCHEMICAL PROFILE

The mild increase in globulins is a reflection of increased production by the immune system which is occasionally noted in immune-mediated processes well as any chronic inflammatory response.

BONE MARROW EXAMINATION OCTOBER 1

$M:E = 0.3$ to 1.0. Hypercellularity with increased numbers of megakaryocytes with immature forms is present. Myeloid series present with a paucity of the segmented forms observed. There may be a mild increase in the erythroid precursors with appropriate maturation through the metarubricyte stage with virtual absence of polychromatophils. Most notable is the presence of numerous macrophages that contain nucleated erythrocyte precursors; some contain mature erythrocytes as well (erythrophagocytosis).

Opinion

Immune-mediated erythrocyte destruction directed at the bone marrow. Probable immune-mediated thrombocytopenia with megakaryocytic response. Depletion of the segmented neutrophil storage pool as a result of peripheral destruction, utilization, or splenic sequestration. Recommend Coombs' test and ANA.

Coombs' test (October 3)	Strong positive ↑
ANA (October 3)	+1 : 1280 ↑

The positive Coombs' and ANA tests support the presence of immune-mediated disease. Disease in other organ systems should be evaluated since a positive test for antinuclear antibody is supportive of a multiorgan system immune-mediated process such as lupus erythematosus.

In this case, even though the Coombs' test was positive supporting an immune-mediated process directed at the erythrocyte, it should be remembered that approximately one third of these patients may be Coombs' test negative.

TREATMENT

Started prednisone and tetracycline October 1 (until the *Ehrlichia* titer came back negative); WBC count returned to normal by October 3, but platelets were $13,000/\mu L$, PCV = 23 with 0.2% reticulocyte count (uncorrected). Started cyclophosphamide and danazol orally and gave vincristine intravenously once.

The identification of macrophages filled with both nucleated erythrocytes as well as mature erythrocytes is supportive of an immune-mediated process directed at the erythrocytes of the bone marrow. Based on these observations one can more comfortably recommend immunotherapy knowing that the bone marrow has the potential to respond. Experience indicates that response to therapy may be slow. In this case it took 3 weeks before an erythrocyte response was noted. A Coombs' test can be run periodically to evaluate suppression of the immune-system. When medication has been decreased to a maintenance level a consistently negative Coombs' test supports discontinuation of all medication. It is also prudent to run it 2 to 3 weeks later as a reflection of recurrence of the immune mediated process.

Thrombocytopenia along with increased megakaryocytes in bone marrow suggest platelet destruction.

An interesting component of this case is the leukopenia, which is reflected by a mature neutropenia with a depletion in the storage pool of the late stages of the granulocytic series. We can only speculate as to what is occurring: (1) an immune-mediated process directed at the neutrophils, or (2) neutrophils are somehow sequestered in the spleen because of either mechanics or an immune-mediated process. There are currently no good tests for antibody directed to neutrophils.

DIAGNOSIS

Immune mediated disease affecting bone marrow production of erythrocytes and causing destruction of platelets.

Patient: Dog, cocker spaniel, male, 4 years old.

Presenting Signs and Complaints: Getting weaker for the past several days; inappetence, and seems to have a yellow look to the eyes.

Physical Examination: Weak; pale, icteric mucous membranes.

Problem List: 1. Icterus. 2. Anemia. 3. Generalized weakness.

Hematology		Serum Chemistry	
↓ **RBC × 10⁶/μL**	1.2 (1.2 × 10¹²/L)	↑ AST (SGOT) (IU/L)	120 (128 U/L)
↓ **Hemoglobin (g/dL)**	3.3 (2.05 mmol/L)	↓ ALT (SGPT) (IU/L)	300 (300 U/L)
↓ **PCV (%)**	10.9 (0.11 volume fraction)	↑ ALP (IU/L)	773 (773 U/L)
Plasma protein (g/dL)	7.2 (72 g/L)	↑ GGT (IU/L)	31 (31 U/L)
↑ **MCV (fL)**	90.8	↑ Total bilirubin (mg/dL)	23.7 (405 mmol/L)
↓ **MCHC (g/dL)**	30.2 (18.72 mmol/L)	↑ Conjugated bilirubin (mg/dL)	13.2 (226 mmol/L)
↑ **Reticulocytes (%)**	18 (0.18 number fraction)	↑ Unconjugated bilirubin (mg/dL)	10.5 (180 mmol/L)
↑ **Corrected reticulocytes (%)**	4.4 (0.044 number fraction)	Total protein (g/dL)	6.8 (68 g/L)
↑ **Reticulocytes/μL**	218,000 (0.22 × 10¹²/L)	Albumin (g/dL)	3.3 (33 g/L)
↑ **NRBC/100 WBC**	29	Globulin (g/dL)	3.5 (35 g/L)
RBC morphology		Amylase (IU/L)	1,200 (1200 U/L)
Blood parasites	None seen	Lipase (IU/L)	75 (75 U/L)
↑ **Polychromasia**	4+	Glucose (mg/dL)	117 (64 mmol/L)
↑ **Spherocytes**	3+	Urea nitrogen (mg/dL)	20 (7.14 mmol/L)
↑ **Anisocytosis**	3+	Creatinine (mg/dL)	1.3 (114.9 μmol/L)
Poikilocytosis	Rare	Carbon dioxide (mEq/L)	20 (20 mmol/L)
↑ **WBC × 10³/μL**	76.6 (76.6 × 10⁹/L)	Chloride (mEq/L)	101 (101 mmol/L)
		Sodium (mEq/L)	148 (148 mmol/L)
Myelocytes/μL	0 (0 × 10⁹/L)	Potassium (mEq/L)	4.2 (4.2 mmol/L)
Metamyelocytes/μL	0 (0 × 10⁹/L)	Na : K ratio	35.2 (35.2)
↑ **Band neutrophils/μL**	4,596 (4.6 × 10⁹/L)	Calcium (mg/dL)	9.2 (2.3 mmol/L)
↑ **Segmented neutrophils/μL**	65,876 (65.9 × 10⁹/L)	Phosphorus (mg/dL)	4.2 (1.4 mmol/L)
Lymphocytes/μL	1,532 (1.5 × 10⁹/L)	↑ Cholesterol (mg/dL)	389 (10.1 mmol/L)
↑ **Monocytes/μL**	4,506 (4.5 × 10⁹/L)	↓ Total T₃ (μg/dL)	50 (0.77 nmol/L)
↓ **Eosinophils/μL**	0 (0 × 10⁹/L)	↓ Total T₄ (μg/dL)	0.8 (10.4 nmol/L)
Basophils/μL	0	LDH (IU/L)	331 (331 U/L)
Toxic neutrophils	None seen	Creatine kinase (IU/L)	492 (492 U/L)
Platelets × 10³/μL	300 (0.3 × 10¹²/L)		
Fibrinogen (mg/dL)	300 (3 g/L)		
↑ **Coombs' test**	**Positive**		

Urinalysis (Cystocentesis)	
Appearance	Dark yellow
Specific gravity	1.032
pH	6.5
Protein	Negative
Glucose	Negative
Ketones	Negative
Blood	Negative
↑ **Bilirubin**	**3+**
Sediment	
WBC/hpf	0–2
RBC/hpf	1–4
Casts	Negative
↑ **Crystals**	**3+ Bilirubin**
Bacteria	Negative

HEMOGRAM

The macrocytic hypochromic, spherocytic, regenerative anemia that is Coombs' test positive supports a diagnosis of immune-mediated hemolytic anemia. Leukocytosis, neutrophilia, and occasionally a left shift may occur in patients with immune-mediated anemia as a nonspecific responsive marrow stimulation. The normal fibrinogen further supports the noninflammatory process. If the leukocytosis persists after the anemia is resolved one should suspect inflammation and/or necrosis.

BIOCHEMICAL PROFILE

Increased ALT and AST activities support hepatocellular membrane leakage, in this case most likely as a result of the acute anemia-related anoxic insult in the centrolobular area of the liver. The increased alkaline phosphatase and GGT are not readily explained in this case but may be increased secondary to the anoxia-induced vacuolar changes that have also interrupted the microcanicular system causing focal areas of cholestasis. The glucocorticoid increase associated with stress may also cause enzyme induction, adding further to these values. The determination of the direct and indirect bilirubin is of little value in the separation of hemolytic disorders from primary liver disorders and of little benefit in separating intrahepatic from extrahepatic cholestatic problems.

Low resting T_3 and T_4 and hypercholesterolemia suggest decreased thyroid function.

DIAGNOSIS

Immune-mediated hemolytic anemia and hypothyroidism.

COMMENT

Information now suggests that there may be a relationship between hypothyroidism and immune-mediated hematopoietic diseases (see also Case 3).

Patient: Cat, domestic shorthair, male, 18 months old.

Presenting Signs and Complaints: Has not been doing well for last several weeks; inappetence.

Physical Examination: Weak; pale mucous membranes; increased pulse and respiratory rates.

Problem List: 1. Anemia. 2. Thin. 3. Lethargic.

Hematology	
↓ **RBC × 10⁶ µL**	**1.0 (1.0 × 10¹²/L)**
↓ **Hemoglobin (g/dL)**	**1.5 (0.93 mmol/L)**
↓ **PCV (%)**	**5.4 (0.54 volume fraction)**
↑ **MCV (fL)**	**54 (54 fl)**
MCHC (g/dL)	34.3 (21.3 mmol/L)
Reticulocytes (%)	0.1 aggregate (0.001 number fraction)
Reticulocytes/µL	10,000 (0.01 × 10¹²/L)
↑ **NRBC/100 WBC**	**55**
Some NRBCs are immature	
Erythrocyte morphology	Normal
WBC × 10³/µL	8.0 (8.0 × 10⁹/L)
Corrected WBC × 10³/µL	5.161 (5.161 × 10⁹/L)
Band neutrophils/µL	0 (0 × 10⁹/L)
↓ **Segmented neutrophils/µL**	**1,445 (1.4 × 10⁹/L)**
Lymphocytes/µL	3,664 (3.6 × 10⁹/L)
Monocytes/µL	0 (0 × 10⁹/L)
Eosinophils/µL	52 (0.052 × 10⁹/L)
Basophils/µL	0 (0 × 10⁹/L)
Toxic neutrophils	None seen
Platelet estimate	Adequate
Blood parasites	None seen
↑ **FeLV (ELISA)**	**Negative**

HEMOGRAM

There is a macrocytic normochromic anemia with a marked increase in nucleated erythroid elements in the peripheral blood. Initially one might categorize this as a regenerative anemia. The lack of an increased reticulocyte count indicates that the anemia is nonregenerative. When a cat has a macrocytic nonregenerative anemia one must consider the potential presence of FeLV in the bone marrow causing dyserythropoiesis. This probability is supported further by the presence of immature nucleated erythrocytes in the peripheral blood.

When there are only a few nucleated erythrocytes present, correction of the leukocyte count is not critical; however, when, as in this case, there is a marked increase it does impact on the total leukocyte count. In this patient what was apparently a normal leukocyte count is now a borderline leukopenia. The mature neutropenia is suggestive of a bone marrow disorder. If a differential count had not been completed one might assume that the leukogram was normal. A total leukocyte count without a differential count is nonproductive.

BONE MARROW EXAMINATION

As peripheral blood findings of a nonregenerative anemia and mature neutropenia suggested production problems, a bone marrow aspirate was completed with the following results. The bone marrow specimen was cellular with adequate numbers of megakaryocytes. The erythroid series was present and complete through the metarubricyte stage with an absence of polychromatophils on the Romanowsky-stained specimen. There were some abnormal morphologic forms of nucleated erythrocytes demonstrating inappropriate maturation. The myeloid series was present and complete through the metamyelocyte stage, and there were sparse band and segmented neutrophils.

Opinion

Myelodysplasia as evidenced by dysgranulopoiesis and dyserythropoiesis compatible with FeLV infection. One of the *unfixed bone marrow slides* was tested for FeLV using an indirect immunofluorescence test.

FeLV (FA on Marrow)   Positive

Some cats with an FeLV infection and a nonregenerative anemia are FeLV ELISA test negative, yet an immunofluorescence test on the marrow will be positive.

DIAGNOSIS

FeLV infection (see also Case 1).

Patient: Cat, domestic shorthair, female, 3 years old.

Presenting Signs and Complaints: Weak and depressed for 4 or 5 days; previously treated for coccidiosis.

Physical Examination: Pale mucous membranes; slight icterus; serous discharge from left nostril.

Problem List: 1. Anemia. 2. Icterus. 3. Depression. 4. Weak.

Hematology		Serum Chemistry	
↓ **RBC × 10⁶/μL**	**1.95 (1.95 × 10¹²/L)**	↑ **AST (SGOT) (IU/L)**	**143 (U/L)**
↓ **Hemoglobin (g/dL)**	**3.3 (2.05 mmol/L)**	↑ **ALT (SGPT) (IU/L)**	**122 (122 U/L)**
↓ **PCV (%)**	**10.5 (0.105 volume fraction)**	ALP (IU/L)	23 (23 U/L)
Plasma protein (g/dL)	7.2 (72 g/L)	GGT (IU/L)	3 (3 U/L)
↑ **MCV (fL)**	**56.4 (56.4 fl)**	↑ **Total bilirubin (mg/dL)**	**3.2 (55 μmol/L)**
↓ **MCHC (g/dL)**	**31.4 (19.5 mmol/L)**	↑ **Conjugated bilirubin (mg/dL)**	**2.8 (48 μmol/L)**
↑ **Aggregate reticulocytes (%)**	**10 (0.1 number fraction)**	↑ **Unconjugated bilirubin (mg/dL)**	**0.4 (6.8 μmol/L)**
Punctate reticulocytes (%)	11 (0.11 number fraction)	Total protein (g/dL)	6.8 (68 g/L)
↑ **Corrected reticulocytes (aggregate)**	**2.8% (0.028% fraction)**	Albumin (g/dL)	3.2 (32 g/L)
↑ **Reticulocytes (aggregate)/μL**	**195,000 (195 × 10⁹/L)**	Globulin (g/dL)	3.6 (36 g/L)
NRBC/100 WBC	66	↑ **Glucose (mg/dL)**	**225 (14 mmol/L)**
Erythrocyte morphology		↑ **Urea nitrogen (mg/dL)**	**42 (15 mmol/L)**
↑ **Blood parasites**	*H. felis*	↑ **Creatinine (mg/dL)**	**2.1 (186 μmol/L)**
↑ **Polychromasia**	**2+**	Carbon dioxide (mEq/L)	23 (23 mmol/L)
↑ **Anisocytosis**	**2+**	Chloride (mEq/L)	102 (102 mmol/L)
Poikilocytosis	None	Sodium (mEq/L)	148 (148 mmol/L)
↑ **Basophilic stippling**	**+**	Potassium (mEq/L)	4.1 (4.1 mmol/L)
↑ **WBC × 10³/μL**	**39.5 (39.5 × 10⁹/L)**	Na : K ratio	36
Myelocytes/μL	0 (0 × 10⁹/L)	Calcium (mg/dL)	8.7 (2.2 mmol/L)
Metamyelocytes/μL	0 (0 × 10⁹/L)	Phosphorus (mg/dL)	4.2 (1.4 mmol/L)
↑ **Band neutrophils/μL**	**1,760 (1.76 × 10⁹/L)**		
↑ **Segmented neutrophils/μL**	**24,260 (24.3 × 10⁹/L)**		
Lymphocytes/μL	5,390 (5.4 × 10⁹/L)		
↑ **Monocytes/μL**	**5,390 (5.4 × 10⁹/L)**		
↑ **Monocytes/μL**	**2,020 (2.02 × 10⁹/L)**		
Eosinophils/μL	670 (0.67 × 10⁹/L)		
Basophils/μL	0		
Toxic neutrophils	None seen		
Platelet estimate	Adequate		
↑ **Coombs' test**	**+**		
Fibrinogen (mg/dL)	200 (2 g/L)		
↑ **FeLV (ELISA)**	**+**		

Urinalysis (Cystocentesis)	
Appearance	Clear, yellow
Specific gravity	1.045
pH	6.5
Protein	Negative
Glucose	Negative
Ketones	Negative
Blood	Negative
↑ **Bilirubin**	**3+**
Sediment	
WBC/hpf	0–3
RBC/hpf	0–1
Casts	None seen
Crystals	Bilirubin
Bacteria	Negative

HEMOGRAM

There is a moderately regenerative anemia as indicated by a significant polychromasia and aggregate reticulocytosis. The absolute aggregated reticulocyte count of 195,000/μL represents a moderate response as a count over 40,000/μL represents an increase. Aggregate reticulocytosis in a cat with a normal per cent of punctate reticulocytes suggests an acute and good response by the bone marrow. Basophilic stippling in the cat, as in the ruminant, is normal in a responsive anemia.

The presence of *Haemobartonella* on the blood film identifies the etiopathogenesis of the anemia.

The leukocytosis, attributed to a neutrophilia and left shift, may be a reflection of a response to an acute inflammatory process, especially one of a bacterial origin. However, in a situation in which there is a markedly active bone marrow this may be a nonspecific response related to the increased erythrogenesis. This may represent a type of inflammatory response caused by the hemolytic process. Monocyte counts are frequently increased in cats with haemobartonellosis. Erythrophagocytosis may be observed.

FeLV infection can predispose to the clinical manifestation of *Haemobartonella*-induced anemia in cats and should be evaluated. In this case the patient is positive for FeLV.

Primary immune-mediated hemolytic anemia is uncommon in the cat, and the positive Coombs' test supports a secondary immune-mediated component associated with the *Haemobartonella* infection. A Coombs' positive in the anemic cat should always be followed by a search for the underlying cause, particularly haemobartonellosis or FeLV infection. It is for this reason that prednisolone is recommended along with tetracyclines in the medical management of cats with haemobartonellosis.

BIOCHEMICAL PROFILE

The increase in serum urea nitrogen and creatinine with a concentrated urine signals the presence of prerenal azotemia with reduced GFR.

The slightly elevated transaminase (AST and ALT) activity suggests increased cell membrane permeability of hepatocytes, probably secondary to hypoxia of the centrolobular area of the liver. When there is an insult to the liver the ALT is usually higher than the AST. However, an occasional AST higher than the ALT with an acute hepatic insult has been noted. As the lesion subsides the AST will decrease more rapidly than the ALT. The increased serum bilirubin is most likely related to the increased hemoglobin metabolism associated with the hemolytic process. There is little value in separating bilirubin into conjugated and unconjugated fractions to classify icterus as prehepatic, intrahepatic, or extrahepatic. If the traditional considerations were valid in animals, one would have expected the unconjugated bilirubin in this patient to exceed conjugated bilirubin, and it does not. Recent studies indicate that conjugated bilirubin may predominate for poorly understood reasons.

Stressed cats often have an increase in serum glucose which is not associated with pancreatic endocrine problems. Since glucose is increased, several glucose determinations should be run to determine if the hyperglycemia is persistent.

Hyperglycemia with no urine glucose suggests that the urine was formed prior to the increase in serum glucose or a false negative urine glucose secondary to ascorbic acid in urine or the use of outdated reagents.

DIAGNOSIS

Haemobartonella-induced hemolytic disease, potentiated by FeLV.

Patient: Cat, domestic shorthair, female, 1 year old.

Presenting Signs and Complaints: Inappetent for 5 days; severely ill on day of admission.

Physical Examination: Pale, yellow mucous membranes; increased pulse and respiratory rates.

Problem List: 1. Anemia. 2. Icterus.

Hematology		Serum Chemistry	
↓ RBC × 10⁶/µL	2.7 (2.7 × 10¹²/L)	↑ AST (SGOT) (IU/L)	352 (352 U/L)
↓ Hemoglobin (g/dL)	7.7 (4.77 mmol/L)	↑ ALT (SGPT) (IU/L)	123 (123 U/L)
↓ PCV (%)	12.9 (0.13 volume fraction)	↑ ALP (IU/L)	93 (93 U/L)
Plasma protein (g/dL)	7.8 (78 g/L)	GGT (IU/L)	1.5 (1.5 U/L)
MCV (fL)	49	↑ Total bilirubin (mg/dL)	4.9 (83.8 µmol/L)
↑ MCHC (gm/dL)	59.4 (36.8 mmol/L)	↑ Conjugated bilirubin (mg/dL)	1.0 (17.1 µmol/L)
Punctate reticulocytes (%)	2.5 (0.025 number fraction)	↑ Unconjugated bilirubin (mg/dL)	3.9 (66.7 µmol/L)
↑ Aggregate reticulocytes (%)	6.0 (0.06 number fraction)	Total protein (g/dL)	7.5 (75 g/L)
↑ Corrected aggregate reticulocytes	2.1% (0.021 number fraction)	Albumin (g/dL)	3.0 (30 g/L)
↑ Aggregate reticulocytes/µL	162,000 (162 × 10⁹/L)	Globulins (g/dL)	4.5 (45 g/L)
↑ NRBC/100 WBC	21	Amylase (IU/L)	1500 (1500 U/L)
Erythrocyte morphology		Lipase (IU/L)	25 (25 U/L)
Blood parasites	None	Glucose (mg/dL)	109 (6.0 mmol/L)
↑ Polychromasia	2+	Urea nitrogen (mg/dL)	30 (10.7 mmol/L)
↑ Anisocytosis	2+	Creatinine (mg/dL)	0.8 (70.7 µmol/L)
↑ Poikilocytosis	Heinz bodies 2+	Carbon dioxide (mEq/L)	21 (21 mmol/L)
WBC × 10³/µL	15.2 (15.2 × 10⁹/L)	Chloride (mEq/L)	122 (122 mmol/L)
Myelocytes/µL	0	Sodium (mEq/L)	151 (151 mmol/L)
Metamyelocytes/µL	0	Potassium (mEq/L)	4.5 (4.5 mmol/L)
Band neutrophils/µL	228 (0.23 × 10⁹/L)	Na : K ratio	33.5
Segmented neutrophils/µL	11,628 (11.6 × 10⁹/L)	Calcium (mg/dL)	10.2 (2.55 mmol/L)
Lymphocytes/µL	2,432 (2.4 × 10⁹/L)	Phosphorus (mg/dL)	5.6 (1.8 mmol/L)
Monocytes/µL	760 (0.76 × 10⁹/L)	Creatine kinase (IU/L)	175 (175 U/L)
Eosinophils/µL	152 (0.15 × 10⁹/L)		
Basophils/µL	0		
Toxic neutrophils	None seen		
Platelet estimate	Adequate		
Fibrinogen (mg/dL)	200 (2 g/L)		

Urinalysis (Cystocentesis)	
Appearance	Opaque, brown
Specific gravity	1.035
pH	6.5
↑ Protein	3+
Glucose	Trace
Ketones	Negative
↑ Blood	3+
↑ Bilirubin	3+
Sediment	
↑ WBC/hpf	30–40
↑ RBC/hpf	150
Casts	None seen
Crystals	Bilirubin
Bacteria	Negative

HEMOGRAM

The erythrocytes are normocytic, and there is an increase in the MCHC. Hyperchromia (high MCHC) is not physiologically possible and is considered an artifact. It occurs in samples that are hemolyzed, lipemic, or have large numbers of Heinz bodies. In this case the presence of a large number of Heinz bodies, which are not destroyed by the lysing agent, increased the optical density, resulting in a false high value for hemoglobin and MCHC. Heinz bodies can be observed with chemical poisons such as methylene blue and benzocaine and plant poisons such as onions and kale. A retrospective history revealed that the owner had fed the cat fried onions as the cat begged for food while liver and onions were being cooked.

The reticulocytosis (polychromasia) with a normal number of punctate suggests that the anemia is recent and regenerative. In this case the anemia is normocytic even though it is regenerative as indicated by an almost four-fold increase in aggregate reticulocytes. This is because the response was detected early before sufficient numbers of macrocytes had been released from the bone marrow. The important point to remember is that reticulocyte numeration is a more sensitive indicator of whether an anemia is regenerative or nonregenerative. The MCV is a less sensitive indicator in separating regenerative and nonregenerative anemias and should only be used as an initial screen since it is automatically included in hemograms. Nucleated erythrocytes (21/100 WBC) may be associated with RBC regeneration but also appear in the peripheral circulation after sudden hypoxia.

BIOCHEMICAL PROFILE

Hyperbilirubinemia is secondary to the increased hemoglobin turnover associated with the Heinz body-induced hemolytic anemia. The increased ALT and AST with a slightly greater increase in AST may occur as a result of an acute insult to the liver in the cat. Sudden anoxia, such as can occur with a rapid destruction of erythrocytes, may alter the integrity of the hepatocyte membrane in the centrolobular area. As the lesion resolves the AST will return toward normal faster than will the ALT.

URINALYSIS

The pyuria, hematuria, and proteinuria support the presence of inflammatory renal or urinary tract disease. The urine should be cultured.

DIAGNOSIS

Heinz body anemia as a result of onion toxicity with secondary anoxic insult to the liver. Suppurative cystitis.

Case 9

Patient: Cat, Persian, male, 4 years old.

Presenting Signs and Complaints: Hair loss; inappetence; weight loss and lethargic.

Physical Examination: Thin and lethargic; many fleas; hair loss; nodules are present on the abdomen; pale mucous membranes; enlarged spleen and liver on palpation.

Problem List: 1. Massive flea infestation. 2. Dorsal alopecia with generalized crusting. 3. Very thin. 4. Crusting around nares. 5. Anemia. 6. Lethargy. 7. Hepatomegaly. 8. Splenomegaly. 9. Small diffuse subcutaneous nodules on ventral abdomen.

Hematology		Serum Chemistry	
↓ RBC × 10⁶/μL	2.49 (2.4/L)	↑ AST (SGOT) (IU/L)	242 (242 U/L)
↓ Hemoglobin (g/dL)	2.5 (1.55 mmol/L)	↑ ALT (SGPT) (IU/L)	253 (253 U/L)
↓ PCV (%)	8.1 (0.08 volume fraction)	↑ ALP (IU/L)	150 (150 U/L)
Plasma protein (g/dL)	6.9 (69 g/L)	↑ GGT (IU/L)	26 (26 U/L)
↓ MCV (fL)	32	Total bilirubin (mg/dL)	0.3 (5.1 μmol/L)
MCHC (g/dL)	31 (19.2 mmol/L)	Total protein (g/dL)	6.0 (60 g/L)
Reticulocytes (%)	0.5 (0.005 number fraction)	Albumin (g/dL)	3.7 (37 g/L)
Reticulocytes/μL	12,450 (12.45 × 10¹⁹/L)	Globulin (g/dL)	2.3 (23 g/L)
NRBC/100 WBC	0	↑ Glucose (mg/dL)	323 (17.8 mmol/L)
RBC morphology		↑ Urea nitrogen (mg/dL)	34 (12.1 mmol/L)
Blood parasites	None	Creatinine (mg/dL)	1.7 (150.3 μmol/L)
Polychromasia	Slight	↓ Carbon dioxide (mEq/L)	12 (12 mmol/L)
Anisocytosis	Moderate	Chloride (mEq/L)	107 (107 mmol/L)
↓ Poikilocytosis	Moderate	Sodium (mEq/L)	139 (139 mmol/L)
WBC × 10³/μL	2.6 (2.6 × 10⁹/L)	Potassium (mEq/L)	5.5 (5.5 mmol/L)
Differential		Na : K ratio	25.3
Myelocytes/μL	0	↑ LDH (IU/L)	1144 (1144 U/L)
Metamyelocytes/μL	0	Calcium (mg/dL)	9.0 (2.25 mmol/L)
↑ Band neutrophils/μL	0	Phosphorus (mg/dL)	4.6 (1.5 mmol/L)
↓ Segmented neutrophils/μL	1900 (1.9 × 10⁹/L)	Cholesterol (mg/dL)	136 (3.6 mmol/L)
Lymphocytes/μL	600 (0.6 × 10⁹/L)	↓ Serum iron (μg/dL)	19 (3.4 μmol/L)
Monocytes/μL	104 (0.1 × 10⁹/L)		
Eosinophils/μL	26 (0.03 × 10⁹/L)		
Basophils/μL	0 (0 × 10⁹/L)		
Toxic neutrophils	None seen		
Platelets	Adequate		
Fibrinogen (mg/dL)	200 (2 g/L)		
FeLV (ELISA)	Negative		

Urinalysis (Cystocentesis)	
Appearance	Medium yellow
Specific gravity	1.040
pH	7.5
Protein	Trace
Glucose	Negative
Ketones	Negative
Blood	Negative
Bilirubin	Negative
Sediment	
WBC/hpf	0–1
RBC/hpf	0–2
Casts	Negative
Crystals	Negative
Bacteria	Negative

HEMOGRAM

There is a microcytic normochromic anemia. On examination of the blood film moderate poikilocytosis was noted. These findings are compatible with an iron deficiency anemia. The low serum iron supports such a diagnosis. The MCV is a crude parameter reflecting an overall change in erythrocyte size, in this case to smaller than normal. This process, secondary to iron deficiency, takes weeks to months to develop, indicating that the reason for iron loss has occurred over a long period of time, in this case, probably secondary to the flea infestation. Iron supplementation will correct the hypoferremia; however, the MCV may not return to normal for weeks to months. Changes in the MCHC occur after changes in MCV because it is less sensitive.

BIOCHEMICAL PROFILE

The increase in transaminases indicates altered hepatocyte membrane integrity by whatever pathologic process. The increases in alkaline phosphatase and GGT indicate that we are dealing with impaired bile flow (cholestasis); however, cholestasis is not sufficiently severe to cause an increase in total bilirubin concentration. Alkaline phosphatase is an indicator of cholestasis in the cat and will increase before total bilirubin becomes abnormal. Studies have found that the GGT is a more sensitive parameter of liver disease in the cat than is alkaline phosphatase.

The question of whether an additional liver function test such as fasting serum bile acids or plasma ammonia is appropriate to evaluate the liver further can be posed at this point. In this patient, a liver function test would provide no further useful additional information. In this case a *fasting serum bile acid* was determined and was 89 mmol/L (notably increased), indicating a marked liver insufficiency along with the previously identified abnormalities of altered membrane and cholestasis. This tends to mitigate any indecision relative to whether or not to obtain tissue for microscopic examination. This decision could have been made without a liver function test.

Because of the history of prolonged anorexia and the suspicion of underlying hepatic lipidosis, a fine needle liver aspirate was completed, and a diffuse population of vacuolated hepatocytes confirmed the suspected clinical diagnosis of hepatic lipidosis.

DIAGNOSIS

Hepatic lipidosis syndrome.

COMMENT

A gastroscopy tube was placed in the cat and conservatively managed for 8 days until spontaneous appetite resumed. The liver enzyme tests returned to normal 2 weeks later, and the fasting serum bile acids returned to normal 3 weeks later.

Patient: Dog, greyhound, spayed female, 11 years old.

Presenting Signs and Complaints: Escaped from a fenced-in backyard and was gone for 5 days; returned weak and depressed.

Physical Examination: Depressed; markedly dehydrated; poor capillary refill.

Problem List: 1. Thin. 2. Dehydrated.

Hematology		Serum Chemistry	
↑ **RBC × 10⁶/μL**	**9.19 (9.19 × 10¹²/L)**	SGOT (AST) (IU/L)	38 (38 U/L)
↑ **Hemoglobin (g/dL)**	**22.4 (13.9 mmol/L)**	SGPT (ALT) (IU/L)	134 (134 U/L)
↑ **PCV (%)**	**63.9 (0.64 volume fraction)**	Total bilirubin (mg/dL)	0.3 (5.1 μmol/L)
MCV (fL)	68	Direct bilirubin (mg/dL)	0.1 (1.7 μmol/L)
Plasma protein (g/dL)	10.5 (105 gm/L)	Indirect bilirubin (mg/dL)	0.2 (3.4 μmol/L)
MCHC (g/dL)	35.7 (22.1 mmol/L)	↑ **Urea nitrogen (mg/dL)**	**39 (13.9 mmol/L)**
NRBC/100 WBC	0	↑ **Creatinine (mg/dL)**	**2.9 (256.4 μmol/L)**
RBC morphology	Normal	Cholesterol (mg/dL)	350 (9.1 mmol/L)
WBC × 10³/μL	9.0 (9 × 10⁹/L)	ALP (IU/L)	71 (71 U/L)
Myelocytes/μL	0 (0 × 10⁹/L)	Glucose (mg/dL)	52 (2.9 mmol/L)
Metamyelocytes/μL	0 (0 × 10⁹/L)	Phosphate (mg/dL)	6.2 (2.0 mmol/L)
Band neutrophils/μL	0 (0 × 10⁹/L)	↑ **Calcium (mg/dL)**	**13.8 (3.5 mmol/L)**
Segmented neutrophils/μL	8640 (8.6 × 10⁹/L)	Corrected calcium (mg/dL)	10.5 (2.6 mmol/L)
↓ **Lymphocytes/μL**	**270 (0.27 × 10⁹/L)**	↑ **Total protein (gm/dL)**	**10.2 (102 g/L)**
Monocytes/μL	90 (0.09 × 10⁹/L)	↑ **Albumin (g/dL)**	**6.8 (68 g/L)**
Eosinophils/μL	0 (0 × 10⁹/L)	↑ **Globulin (g/dL)**	**5.4 (54 g/L)**
Basophils/μL	0 (0 × 10⁹/L)	↑ **Sodium (mEq/L)**	**167 (167 mmol/L)**
Toxic neutrophils	None	↑ **Potassium (mEq/L)**	**6.6 (6.6 mmol/L)**
Platelet estimate	Adequate	↑ **Chloride (mEq/L)**	**123 (123 mmol/L)**
		Carbon dioxide (mEq/L)	25 (25 mmol/L)

Urinalysis	(Cystocentesis)
Appearance	Clear, yellow
Specific gravity	**1.068**
pH	6
Protein	Negative
Glucose	Negative
Ketones	Negative
Blood	Negative
Bilirubin	Negative
Sediment	
WBC/hpf	**0–1**
RBC/hpf	1–2
Casts	None seen
Bacteria	Negative

HEMOGRAM

Increased RBC parameters reflect dehydration; the lymphopenia is compatible with stress.

BIOCHEMICAL PROFILE

The hyperproteinemia (albumin and globulin), hypernatremia, hyperkalemia, and hyperchloridemia are compatible with loss of body water. The uncorrected serum calcium is normal when corrected for the hyperalbuminemia.

The azotemia is prerenal, supported by the markedly concentrated urine specific gravity, and attributable to dehydration and the accompanying decrease in glomerular filtration rate.

DIAGNOSIS

Loss of body water.

COMMENT

The patient was rehydrated using appropriate fluid therapy, and within 48 hours all hematologic and biochemical parameters returned to normal.

Patient: Dog, cocker spaniel, female, 2 years old.

Presenting Signs and Complaints: Hematoma spontaneously developed on the shoulder; veterinarian surgically drained it and bleeding persisted for several hours; presented to the emergency clinic.

Physical Examination: Bleeding wound on right shoulder; pale mucous membranes.

Problem List: 1. Anemia. 2. Persistent bleeding.

Hematology	
↓ **RBC × 10⁶/μL**	**3.21 (3.21 × 10¹²/L)**
↓ **Hemoglobin (g/dL)**	**7.9 (4.9 mmol/L)**
↓ **PCV (%)**	**22.5 (0.225 volume fraction)**
↓ **Plasma protein (g/dL)**	**4.9 (49 g/L)**
MCV (fL)	70
MCHC (gm/dL)	35.3 (21.9 mmol/L)
NRBC/100 WBC	0
RBC morphology	Normal
Reticulocytes (%)	3.6 (0.036 number fraction)
Corrected reticulocytes (%)	1.4 (0.014 number fraction)
Reticulocytes/μL	115,000 (115 × 10⁹/L)
WBC × 10³/μL	10.4 (10.4 × 10⁹/L)
Band neutrophils/μL	104 (0.1 × 10⁹/L)
Segmented neutrophils/μL	8,216 (8.2 × 10⁹/L)
Lymphocytes/μL	936 (0.94 × 10⁹/L)
Monocytes/μL	1,040 (1.04 × 10⁹/L)
Eosinophils/μL	104 (0.1 × 10⁹/L)
Basophils/μL	0 (0 × 10⁹/L)
Toxic neutrophils	None
Platelets × 10³/μL	470 (0.47 × 10⁹/L)
Platelet estimate	Adequate
↑ **PT (sec)**	**30.7**
↑ **APTT (sec)**	**58.4**
Thrombin time (sec)	6.1
Fibrinogen (mg/dL)	224 (2.2 g/L)

HEMOGRAM

The anemia is classified as non/poorly regenerative. With the history of recent blood loss this is not surprising as there has not been time for a bone marrow response to be noted.

The lymphopenia and monocytosis suggest a reaction to excess glucocorticoids/ stress.

COAGULATION PROFILE

The prolonged prothrombin time and activated partial thromboplastin time with a normal thrombin time, platelet count, and plasma fibrinogen suggest the possibility of intoxication with a coumarin-containing rodenticide.

DIAGNOSIS

The patient was treated with subcutaneous K_1. There was no further hematoma enlargement, and the PT and APTT returned to normal the following morning, supporting the diagnosis of rodenticide intoxication.

Patient: Dog, Labrador-shepherd cross, neutered male, 9 years old.

Presenting Signs and Complaints: Presented as an emergency for vomiting three or four times during the night. Leftovers from a picnic appeared in the vomited material.

Past history: The owner thought that the dog was a little more lethargic and depressed during the preceding 2 months but attributed it to old age and hot weather.

Physical Examination: Mildly depressed and dehydrated, fetid odor to breath, and increased amounts of fluid and gas were noted in the intestinal loops upon abdominal palpation. Radiographic examination of the abdomen was unremarkable. A blood count was taken, and the animal was sent home with conservative management for gastroenteritis. The patient was reexamined 5 days later. Four days later the dog collapsed approximately 30 minutes after jumping up to greet the owner. The dog was presented on an emergency basis. The dog was weak, had weak pulses, and poor capillary refill time with a heart rate of 188. A blood sample was taken, and the patient was placed on intravenous fluids and kept for observation. The next morning the dog was stronger, able to walk, and was referred to another hospital for further examination. Abdominal fluid was suspected on physical examination. Radiographic examination of the abdomen confirmed the presence of fluid, and ultrasound indicated an irregular mass on the spleen with multiple hypoehcoic areas compatible with a cavernous lesion. Abdominocentesis yielded blood with a PCV of 20%. These findings along with the hematology results suggested a hemangiosarcoma. The patient was taken to surgery, the spleen removed, and histologic confirmation of hemangiosarcoma was made.

Hematology	07/04	07/08	07/09
↓ RBC × 10⁶/μL	4.1 (4.1 × 10¹²/L)	2.1 (2.1 × 10¹²/L)	2.9 (2.9 × 10¹²/L)
↓ Hemoglobin (g/dL)	9.4 (5.8 mmol/L)	4.9 (3.0 mmol/L)	7.4 (4.6 mmol/L)
↓ PCV (%)	29.5 (0.295 volume fraction)	15 (0.15 volume fraction)	21 (0.22 volume fraction)
MCV (fL)	72	71.4	72.4
Plasma protein (g/dL)	7.1 (71 g/L)	5.1 (51 g/L)	5.8 (58 g/L)
MCHC (g/dL)	34 (21.1 mmol/L)	34 (20.4 mmol/L)	33 (19.8 mmol/L)
Reticulocytes (%)			5.2 (0.052 number fraction)
Corrected reticulocytes (%)			2.6
Absolute reticulocytes/μL			156,000 (156 × 10⁹/L)
NRBC/100 WBC	7	9	2
RBC morphology			
Poikilocytes	2+ᵃ	2+ᵃ	2+ᵃ
WBC × 10³/μL	11.6 (11.6 × 10⁹/L)	19.9 (19.9 × 10⁹/L)	19.5 (19.5 10⁹/L)
Metamyelocytes/μL	0 (0 × 10⁹/L)	0 (0 × 10⁹/L)	0 (0 × 10⁹/L)
Band neutrophils/μL	116 (0.12 × 10⁹/L)	0 (0.11 × 10⁹/L	175 (0.18 × 10⁹/L)
Segmented neutrophils/μL	7,656 (7.66 × 10⁹/L)	15,552 (15.6 × 10⁹/L)	13,825 (13.8 × 10⁹/L)
Lymphocytes/μL	1,740 (1.74 × 10⁹/L)	995 (1.0 × 10⁹/L)	1,400 (1.4 × 10⁹/L)
Monocytes/μL	2.088 (2.01 × 10⁹/L)	3,383 (3.4 × 10⁹/L)	2,100 (2.1 × 10⁹/L)
Eosinophils/μL	0 (0 × 10⁹/L)	0 (0 × 10⁹/L)	0 (0 × 10⁹/L)
Basophils/μL	0 (0 × 10⁹/L)	0 (0 × 10⁹/L)	0 (0 × 10⁹/L)
Toxic neutrophils	None	None	None
Platelets × 10³/μL	210 (0.21 × 10¹²/L)	110 (0.11 × 10¹²/L)	160ᵇ (0.16 × 10¹²/L)
Fibrinogen (mg/dL)	200 (2.0 g/L)	200 (2.0 gm/L)	400 (4.0 g/L)

ᵃ **Acanthocytes.**
ᵇ Some large forms.

HEMOGRAM

On July 4, the first day of admission, there was a mild anemia which was classified as nonregenerative. The presence of acanthocytes and the inappropriate numbers of nucleated erythrocytes are notable and suggestive of hemangiosarcoma.

Examination of the hemogram on the night the dog collapsed (July 8) was notable for an apparent blood loss anemia based on the decreased PCV and plasma protein. With no external evidence of hemorrhage or fluid noted in the abdominal film, an intraorgan bleed could be suspected. Again, acanthocytes and inappropriate numbers of nucleated erythrocytes were present on the blood film. There was also a mild decrease in platelets and variability in size, suggesting increased turnover.

The last hemogram, taken approximately 24 hours later (July 9) was remarkable for the dramatic increase in the PCV and plasma protein. This could not be attributed to a responsive bone marrow for two reasons. First, there was only slight reticulocytosis, and bone marrow can only respond to a maximum of approximately one to two points per day in the PCV when there is marked erythropoiesis. This dramatic increase in the PCV as well as protein lent further support to an intraorgan bleed that had undergone resorption of some of the blood components. The presence of acanthocytes and nucleated erythrocytes were again noted as well as the fact that the bone marrow was responding to platelet consumption by releasing larger forms of platelets.

The initial hemogram was typical for an underlying hemangiosarcoma and a mild to moderate anemia with inappropriate numbers of nucleated erythrocytes in relation to the polychromasia. The subsequent hemograms were typical for a cavitational neoplasm such as hemangiosarcoma that has undergone a spontaneous bleed and resorption of the blood components. We have seen cases in which this has gone on for weeks to months before having a catastrophe with hemoperitoneum. This case illustrates the value of the reticulocyte count for classifying anemia; had it been done earlier endogenous blood loss would have been suggested right away.

The leukograms were characteristic for a stress pattern on the second admission.

DIAGNOSIS

Hemangiosarcoma of the spleen with rupture.

Patient: Dog, springer, spayed female, 12 years old.

Presenting Signs and Complaints: Weight loss; poor appetite; lack of energy.

Physical Examination: Pale mucous membranes; depressed and does not respond to surroundings; 10% dehydrated.

Problems List: 1. Depression. 2. Anemia. 3. Dehydration.

Hematology		Serum Chemistry	
↓ **RBC × 10⁶/µL**	**3.7 (3.7 × 10¹²/L)**	AST (SGOT) (IU/L)	55 (55 U/L)
↓ **Hemoglobin (g/dL)**	**8.0 (4.97 mmol/L)**	ALT (SGPT) (IU/L)	62 (62 U/L)
↓ **PCV (%)**	**24 (0.24 volume fraction)**	ALP (IU/L)	135 (135 U/L)
MCV (fL)	64.9 (20.6 mmol/L)	GGT (IU/L)	10 (10 U/L)
MCHC (g/dL)	33.3 (20.6 mmol/L)	Total bilirubin (mg/dL)	0.2 (3.4 µmol/L)
Reticulocytes (%)	0.5 (0.005 number fraction)	Conjugated bilirubin (mg/dL)	0.1 (1.7 µmol/L)
Corrected reticulocytes (%)	2.6 (0.26 number fraction)	↑ **Total protein (g/dL)**	**11.8 (118 g/L)**
Reticulocytes/µL	18,500 (18.5 × 10⁹/L)	↑ **Albumin (g/dL)**	**1.5 (15 g/L)**
NRBC/100 WBC	0	↑ **Globulin (g/dL)**	**10.3 (103 g/L)**
RBC morphology	Normal	Amylase (IU/L)	525 (525 U/L)
Platelet estimate	Adequate	Lipase (IU/L)	25 (25 U/L)
↓ **WBC × 10³/µL**	**3.8 (3.8 × 10⁹/L)**	Glucose (mg/dL)	97 (5.3 mmol/L)
Differential		↑ **Urea nitrogen (mg/dL)**	**45 (16.1 mmol/L)**
Myelocytes/µL	0 (0 × 10⁹/L)	↑ **Creatinine (mg/dL)**	**2.4 (212.2 µmol/L)**
Metamyelocytes/µL	0 (0 × 10⁹/L)	Calcium (mg/dL)	8.5 (2.13 mmol/L)
Band neutrophils/µL	0 (0 × 10⁹/L)	Phosphorus (mg/dL)	4.5 (1.5 mmol/L)
↓ **Segmented neutrophils/µL**	**2,640 (2.6 × 10⁹/L)**	Sodium (mEq/L)	145 (145 mmol/L)
Lymphocytes/µL	1,044 (1.04 × 10⁹/L)	Potassium (mEq/L)	4.3 (4.3 mmol/L)
Monocytes/µL	116 (0.12 × 10⁹/L)	Chloride (mEq/L)	98 (98 mmol/L)
↓ **Eosinophils/µL**	**0 (0 × 10⁹/L)**	Carbon dioxide (mEq/L)	21 (21 mmol/L)
Basophils/µL	0 (0 × 10⁹/L)	LDH (IU/L)	138 (138 U/L)
Toxic neutrophils	None	Creatine kinase (IU/L)	130 (130 U/L)
↑ **Plasma protein (g/dL)**	**12.0 (120 g/L)**	↓ **Total T₄ (µg/dL)**	**0.8 (10.3 nmol/L)**
Fibrinogen (mg/dL)	300 (3 g/L)	↓ **Total T₃ (ng/dL)**	**55 (0.85 nmol/L)**
		↓ **Free T₄ (ng/dL)**	**0.5 (39.5 pmol/L)**

Protein Electrophoresis	
Albumin (g/dL)	1.7 (17 g/L)
α_1 (g/dL)	0.5 (5 g/L)
α_2 (g/dL)	1.5 (15 g/L)
β (g/dL)	0.9 (9 g/L)
↑ **γ (g/dL)**	**7.2 (72 g/L)**

Pathologist's comment: **Monoclonal gammopathy**

Urinalysis (Cystocentesis)[a]	
Appearance	Clear, yellow
Specific gravity	1.020
pH	6.5
↑ **Protein (dipstick)**	+
↑ **Protein (sulfosalicylic acid)**	3+
Glucose	Negative
Ketones	Negative
Blood	Negative
Bilirubin	Negative
Sediment	
WBC/hpf	0–2
RBC/hpf	1–3
Casts	Rare hyaline
Crystals	None
Bacteria	Negative

[a] Heating the urine in a 56° C water bath caused it to become turbid. Urine electrophoresis after concentration was *positive for Bence Jones protein.*

HEMOGRAM

There is a normocytic, normochromic, nonregenerative anemia accompanied by a leukopenia caused by a mature neutropenia. These findings suggest a problem of production and/or release of cells to the peripheral blood from the bone marrow.

Examination of the bone marrow is an appropriate next step in defining these abnormalities.

BIOCHEMICAL PROFILE

There is a hyperproteinemia characterized by hyperglobulinemia and hypoalbuminemia. Hyperglobulinemia can be secondary to inflammatory or neoplastic disorders. When there is a hyperglobulinemia of any cause a mechanism is invoked which sends a signal to the liver to decrease albumin production. Protein electrophoresis is the next step in defining the hyperglobulinemia, a polyclonal gammopathy is often associated with a chronic inflammatory condition and monoclonal gammopathy with neoplastic conditions such as plasma cell myeloma or lymphosarcoma. Infectious agents such as ehrlichiosis occasionally cause a monoclonal gammopathy. In endemic areas, appropriate serology should also be evaluated.

There is an azotemia with an increase in creatinine indicative of decreased glomerular filtration, either prerenal or renal. Examination of urine specific gravity will aid in differentiating the cause of the azotemia. Because the specific gravity does not indicate marked concentration as would be expected in dehydration this is probably not prerenal azotemia; therefore a primary renal disease is suspected. The dipstick was slightly positive, but the sulfosalicylic acid method (Bumitest, Ames Co., Elkhart Indiana) was strongly positive for protein. The dipstick is more sensitive for albumin whereas the sulfosalicylic acid procedure will detect all types of protein. The dichotomy between the dipstick and the sulfosalicylic method is characteristic of Bence Jones proteinuria, which is the presence of immunoglobulin light chains produced by plasma cell tumors. The

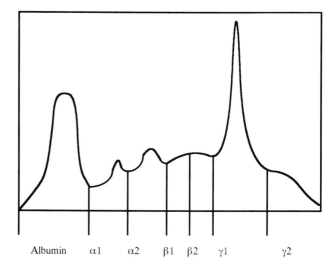

CASE 13. Protein electrophoresis tracing. Note the single high γ_1 peak.

Albumin   α1   α2   β1   β2   γ1   γ2

best method for confirming the presence of Bence Jones proteins in the urine is by protein electrophoresis of the urine. However, a preliminary test can be completed by placing 4 mL of clear urine in a test tube and heating the test tube in a 56° C water bath for 15 minutes. Any precipitation is an indication of Bence Jones protein. If there is turbidity or precipitate, heating the same tube in a boiling water bath for 3 minutes should produce a decrease in the amount of turbidity or precipitate, supporting further the presence of immunoglobulin light chains. If the turbidity increases on boiling it is indicative of albumin or other globulins which are leaking through the damaged glomerular membrane.

Based on the nonregenerative anemia, mature neutropenia, and hyperglobulinemia, a plasma cell tumor in the bone marrow is suspected. The finding of a monoclonal gammopathy on protein electrophoresis along with the positive precipitation upon heating the urine and the positive protein electrophoresis test for Bence Jones proteinuria support the presence of a plasma cell tumor further.

BONE MARROW EXAMINATION

The bone marrow is hypercellular. Myeloid and erythroid series is complete, and development appears orderly. Megakaryocytes are present and appear adequate. Most notable is that 70% of the marrow elements are comprised of plasma cells confirming the diagnosis of plasma cell myeloma.

DIAGNOSIS

Plasma cell myeloma.

Patient: Dog, spaniel, spayed female, 9 years old.

Presenting Signs and Complaints: Lethargic; coughs frequently; seems to have difficulty breathing; weight loss.

Physical Examination: Coughs almost continually after minimal exercise; moist rales on ascultation; thin.

Problem List: 1. Dyspnea. 2. Coughing. 3. Pulmonary fluid. 4. Thin.

Hematology		Serum Chemistry	
RBC × 10⁶/µL	6.17 (6.17 × 10¹²/L)	AST (SGOT) (IU/L)	66 (66 U/L)
Hemoglobin (g/dL)	15.9 (9.87 mmol/L)	ALT (SGPT) (IU/L)	118 (118 U/L)
PCV (%)	43 (0.43 volume fraction)	Alkaline phosphatase (IU/L)	54 (54 U/L)
MCV (fL)	70	GGT (IU/L)	1 (1 U/L)
MCHC (g/dL)	37 (22.9 mmol/L)	Total bilirubin (mg/dL)	0.2 (3.4 µmol/L)
Reticulocytes (%)	0.1 (0.01 number fraction)	Conjugated bilirubin (mg/dL)	0 (0 µmol/L)
NRBC/100 WBC	0	↑ Total protein (g/dL)	8.2 (82 g/L)
RBC morphology	Normal	↓ Albumin (g/dL)	2.1 ↓ (21 g/L)
↑ WBC × 10³/µL	64.2 ↑ (64.2 × 10⁹/L)	↑ Globulin (g/dL)	6.1 ↑ (61 g/L)
		Amylase (IU/L)	799 (799 U/L)
Myelocytes/µL	0 (0 × 10⁹/L)	Lipase IU/L)	61 (61 U/L)
Metamyelocytes/µL	0 (0 × 10⁹/L)	Glucose (mg/dL)	92 (5.1 mmol/L)
↑ Band neutrophils/µL	4,494 (4.5 × 10⁹/L)	Urea nitrogen (mg/dL)	10 (3.6 mmol/L)
↑ Segmented neutrophils/µL	26,322 (26.3 × 10⁹/L)	Creatinine (mg/dL)	1.0 (88.4 µmol/L)
Lymphocytes/µL	1,284 (1.3 × 10⁹/L)	Calcium (mg/dL)	7.7 (1.9 mmol/L)
↑ Monocytes/µL	4,494 (4.5 × 10⁹/L)	Phosphorus (mg/dL)	4.2 (1.4 mmol/L)
↑ Eosinophils/µL	25,680 (25.7 × 10⁹/L)	Sodium (mEq/L)	144 (144 mmol/L)
↑ Basophils/µL	1,926 (1.9 × 10⁹/L)	Potassium (mEq/L)	4.2 (4.2 mmol/L)
Toxic neutrophils	None seen	Chloride (mEq/L)	102 (102 mmol/L)
Platelets estimate	Adequate	Carbon dioxide (mEq/L)	20 (20 mmol/L)
Heartworms	**Positive for *D. immitis***	LDH (IU/L)	268 (268 U/L)
Plasma protein (g/dl)	**8.8 (88 g/L)**	Creatine kinase (IU/L)	72 (72 U/L)
Fibrinogen (mg/dL)	**600 (6 g/L)**	Total T₄ (mg/dL)	2.1 (27.02 nmol/L)

Urinalysis (Cystocentesis)[a]	
Appearance	Yellow, clear
Specific gravity	1.038
pH	6.5
↑ Protein	Negative
Glucose	Negative
Ketones	Negative
Blood	Negative
Bilirubin	Negative
Sediment	
WBC/hpf	1–3
RBC/hpf	3–5
Casts	Negative
Crystals	Negative
Bacteria	Negative

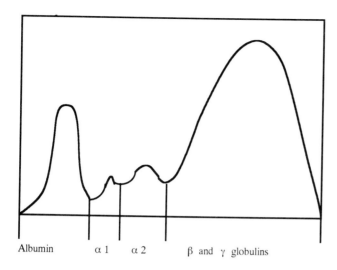

Albumin   α 1   α 2   β and γ globulins

CASE 14. Serum protein electrophoresis with polyclonal gammopathy. Note the broad β-γ peak.

HEMOGRAM

The leukogram depicts a leukocytosis and neutrophilia with a left shift and hyperfibrinogenemia indicating an inflammatory process. There are also an eosinophilia and basophilia which support a parasitic infection, especially dirofilariasis, which was confirmed by finding microfilaria. Based on these latter two hematologic findings if microfilaria are not found it is appropriate to do an occult heartworm test.

BIOCHEMICAL PROFILE

Significant biochemical findings include a hyperglobulinemia and mild hypoalbuminemia culminating in hyperproteinemia. Any chronic antigenic stimulation to the immune system can result in an increased globulin production. An increase in globulins sends a signal to the liver to decrease albumin production which is reflected in this case. Hyperglobulinemia secondary to chronic antigenic stimulation is usually a polyclonal gammopathy as demonstrated on the protein electrophoresis.

DIAGNOSIS

Heartworm, infection.

Patient: Bovine, Holstein, female, 2 years old.

Presenting Signs and Complaints: Had mastitis about 3 weeks ago; responded to antibiotic therapy and now back in milking string; inappetent and weak for 2 days; seems weak today.

Physical Examination: Temperature 104.2° F, increased pulse and respiratory rates, abnormal milk from three quarters, no rumen motility.

Problem List: 1. Anorexia. 2. Pyrexia. 3. Mastitis. 4. Rumen atony.

Hematology	
RBC × 10⁶/μL	5.42 (5.42 × 10^{12}/L)
Hemoglobin (g/dL)	9.2 (5.71 mmol/L)
PCV (%)	25 (0.25 volume fraction)
MCV (fL)	46.1
Plasma protein (g/dL)	8.080 (g/L)
MCHC (g/dL)	36.8 (22.8 mmol/L)
NRBC/100 WBC	0
Erythrocyte morphology	Normal
↑ WBC × 10³/μL	**2.5 (2.5 × 10^9/L)**
↑ Metamyelocytes/μL	**150 (0.15 × 10^9/L)**
↑ Band neutrophils/μL	**200 (0.2 × 10^9/L)**
↓ Neutrophils/μL	**250 (0.25 × 10^9/L)**
Segmented	
↓ Lymphocytes/μL	**1700 (1.7 × 10^9/L)**
Monocytes/μL	200 (0.2 × 10^9/L)
Eosinophils/μL	**0 (0 × 10^9/L)**
Basophils/μL	0
↑ Toxic neutrophils	2+
Platelet Estimate	Adequate
↑ Fibrinogen (mg/dL)	**900 (9 g/L)**
Bacteriology of milk	*Escherichia coli* **isolated in pure culture**

HEMOGRAM

Examination of the hemogram reveals a dramatic leukopenia caused by a combination of a marked neutropenia and lymphopenia. It must be remembered that the bovine normally has more lymphocytes than neutrophils. The neutropenia is accompanied by a degenerative left shift through metamyelocytes. The neutrophil series shows toxic morphology along with the left shift, indicating an acute inflammatory process that is supported by the hyperfibrinogenemia.

E. coli was cultured from the milk, indicative of mastitis.

DIAGNOSIS

Mastitis with attendant endotoxemia resulting from the Gram-negative bacterial infection.

Patient: Horse, thoroughbred, female, 11 years old.

Presenting Signs and Complaints: Had abdominal pain about a month ago; another veterinarian prescribed antibiotics; improved but has not returned to normal; poor appetite, weight loss, kicks at abdomen periodically.

Physical Examination: Temperature 104.8° F. Ascites. Mucous membranes appear muddy. Thin and dehydrated.

Problem List: 1. Pyrexia. 2. Weight loss. 3. Ascites. 4. Dehydration (10%).

Hematology		Serum Chemistry	
↓ **RBC × 10⁶/μL**	**4.56 (4.56 × 10¹²/L)**	AST (SGOT) (IU/L)	126 (126 U/L)
↓ **Hemoglobin (g/dL)**	**8.6 (5.3 mmol/L)**	ALT (SGPT) (IU/L)	50 (50 U/L)
↓ **PCV (%)**	**23.5 (0.24 volume fraction)**	Alkaline phosphatase (IU/L)	62 (62 U/L)
↑ **Plasma protein (g/dL)**	**9.4 (94 g/L)**	GGT (IU/L)	1 (1 U/L)
MCV (fL)	51	Total bilirubin (mg/dL)	0.6 (10.3 μmol/L)
MCHC (g/dL)	36.6 (22.7 mmol/L)	Conjugated bilirubin (mg/dL)	0.1 (1.7 μmol/L)
RDW (%)	17.6 (0.176 volume fraction)	Total protein (g/dL)	8.7 (87 g/L)
Reticulocytes (%)	Not done	↑ **Albumin (g/dL)**	**4.7 (47 g/L)**
NRBC/100 WBC	0	Globulins (g/dL)	4.0 (40 g/L)
Erythrocyte morphology	Normal	Cholesterol (mg/dL)	96 (2.5 mmol/L)
WBC × 10³/μL	**68.1 (68.1 × 10⁹/L)**	↑ **Urea nitrogen (mg/dL)**	**36 (12.9 mmol/L)**
Myelocytes/μL	0 (0 × 10⁹/L)	↑ **Creatinine (mg/dL)**	**1.9 (168 μmol/L)**
↑ **Metamyelocytes/μL**	**681 (0.68 × 10⁹/L)**	Glucose (mg/dL)	85 (80.3 mmol/L)
↑ **Band neutrophils/μL**	**4,086 (4.1 × 10⁹/L)**	Sodium (mEq/L)	158 (158 mmol/L)
↑ **Segmented neutrophils/μL**	**45,627 (45.6 × 10⁹/L)**	Potassium (mEq/L)	5.0 (5 mmol/L)
↑ **Lymphocytes/μL**	**12,258ᵃ (12.3 × 10⁹/L)**	Chloride (mEq/L)	107 (107 mmol/L)
↑ **Monocytes/μL**	**5,448 (5.4 × 10⁹/L)**	Carbon dioxide (mEq/L)	25 (25 mmol/L)
↓ **Eosinophils/μL**	**0 (0 × 10⁹/L)**	Calcium (mg/dL)	12.0 (3.0 mmol/L)
Basophils/μL	0 (0 × 10⁹/L)	Phosphorus (mg/dL)	2.6 (0.84 mmol/L)
↑ **Toxic neutrophils**	**2+**	Creatine kinase (IU/L)	168 (168 U/L)
Platelet estimate	Adequate	↑ **LDH (IU/L)**	**1,272 (1,272 U/L)**
↑ **Fibrinogen (mg/dL)**	**700 (7 g/L)**		

ᵃ Majority of lymphocytes are medium to large.

Abdominal Fluid Analysis	
Color	Red
Appearance	Flocculent
Specific gravity	1.017
↑ **Protein (g/dL)**	**4.2 (42 g/L)**
↑ **WBC/μL**	**63,360 (63.4 × 10⁹/L)**
↑ **RBC/μL**	**30,000 (30 × 10⁹/L)**

CYTOLOGY

Many degenerative neutrophils. Bacterial rods numerous. Interpretation: septic infection.

HEMOGRAM

Evaluation of the erythron indicates an anemia. Evaluation of anemia in the horse is difficult because signs of regeneration (reticulocytes and polychromasia) do not appear in the peripheral blood. Consequently, bone marrow examination is required for further characterization of the anemia.

The leukogram is characterized by a marked leukocytosis and neutrophilia with a regenerative left shift to metamyelocytes. The granulocytic cells show toxic morphology. There is a lymphocytosis with the majority of the lymphocytes appearing medium to large. Neutrophilia with a regenerative left shift is suggestive of a severe active inflammatory process, particularly bacterial in origin. Lymphocytosis in the presence of an inflammatory process is inappropriate and leads one to wonder if there is a lymphoproliferative neoplastic process present. Abdominocentesis revealed a flocculent fluid with increased nucleated cells comprised primarily of neutrophils in various stages of karyolysis. Bacteria were noted within neutrophils as well as extracellular confirming the diagnosis of a septic abdomen.

BIOCHEMICAL PROFILE

The biochemical profile is unremarkable except for a slight azotemia that suggests a decreased glomerular filtration rate. The azotemia is probably prerenal because the patient was clinically dehydrated with increased serum albumin.

The increase in LDH, a nonspecific enzyme, may represent tissue necrosis.

Comment

A laparotomy was performed, and mesenteric lymph nodes were enlarged. A mass involved the perforated intestine. Aspiration cytology of the lymph nodes and scrapings of the thickened intestinal mucosa demonstrated neoplastic lymphocytes, providing a diagnosis of lymphosarcoma. It should be noted that lymphosarcoma is frequently present without an accompanying lymphocytosis in the peripheral blood.

DIAGNOSIS

Lymphosarcoma with secondary rupture of intestine causing peritonitis.

Patient: Dog, terrier, spayed female, 4 years old.

Presenting Signs and Complaints (October 15): Vomiting periodically for 3 weeks; does not appear to be related to eating; does not eat well; weight loss; stools are soft and not formed.

Physical Examination (October 15): Thin; dehydrated; soft stool on rectal examination; intestinal walls thickened on palpation; gas and fluid also noted on palpation of intestine.

Problem List (October 15): 1. Chronic diarrhea. 2. Weight loss. 3. Thickening of intestinal walls. Endoscopy was performed and biopsies taken with a histologic diagnosis of lymphocytic plasmacytic enteritis (inflammatory bowel disease). Dog was managed with d/d diet and prednisolone with moderate improvement noted the first 3 weeks. The diarrhea worsened and azathioprine was added for 3 more weeks. The dog presented acutely collapsed.

Physical Examination (December 15): Weak and unable to rise; distended abdomen; dehydration; temperature 104.5° F.

Problem List (December 15) 1. Pyrexia 2. Marked depression. 3. Tense abdomen. 4. Dehydration.

Hematology	October 15	December 2
RBC × 10⁶/μL	6.9 (6.9 × 10^{12}/L)	8.0 (8 × 10^{12}/L)
Hemoglobin (g/dL)	16.11 (0 mmol/L)	19.1 (11.9 mmol/L)
PCV (%)	47 (0.47 volume fraction)	56 (0.56 volume fraction)
MCV (fL)	68.1	70
MCHC (g/dL)	34.2 (20.5 mmol/L)	34 (20.4 mmol/L)
NRBC/100 WBC	0	2
RBC morphology	Normal	Normal
WBC × 10³/μL	11.5 (11.5 × 10^9/L)	↓ **2.8 (2.8 × 10^9/L)**
Myelocytes/μL	0 (0 × 10^9/L)	↑ **28 (0.03 × 10^9/L)**
Metamyelocytes/μL	0 (0 × 10^9/L)	↑ **168 (0.17 × 10^9/L)**
Band neutrophils/μL	0 (0 × 10^9/L)	↑ **560 (0.56 × 10^9/L)**
Segmented neutro-phils/μL	9545 (9.5 × 10^9/L)	↓ **672 (0.67 × 10^9/L)**
Lymphocytes/μL	**575 (0.58 × 10^9/L)**	↓ **504 (0.54 × 10^9/L)**
Monocytes/μL	1380 (1.38 × 10^9/L)	924 (0.92 × 10^9/L)
Eosinophils/μL	**0 (0 × 10^9/L)**	↓ **0 (0 × 10^9/L)**
Basophils/μL	0 (0 × 10^9/L)	0 (0 × 10^9/L)
Toxic neutrophils	None	+
Platelets × 10³/μL	2100 (21 × 10^9/L)	↓ **120 (0.12 × 10^9/L)**
Platelet estimate	Adequate	Adequate
Blood parasites	None	None
Plasma protein (g/dL)	4.2 (42 g/L)	4.5 (45 g/L)
Fibrinogen (mg/dL)	200 (2 g/L)	100 (1 g/L)

Table continued on following page

Serum Chemistry	October 15	December 2
AST (SGOT) (IU/L)	27 (27 U/L)	76 (76 U/L)
ALT (SGPT) (IU/L)	**36 (36 U/L)**	↑ **122 (122 U/L)**
Total bilirubin (mg/dL)	0.2 (3.4 mmol/L)	0.6 (10.3 mmol/L)
Urea nitrogen (mg/dL)	11 (3.9 mmol/L)	↑ 68 (24.3 mmol/L)
Creatinine (mg/dL)	1.2 (106 μmol/L)	↑ **2.7 (239 μmol/L)**
Cholesterol (mg/dL)	78 (2.0 mmol/L)	78 (2.08 mmol/L)
Alkaline phosphatase (IU/L)	16 (16 U/L)	↑ 676,676 U/L
GGT (IU/L)	1 (1 U/L)	12 (12 U/L)
Glucose (mg/dL)	85 (4.68 mmol/L)	↓ **47 (2.59 mmol/L)**
Inorganic phosphate (mg/dL)	4.2 (1.36 mmol/L)	4.7 (1.52 mol/L)
Calcium (mg/dL)	7.9 (1.98 mmol/L)	8.1 (2.0 mmol/L)
Corrected calcium (mg/dL)	9.5 (2.38 mmol/L)	9.4 (2.35 mmol/L)
Total protein (g/dL)	↓ **3.9 (39 g/L)**	↓ **4.5 (45 g/L)**
Albumin (g/dL)	↓ **1.9 (19 g/L)**	↓ **2.2 (22 g/L)**
Globulin (g/dL)	↓ **2 (2.0 g/L)**	↓ **2.3 (2.3 g/L)**
Sodium (mEq/L)	147 (147 mmol/L)	157 (157 mmol/L)
Potassium (mEq/L)	5 (5.0 mmol/L)	4.9 (4.9 mmol/L)
Na : K ratio	32.7	32.0
Chloride (mEq/L)	101 (101 mmol/L)	114 (114 mmol/L)
Carbon dioxide (mEq/L)	31 (31 mmol/L)	16 (16 mmol/L)
Amylase (IU/L)	1200 (1200 U/L)	1498 (1498 U/L)
Lipase (IU/L)	34 (34 U/L)	25 (25 U/L)
TLI (μg/L)	17.2	18.5
Cobalamin (ng/L)		↓ **85**
Folate (μg/L)		↑ **126**

Urinalysis (Cystocentesis)		
	10/15	12/2
Appearance	Clear, yellow	Clear, yellow
Specific gravity	1.039	1.047
pH	6.5	6
Protein	Negative	+
Glucose	Negative	Negative
Ketones	Negative	Negative
Occult blood	Negative	Negative
Bilirubin	Negative	Negative
Sediment		
WBC/hpf	1–2	3–4
RBC/hpf	Occasional	None
Casts/lpf	Negative	Hyaline
Crystals	Negative	Negative
Bacteria	Negative	Negative

HEMOGRAM (OCTOBER 15)

The initial hemogram on October 15 is characterized by lymphopenia and eosinopenia. These may be a reflection of chronic endogenous stress.

BIOCHEMICAL PROFILE (OCTOBER 15)

The biochemical profile is remarkable for hypoalbuminemia and hypoglobulinemia culminating in a hypoproteinemia. That both components of protein are decreased suggests protein loss to the outside of the body such as a protein-losing enteropathy. Clinical signs support this interpretation.

The TLI was normal, ruling out exocrine pancreatic insufficiency as a cause of the diarrhea. Normal TLI, decreased cobalamin (vitamin B_{12}), and increased folate suggest intestinal bacterial overgrowth which is often associated with a number of diverse enteric disease (see Fig. 5–3).

HEMOGRAM (DECEMBER 2)

On December 2 there was a marked leukopenia and neutropenia with a degenerative left shift through myelocytes indicating an intense response to an acute need, most likely bacterial in origin.

BIOCHEMICAL PROFILE (DECEMBER 2)

Examination of the biochemical profile reveals a mild increase in ALT which may be the result of endotoxin leaking across a damaged intestinal barrier into the portal circulation and altering the integrity of hepatocyte membranes. The alkaline phosphatase activity was increased and in this case was probably drug induced as the patient had been treated with prednisolone.

The azotemia indicates decreased glomerular filtration. The urine specific gravity indicates that the kidney was capable of concentrating urine and supporting a prerenal component secondary to dehydration which is supported by the high PCV.

Hypoalbuminemia and hypoglobulinemia are still present, probably secondary to the underlying enteropathy.

There was a hypoglycemia which, in this case, may be related to a septicemic endotoxemic condition.

DIAGNOSIS

The dog died during the night of December 2. Necropsy revealed an acute peritonitis secondary to perforations in the small intestine. The small intestine was thickened in the areas of the perforation. Histologic examination revealed superficial lymphocytic, plasmacytic inflammation with an underlying lymphosarcoma in the deeper layers of the intestinal wall.

Patient: Bovine, Holstein, female, 4 years old.

Presenting Signs and Complaints: Off feed for 2 days; milk production greatly reduced.

Physical Examination: Pain elicited on palpation over xyphoid cartilage; grunts when walking; dehydrated; rumen motility reduced; temperature 103° F.

Problem List: 1. Anorexia. 2. Dehydration. 3. Weak rumen motility. 4. Pyrexia.

Hematology	
RBC × 10⁶/μL	5.6 (5.6 × 10¹²/L)
Hemoglobin (g/dL)	9.8 (6.1 mmol/L)
PCV (%)	29 (0.29 volume fraction)
MCV (fL)	51.8
Plasma protein (g/dL)	7.9 (79 g/L)
MCHC (g/dL)	33.8 (21 mmol/L)
Erythrocyte morphology	Normal
WBC × 10³/μL	10.8 (10.8 × 10⁹/L)
↑ **Band neutrophils/μL**	**216 (0.21 × 10⁹/L)**
↑ **Segmented neutrophils/μL**	**8200 (8.2 × 10⁹/L)**
↓ **Lymphocytes/μL**	**2160 (2.2 × 10⁹/L)**
Monocytes/μL	108 (0.01 × 10⁹/L)
Eosinophils/μL	108 (0.01 × 10⁹/L)
Basophils/μL	0
Toxic neutrophils	Present
Platelet estimate	Adequate
Blood parasites	None seen
Plasma protein (g/dL)	7.9 (79 g/L)
↑ **Fibrinogen (mg/dL)**	**1000 (10 g/L)**

HEMOGRAM

Evaluation of the leukogram discloses a neutrophilia, left shift, and lymphopenia indicative of an inflammatory process and stress. Leukogram changes in the bovine are frequently subtle and not as dramatic as in carnivorous or equine species. Total leukocyte counts often remain within the normal range but with an increase in neutrophils. As the cow normally has a higher lymphocyte count than other species, stress causes a marked reduction in lymphocytes and although there is an increase in neutrophils there is little or no increase in the total leukocyte count. It is possible for a cow to have fewer total leukocytes than normal but still have evidence of an infection or stress as manifested by neutrophilia.

The fibrinogen is markedly increased. In the bovine the fibrinogen concentration is often a better indicator of an inflammatory process than a leukogram (see the section on fibrinogen in Chapter 3).

DIAGNOSIS

A standing laparotomy revealed the presence of traumatic reticulopericarditis.

Patient: Dog, mixed breed, male, 5 years old.

Presenting Signs and Complaints: Collapses when exercised. Inappetence and weight loss for 3 months.

Physical Examination: Enlarged prescapular, popliteal, femoral and submandibular lymph nodes; petechia on abdomen and mucous membranes.

Problem List: 1. Inappetence. 2. Weight loss. 3. Peripheral lymphadenopathy. 4. Petechia.

Hematology		Serum Chemistry	
RBC × 10⁶/μL	5.2 (5.2 × 10¹²/L)	AST (SGOT) (IU/L)	26 (26 U/L)
Hemoglobin (g/dL)	11.4 (7.07 mmol/L)	ALT (SGPT) (IU/L)	36 (36 U/L)
PCV (%)	31.8 (0.318 volume fraction)	ALP (IU/L)	0 (0 U/L)
MCV (fL)	611	Total bilirubin (mg/dL)	0.5 (8.5 μmol/L)
MCHC (g/dL)	35.5 (22.01 mmol/L)	Direct bilirubin (mg/dL)	0.3 (5.1 μmol/L)
Reticulocytes (%)	0.8 (0.008 number fraction)	Indirect bilirubin (mg/dL)	0.2 (3.4 μmol/L)
NRBC/100 WBC	0	↑ **Total protein (g/dL)**	**9.9 (99 g/L)**
RBC morphology	Normal	Albumin (g/dL)	2.4 (24 g/L)
WBC × 10³/μL	5.8 (5.8 × 10⁹/L)	↑ **Globulin (g/dL)**	**7.5 (75 g/L)**
		Amylase (IU/L)	750 (750 U/L)
Myelocytes/μL	0 (0 × 10⁹/L)	Lipase (IU/L)	72 (72 U/L)
Metamyelocytes/μL	0 (0 × 10⁹/L)	Glucose (mg/dL)	115 (6.3 mmol/L)
Band neutrophils/μL	0 (0 × 10⁹/L)	Urea nitrogen (mg/dL)	15 (5.4 mmol/L)
Segmented neutrophils/μL	3886 (3.88 × 10⁹/L)	Creatinine (mg/dL)	1 (88.4 μmol/L)
Lymphocytes/μL	1334 (1.33 × 10⁹/L)	Calcium (mg/dL)	9.9 (2.48 mmol/L)
Monocytes/μL	464 (0.46 × 10⁹/L)	Phosphorus (mg/dL)	4.5 (1.45 mmol/L)
Eosinophils/μL	174 (0.17 × 10⁹/L)	Sodium (mEq/L)	144 (144 mmol/L)
Basophils/μL	0 (0 × 0⁹/L)	Potassium (mEq/L)	4.1 (4.1 mmol/L)
Toxic neutrophils	None	Chloride (mEq/L)	112 (112 mmol/L)
		Carbon dioxide (mEq/L)	19 (19 mmol/L)
↓ **Platelets × 10³/μL**	**47 (0.047 × 10¹²/L)**	Electrophoresis (total protein = 10.2)	
PT (sec)	8.9	Albumin (g/dL)	2.6 (26 g/L)
APTT (sec)	13.1	α₁-Globulin (g/dL)	0.2 (2 g/L)
Thrombin clot time (sec)	7.8	α₂-globulin (g/dL)	0.3 (3 g/L)
Platelet factor 3 test	Negative	β-Globulins (g/dL)	0.2 (2 g/L)
Other tests		γ₁ (g/dL)	0.2 (2 g/L)
Lymph node biopsy	Reactive node	↑ **γ₂ (g/dL)**[a]	**6.7 (67 g/L)**
↑ **Ehrlichia titer**	**↑ 1 : 1280**		

[a] Pathologist's comment: Compatible with a monoclonal gammopathy

Urinalysis (Cystocentesis)	
Appearance	Cloudy, red
Specific gravity	1.050
pH	6.5
Protein	Trace
Glucose	Negative
Ketones	Negative
↑ **Blood**	**4+**
Bilirubin	Negative
Sediment	
WBC/hpf	1–4
↑ **RBC/hpf**	**TNTC**
Casts	Negative
Crystals	Negative
Bacteria	Negative

HEMOGRAM

Evaluation of the hemogram indicates a nonregenerative anemia and a thrombocytopenia. The hemogram changes as well as the monoclonal gammopathy support the need for a bone marrow examination.

BIOCHEMICAL PROFILE

The biochemical profile reveals hypoalbuminemia and hyperglobulinemia resulting in hyperproteinemia. The hyperglobulinemia may be monoclonal or polyclonal. The hyperglobulinemia sends a signal to the liver to decrease albumin production, resulting in hypoalbuminemia. Protein electrophoresis reveals a monoclonal gammopathy, which is frequently associated with neoplastic lymphoproliferative disorders such as plasma cell myeloma (see case 13 for a tracing representing a monoclonal gammopathy) and on occasion with infections such as ehrlichiosis.

The increase in ALT indicates enzyme leakage from hepatocytes. No cause can be suspected. Once the primary disease process is managed appropriately the ALT can be redetermined; if increased on two or more determinations, further diagnostic tests can be directed toward the liver.

Hemorrhage into the urinary tract is probably related to the thrombocytopenia.

LYMPH NODE ASPIRATE

A fine needle aspirate of one of the enlarged lymph nodes was completed. The predominant cell type is a mature small lymphocyte with increased numbers of variably sized immature lymphocytes ranging from medium to large lymphocytes to lymphoblasts and plasma cells. These findings are compatible with benign lymphoid hyperplasia (reactive lymphoid tissue). No etiology was identified.

BONE MARROW EXAMINATION

Several unit particles were examined from the bone marrow aspirate and were notable for the marked hypocellularity. A rare megakaryocyte was observed, and occasional myeloid and erythroid elements were scattered about. The stroma of the unit particles contained small accumulations of plasma cells. The hypoplastic marrow is compatible with a chronic ehrlichia infection. The observation of the small focal accumulations of plasma cells within the stroma are: (1) probably a reflection of the generalized antigenic response by the immune system to the presence of the ehrlichia agent; and (2) visualized in the bone marrow because of the loss of other cellular elements, making them more obvious. This should not be confused with a plasma cell tumor (refer to Case 12 for comparison).

The *Ehrlichia* serum titer of 1 : 1280 plus hypoplastic marrow support a diagnosis of chronic ehrlichiosis. *Ehrlichia* are difficult to demonstrate in blood, bone marrow, or lymphoid tissues. Hypoplastic marrow can be caused by a number of different etiologies such as drugs, viruses, and unknown toxins. In this case the *Ehrlichia canis* serum titer was used to support the etiopathogenesiss of the aplastic anemia.

DIAGNOSIS

E. canis infection causing aplastic anemia.

COMMENT

Regarding the mild increase in ALT, the liver may develop a nonspecific reaction (hepatitis) when there is a systemic antigenic response. If one biopsied the liver a mild to moderate portal triaditis might be noted. The predominant cell type is the lymphocyte with lesser numbers of macrophages and plasma cells. This is somewhat analogous to the reactive lymph nodes responding to the antigenic stimulation occurring in the body. This can be considered a secondary type of hepatitis and should resolve when the primary disease is managed successfully.

Patient: Dog, English pointer, female, 9 years old.

Presenting Signs and Complaints: Anorectic; black tarry feces; bred a month ago and was given estrogen to prevent pregnancy.

Physical Examination: Bloody mucous discharge from vagina; small hemorrhages on mucous membranes of mouth and vagina.

Problem List: 1. Vaginal bleeding. 2. Multiple petechial hemorrhages.

Hematology		Serum Chemistry	
↓ **RBC × 10⁶/μL**	**3.77 (3.77 × 10¹²/L)**	AST (SGOT) (IU/L)	25 (25 U/L)
↓ **Hemoglobin (g/dL)**	**8.7 (5.4 mmol/L)**	ALT (SGPT) (IU/L)	25 (25 U/L)
↓ **PCV (%)**	**25.4 (0.25 volume fraction)**	ALP (IU/L)	155 (155 U/L)
MCV (fL)	67	GGT (IU/L)	2 (2 U/L)
Plasma protein (g/dL)	5.2 (57 g/L)	Total bilirubin (mg/dL)	0.2 (3.4 μmol/L)
MCHC (g/dL)	34.4 (21.3 mmol/L)	Conjugated bilirubin (mg/dL)	0.1 (1.7 μmol/L)
Reticulocytes (%)	0	Unconjugated bilirubin (mg/dL)	0.1 (1.7 μmol/L)
NRBC/100 WBC	0	Total protein (g/dL)	5.0 (50 g/L)
RBC morphology	Normal	Albumin (g/dL)	2.6 (26 g/L)
↓ **WBC × 10³/μL**	**3.4 (3.4 × 10⁹/L)**	Globulin (g/dL)	2.4 (24 g/L)
Myelocytes/μL	0 (0 × 10⁹/L)	Cholesterol (mg/dL)	135 (3.5 mmol/L)
Metamyelocytes/μL	0 (0 × 10⁹/L)	↑ **Urea nitrogen (mg/dL)**	**45 (16.1 mmol/L)**
Band neutrophils/μL	0 (0 × 10⁹/L)	Creatinine (mg/dL)	0.8 (70.7 μmol/L)
↓ **Segmented neutrophils/μL**	**2372 (2.4 × 10⁹/L)**	Glucose (mg/dL)	107 (5.9 mmol/L)
↓ **Lymphocytes/μL**	**910 (0.91 × 10⁹/L)**	Amylase (IU/L)	350 (360 U/L)
Monocytes/μL	0 (0 × 10⁹/L)	Lipase (IU/L)	25 (25 U/L)
Eosinophils/μL	118 (0.12 × 10⁹/L)	Sodium (mEq/L)	151 (151 mmol/L)
Basophils/μL	0 (0 × 10⁹/L)	Potassium (mEq/L)	3.8 (3.8 mmol/L)
Toxic neutrophils	None	Na : K ratio	39.7
Platelet estimate	Decreased	Chloride (mEq/L)	102 (102 mmol/L)
↓ **Platelets × 10³/μL**	**19 (0.019 × 10¹²/L)**	Carbon dioxide (mEq/L)	19 (19 mmol/L)
Coagulation tests		Calcium (mg/dL)	8.8 (2.2 mmol/L)
PT (sec)	9.8	Phosphorus (mg/dL)	3.8 (1.23 mmol/L)
APTT (sec)	12.1		
Thrombin time (sec)	8.3		
Fibrinogen (mg/dL)	200 (2 g/L)		

Urinalysis (Cystocentesis)	
Appearance	**Reddish brown**
Specific gravity	1.045
pH	6.5
Protein	Negative
Glucose	Negative
Ketones	Negative
↑ **Blood**	4
Bilirubin	Negative
Sediment	
WBC/hpf	0–4
↑ **RBC/hpf**	**20–50**
Casts	None
Crystals	None
Bacteria	None

HEMOGRAM

There is an anemia with a decrease in plasma proteins, suggesting blood loss. There is also a marked leukopenia secondary to an absolute neutropenia along with thrombocytopenia and a normocytic normochromic nonregenerative anemia suggesting marrow aplasia.

BIOCHEMICAL PROFILE

The hypoproteinemia with a decrease of both albumin and globulin along with the anemia suggests blood loss. There is an increased urea nitrogen with a normal creatinine; this inappropriate relationship suggests the presence of gastrointestinal hemorrhage because blood is a rich source of protein. This concentrated protein source is carried to the liver for protein metabolism with urea nitrogen as a by-product (see discussion in Chapter 6).

URINALYSIS

Hemorrhage into the urinary tract is probably caused by the thrombocytopenia, as there is no pyuria or bactiuria that would suggest infection or inflammation of the urinary bladder.

BONE MARROW EXAMINATION

Examination shows that the cellularity is low, and only occasional particles contain hematopoietic cells. The pathologist's opinion is severe marrow hypoplasia of all hematopoietic elements.

Such a marked hypocellularity can be caused by a diversity of insults. However, the history in this case leads us to implicate estrogen toxicity as the etiopathogenesis. Marrow examinations are essential in evaluating patients with multiple cytopenias in the peripheral blood.

Most dogs, after receiving estrogen, probably undergo transient depression of the bone marrow, and it is only the occasional patient that develops an aplastic process such as seen in this dog. Two to 3 weeks after the administration of estrogen there may be a neutrophilia followed by a precipitous drop in neutrophils. Platelets follow a similar pattern, increasing for a week to 10 days and then decreasing rapidly at about 2 weeks.

DIAGNOSIS

Bone marrow aplasia secondary to estrogen toxicity.

Patient: Cat, domestic shorthair, spayed female, 11 years old.

Presenting Signs and Complaints: Inactive lately, weight loss.

Physical Examination: Splenomegaly; thin; lethargic.

Problem List: 1. Weight loss. 2. Lethargy. 3. Splenomegaly.

Hematology		Serum Chemistry	
RBC × 10⁶/μL	6.89 (6.89 × 10¹²/L)	AST (SGOT) (IU/L)	40 (40 U/L)
Hemoglobin (g/dL)	10.5 (6.52 mmol/L)	ALT (SGPT) (IU/L)	40 (40 U/L)
PCV (%)	32.4 (0.324 volume fraction)	ALP (IU/L)	28 (28 U/L)
Plasma protein (g/dL)	7.1 (71 g/L)	Total bilirubin (mg/dL)	0.1 (1.7 μmol/L)
MCV (fL)	47	Total protein (g/dL)	7.0 (70 g/L)
MCHC (g/dL)	32.4 (20 mmol/L)	Albumin (g/dL)	3.8 (38 g/L)
NRBC/100 WBC	0	Globulin (g/dL)	3.2 (32 g/L)
RBC morphology	Normal	Cholesterol (mg/dL)	202 (5.3 mmol/L)
↑ **WBC × 10³/μL**	**42.8 (42.8 × 10⁹/L)**	Urea nitrogen (mg/dL)	21 (7.5 mmol/L)
Myelocytes/μL	0 (0 × 10⁹/L)	Creatinine (mg/dL)	1.9 (168.0 μmol/L)
Metamyelocytes/μL	0 (0 × 10⁹/L)	Glucose (mg/dL)	94 (5.2 mmol/L)
Band neutrophils/μL	0 (0 × 10⁹/L)	Calcium (mg/dL)	10.2 (2.55 mmol/L)
Segmented neutro- phils/μL	13,268 (13.3 × 10⁹/L)	Phosphorus (mg/dL)	5.0 (1.62 mmol/L)
Lymphocytes/μL	5,136 (5.1 × 10⁹/L)		
Monocytes/μL	428 (0.43 × 10⁹/L)		
Eosinophils/μL	1,284 (1.3 × 10⁹/L)		
↑ **Mast cells/μL**	**22,684 (11.7 × 10⁹/L)**		
Toxic neutrophils	None seen		
Platelet estimate	Adequate		
Fibrinogen (mg/dL)	100 (1.0 g/L)		

HEMOGRAM

There is a leukocytosis, and mast cells are numerous. One or two mast cells may occasionally be observed in blood from patients with a variety of disorders such as gastroenteritis and pulmonary disease; however, this dramatic number is diagnostic for mast cell leukemia. A fine needle aspirate of the spleen on the spleen disclosed numerous mast cells.

DIAGNOSIS

Mast cell leukemia.

Patient: Cat, domestic shorthair, female, 11 years old.

Presenting Signs and Complaints: Losing weight for the past month; poor appetite.

Physical Examination: Very thin; membranes pale mucous.

Problem List: 1. Anorexia. 2. Weight loss. 3. Anemia.

Hematology		Serum Chemistry	
RBC × 10⁶/μL	5.62 (5.62 × 10¹²/L)	↑ AST (SGOT) (IU/L)	115 (115 U/L)
Hemoglobin (g/dL)	10.3 (6.4 mmol/L)	↑ ALT (SGPT) (IU/L)	288 (288 U/L)
PCV (%)	31.1 (0.31 volume fraction)	↑ ALP (IU/L)	101 (101 U/L)
MCV (fL)	55	GGT (IU/L)	8 (8 U/L)
MCHC (g/dL)	33 (20.5 mmol/L)	Total bilirubin (mg/dL)	0.2 (3.4 μmol/L)
NRBC/100 WBC	0	Direct bilirubin (mg/dL)	0.1 (1.7 μmol/L)
RBC morphology	Normal	Indirect bilirubin (mg/dL)	0.1 (1.7 μmol/L)
↑ **WBC × 10³/μL**	**73.2 (73.2 × 10⁹/L)**	Total protein (g/dL)	8.0 (80 g/L)
Myelocytes/μL	0 (0 × 10⁹/L)	Albumin (g/dL)	3.9 (39 g/L)
Metamyelocytes/μL	0 (0 × 10⁹/L)	Globulin (g/dL)	4.1 (41 g/L)
Band neutrophils/μL	0 (0 × 10⁹/L)	Cholesterol (mg/dL)	65 (1.7 mmol/L)
↑ **Segmented neutrophils/μL**	**10,248 (10.2 × 10⁹/L)**	Urea nitrogen (mg/dL)	20 (7.14 mmol/L)
↑ **Lymphocytes/μL**[a]	**60,756 (60.8 × 10⁹/L)**	Creatinine (mg/dL)	1.5 (132.6 μmol/L)
Monocytes/μL	732 (0.73 × 10⁹/L)	Glucose (mg/dL)	62 (3.4 mmol/L)
↑ **Eosinophils/μL**	**1,464 (1.5 × 10⁹/L)**	Sodium (mEq/L)	154 (154 mmol/L)
Basophils/μL	0 (0 × 10⁹/L)	Potassium (mEq/L)	4.3 (4.3 mmol/L)
Toxic neutrophils	None seen	Na : K ratio	35.8
Immature cells	None seen	Chloride (mEq/L)	111 (111 mmol/L)
Platelet estimate	Decrease	Carbon dioxide (mEq/L)	21 (21 mmol/L)
Blood parasites	None	Calcium (mg/dL)	9.3 (2.33 mmol/L)
FeLV (ELISA)	Negative	Corrected calcium (mg/dL)	8.9 (2.23 mmol/L)
Plasma protein (g/dL)	8.2 (82 g/L)	Phosphorus (mg/dL)	3.8 (1.23 mmol/L)
Fibrinogen (mg/dL)	100 (1 g/L)	Creatine kinase (IU/L)	105 (105 U/L)
		Total resting T₄ (mg/dL)	1.5 (19.3 nmol/L)

[a] Lymphocytes appear to be normal small lymphocytes. No immature lymphocytes are observed.

HEMOGRAM

This patient is not anemic, but there is a mild macrocytosis. The FeLV may cause abnormal erythrocyte maturation in the bone marrow resulting in the release of macrocytic erythrocytes that are not polychromatophilic.

There is a leukocytosis, and most of the increase is caused by the presence of mature small lymphocytes. Physiologic lymphocytosis is a transient event that is prominent in young, vigorously active cats; however, the absolute lymphocyte count seldom exceeds 10,000 to 12,000. In an aged, sick animal the presence of this number of mature small lymphocytes indicates a neoplastic disorder. The eosinophilia is an observation that we have made occasionally in association with lymphosarcoma. An examination of the bone marrow is appropriate for prognosis as well as staging the neoplasm if the owners consider chemotherapy.

BIOCHEMICAL PROFILE

The elevated ALT and AST imply hepatocellular enzyme leakage, and the moderately increased alkaline phosphatase reflects cholestasis. Because cats do not show increased alkaline phosphatase secondary to stress from the endogenous release of corticosteroids these abnormal liver tests strongly suggest an infiltrative process associated with the neoplasm. When considering chemotherapy to stage the neoplastic process, a biopsy is appropriate. In this case a fine needle liver aspirate was performed, and 10 to 30% of the nucleated cells were lymphocytes, supporting the presence of neoplasia.

BONE MARROW EXAMINATION

A bone marrow aspirate was examined. The specimen was hypercellular with megakaryocytes present and adequate in numbers. The myeloid series was present and complete. The erythroid series was present and complete with morphologic abnormalities noted in some of the nucleated erythrocytes. Approximately 50% of the cellular elements were mature small lymphocytes.

Opinion

Lymphocytic leukemia.

The ELISA test for the FeLV was negative. Most cats with lymphocytic leukemia are FeLV test positive, but some remain negative throughout the course of the disease. Indirect immunofluorescence (FA) tests on bone marrow may be positive in such patients (see Case 23). In this case the FeLV immunofluorescence test on *unfixed marrow slides* was negative.

DIAGNOSIS

Lymphocytic leukemia with infiltration of bone marrow and liver.

Patient: Cat, domestic shorthair, neutered male, 2 years old.

Presenting Signs and Complaints: Depressed; has been on amoxicillin drops for 5 days for a fever when examined on June 23; was active until this morning.

Physical Examination: Temperature 107° F; some fleas.

Problem List: 1. Pyrexia. 2. Flea infestation.

Hematology	June 23	June 28
RBC × 10⁶/μL	7.45 (7.45 × 10¹²/L)	↓ **5.13 (5.13 × 10¹²/L)**
Hemoglobin (g/dL)	11.0 (6.83 mmol/L)	↓ **7.6 (4.72 mmol/L)**
PCV (%)	31.2 (0.31 volume fraction)	↓ **22.6 (0.23 concentrated fraction)**
MCV (fL)	42	43
MCHC (g/dL)	35 (21.7 mmol/L)	34 (20.4 mmol/L)
NRBC/100 WBC	6	0
RBC morphology	Normal	Normal
WBC × 10³/μL	4.8 (4.8 × 10⁹/L)	↓ **2.0 (2.0 × 10⁹/L)**
Myelocytes/μL	0 (0 × 10⁹/L)	0 (0 × 10⁹/L)
↑ **Metamyelocytes/μL**	**240 (0.24 × 10⁹/L)**	0 (0 × 10⁹/L)
↑ **Band neutrophils/μL**	**624 (0.6 × 10⁹/L)**	0 (0 × 10⁹/L)
↓ **Segmented neutrophils/μL**	**1296 (1.3 × 10⁹/L)**	↓ **0 (0 × 10⁹/L)**
Lymphocytes/μL	2016 (2.0 × 10⁹/L)	1930ᵃ (1.9 × 10⁹/L
Monocytes/μL	336 (0.3 × 10⁹/L)	70 0.07 × 10⁹/L)
Eosinophils/μL	240 (0.24 × 10⁹/L)	↓ **0 (0 × 10⁹/L)**
Basophils/μL	0 (0 × 10⁹/L)	0 (0 × 10⁹/L)
↑ **Toxic neutrophils**	**2+**	None
↓ **Platelets**	**Slight decrease**	↓ **Marked decrease**
Plasma protein (g/dL)	7.9 (79 g/L)	7.3 (73 g/L)
Fibrinogen (mg/dL)	300 (3 g/L)	↑ **400 (4 g/L)**

ᵃ Occasional large atypical lymphocyte.

HEMOGRAM (JUNE 23)

This hemogram is remarkable for a neutropenia with a left shift to myelocytes and toxic neutrophils supportive of an acute severe response to a bacterial infection. In carnivorous species the fibrinogen concentration is a less reliable indicator of inflammation. There was a slight decrease in platelets.

HEMOGRAM (JUNE 28)

Five days later, with no clinical improvement, the hemogram is again remarkable for neutropenia, this time there is no left shift, and the platelets are now markedly decreased and anemia is present. There were a few atypical lymphocytes, which suggests response to an antigenic stimulation and should not be confused with lymphocytic leukemia.

BONE MARROW EXAMINATION

With a persistent neutropenia and the development of a marked thrombocytopenia, examination of bone marrow is appropriate. The marrow aspirate was cellular with rare megakaryocytes present. The M : E ratio was 20 : 1.0. The erythroid series was present and complete. The myeloid series predominated, and maturation stopped at the myelocyte stage with only a few metamyelocyte, band, or segmented neutrophils noted.

An immunofluorescence test for FeLV was positive on an unfixed bone marrow aspirate smear.

Opinion

Ineffective granulopoiesis, megakaryocyte aplasia, probably a reflection of FeLV induced myelodysplasia.

DIAGNOSIS

FeLV-induced myelodysplasia.

Patient: Dog, Pekingese, male, 4 months old.

Presenting Signs and Complaints: Developed nosebleed and a red eye after playing with a littermate.

Physical Examination: Blood from nares; pale mucous membranes; blood in left eye.

Problem List: 1. Epistaxis. 2. Hyphemia. 3. Anemia.

Hematology	
↓ **Hemoglobin (g/dL)**	**5.7 (3.54 mmol/L)**
↓ **PCV (%)**	**17 (0.17 volume fraction)**
MCV (fL)	65.4
MCHC (g/dL)	33.5 (20.8 mmol/L)
Reticulocytes (%)	0.1 (0.01 number fraction)
NRBC/100 WBC	0
RBC morphology	Normal
↑ **WBC × 10³/μL**	**24.3 (24.3 × 10⁹/L)**
Myelocytes/μL	0 (0 × 10⁹/L)
Metamyelocytes/μL	0 (0 × 10⁹/L)
Band neutrophils/μL	118 (0.12 × 10⁹/L)
↑ **Segmented neutrophils/μL**	**23,147 (23.1 × 10⁹/L)**
↓ **Lymphocytes/μL**	**705 (0.71 × 10⁹/L)**
Monocytes/μL	470 (0.47 × 10⁹/L)
↓ **Eosinophils/μL**	**0 (0 × 10⁹/L)**
Basophils/μL	0 (0 × 10⁹/L)
Toxic neutrophils	None
Platelets × 10³/μL	350 (0.35 × 10¹²/L)
↓ **Plasma protein (g/dL)**	**3.6 (36 g/L)**
Fibrinogen (mg/dL)	250 (2.5 g/L)

Coagulation Tests	Patient	Control
PT (sec)	7.3	7.5
↑ **APTT (sec)**	**48.3**	15.2
TCT (sec)	7.1	7.0

HEMOGRAM

There is a normocytic normochromic nonregenerative anemia. Blood loss is suspected as the cause of the anemia based on the history as well as the low plasma protein. If the blood loss is of short duration, as indicated by the history, an erythrocyte regeneration response would not be expected.

There is a leukocytosis, mature neutrophilia, lymphopenia, and eosinopenia compatible with a "stress leukogram."

COAGULATION PROFILE

The prolonged APTT with normal prothrombin and thrombin times and adequate fibrinogen indicates a coagulation factor deficiency in the intrinsic pathway which contains coagulation factors VIII, IX, XI, and XII. In a male with bleeding history, hemophilia is most likely. Hemophilia A (factor VIII:C deficiency) and hemophilia B (factor IX deficiency) are the most common. Factor X or XI deficiency could also present this pattern in either sex but is rare. For further identification of the specific factor deficiency blood needs to be sent to the appropriate laboratory for analysis.

DIAGNOSIS

Congenital coagulopathy (hemophilia).

Patient: Dog, English pointer, female, 5 years old.

Presenting Signs and Complaints: Enlarged mammary glands on left side; bleeding from the nose for the last 10 days.

Physical Examination and Problem List: 1. Subcutaneous fluid along right ventral anterior abdomen and thorax. 2. Mass (3 cm) in right posterior mammary gland. 3. Dark thick purulent material from abscess in middle left mammary gland. 4. Epistaxis.

Hematology		Serum Chemistry	
↓ RBC × 10⁶/µL	3.1 (3.1 × 10¹²/L)	↑ AST (SGOT) (IU/L)	342 (342 U/L)
↓ Hemoglobin (g/dL)	6.5 (4.0 mmol/L)	ALT (SGPT) (IU/L)	88 (88 U/L)
↓ PCV (%)	19 (0.19 volume fraction)	↑ ALP (IU/L)	480 (480 U/L)
MCV (fL)	61.3	GGT (IU/L)	3 (3 U/L)
MCHC (g/dL)	34.2 (21.2 mmol/L)	Total bilirubin (mg/dL)	0.2 (3.4 µmol/L)
↑ Reticulocytes (%)	8 (0.08 number fraction)	Conjugated bilirubin (mg/dL)	0.1 (1.7 µmol/L)
↑ Corrected Reticulocytes (%)	3.4 (0.034 number fraction)	Unconjugated bilirubin (mg/dL)	0.1 (1.7 µmol/L)
↑ Reticulocytes/µL	248,000 (248 × 10⁹/L)	Total protein (g/dL)	6.3 (63 g/L)
↑ NRBC/100 WBC	7	Albumin (g/dL)	2.5 (25 g/L)
RBC morphology		Globulin (g/dL)	3.8 (38 g/L)
↑ Polychromasia	2+	Cholesterol (mg/dL)	165 (4.3 mmol/L)
↑ Anisocytosis	3+	Urea nitrogen (mg/dL)	21 (7.5 mmol/L)
↑ Poikilocytosis	2+Fragmentation	Creatinine (mg/dL)	1.1 (97.2 µmol/L)
↑ WBC × 10³/µL	46.1 (46.1 × 10⁹/L)	Glucose (mg/dL)	98 (5.4 mmol/L)
↑ Myelocytes/µL	460 (0.46 × 10⁹/L)	Amylase (IU/L)	1250 (1250 U/L)
↑ Metamyelocyte/µL	1,380 (1.4 × 10⁹/L)	Lipase (IU/L)	75 (75 U/L)
↑ Band neutrophils/µL	10,140 (10.1 × 10⁹/L)	Sodium (mEq/L)	148 (148 mmol/L)
↑ Segmented neutrophils/µL	26,740 (267 × 10⁹/L)	Potassium (mEq/L)	4.1 (4.1 mmol/L)
Lymphocytes/µL	5,070 (5.0 × 10⁹/L)	Na : K ratio	36.1
↑ Monocytes/µL	1,840 (1.8 × 10⁹/L)	Chloride (mEq/L)	102 (102 mmol/L)
Eosinophils/µL	460 (0.46 × 10⁹/L)	Carbon dioxide (mEq/L)	23 (23 mmol/L)
Basophils/µL	0 (0 × 10⁹/L)	Calcium (mg/dL)	8.7 (2.18 mmol/L)
↑ Toxic neutrophils	2+	Phosphorus (mg/dL)	4.2 (1.4 mmol/L)
↓ Platelet × 10³/µL	15 (0.15 × 10¹²/L)	↓ Serum iron (µg/dL)	63 (11.3 µmol/L)
Plasma protein (g/dL)	6.3 (63 g/L)		
Coagulation tests	Patient/Control		
PT (sec)	13/8.6		
↑ APTT (sec)	No clot/16.5		
↑ TCT (sec)	>60/6.9		
↑ Fibrinogen (mg/dL)	<50/350		
↑ FSPᵃ	+1 : 40/Negative		

ᵃ Fibrin split products.

Urinalysis	
Appearance	Clear, yellow
Specific gravity	1.038
pH	6.5
Protein	Negative
Glucose	Negative
Ketones	Negative
Blood	Negative
Bilirubin	Negative
Sediment	
WBC/hpf	0–2
RBC/hpf	3–5
Casts	Negative
Crystals	Negative
Bacteria	Negative

HEMOGRAM

There is a normocytic normochromic anemia with mild polychromasia and reticulocytosis. With evidence of mild regeneration one would expect the MCV to be increased or in the high normal range. The presence of a low normal MCV suggests that there has been some chronic iron loss impairing the bone marrow response to anemia. This is supported by the low serum iron concentration. Poikilocytes of a variety of forms including fragmentation were observed, suggestive of a microangiopathic process. There is a leukocytosis and neutrophilia with an appropriate left shift to myelocytes, indicating an intense response to an inflammatory process, most likely the presence of a bacterial component. The toxic morphologic changes to the neutrophils support a bacterial component to the inflammatory process.

There is a marked thrombocytopenia with all coagulation parameters abnormal. The constellation of fragmentation, thrombocytopenia, and abnormal PT, APTT, TCT, and hypofibrinogenemia suggest DIC. The positive test for fibrin split products is further evidence of DIC.

BIOCHEMICAL PROFILE

The elevation in AST with a normal ALT suggests muscle damage. A creatine kinase assay can be used to confirm.

The increased serum alkaline phosphatase (SAP) may be stress induced or reflect metastatic disease of liver or bone. The normal GGT (with increased SAP) suggests that a search for a nonhepatic lesion involving the bone should be undertaken because the liver contains both GGT and ALP, but bone only contains ALP and does not have GGT. Radiographs were taken and metastatic disease in the pulmonary area as well as multiple lytic lesions in the bone were observed.

DIAGNOSIS

DIC secondary to mammary adenocarcinoma with metastasis to bone.

Patient: Dog, basset hound, male, 1 year old.

Presenting Signs and Complaints: Whole body tremors; excessive bleeding noted between 4 and 6 months of age when teething, vitamin K injections were given; bled excessively from a small cut on left front foot 2 days prior to referral.

Physical Examination: Apparently healthy dog with a wrap around the left front foot to protect the cut. When the bandage was removed the wound began to seep blood.

Problem List: 1. Prolonged bleeding. 2. Whole body tremors.

Hematology	
RBC × 10⁶/µl	8.16 (8.16 × 10^{12}/L)
↑ **Hemoglobin (g/dL)**	**20.4 (12.7 mmol/L)**
↑ **PCV (%)**	**54.3 (0.54 volume fraction)**
MCV (fL)	67
MCHC (g/dL)	37 (22.9 mmol/L)
NRBC/100 WBC	0
RBC morphology	Normal
WBC × 10³/µl	15.0 (15 × 10^9/L)
Myelocytes/µL	0
Metamyelocytes/µL	0
Bands neutrophils/µL	150 (0.15 × 10^9/L)
Segmented neutrophils/µl	10,350 (10.4 × 10^9/L)
Lymphocytes/µL	3,000 (3.0 × 10^9/L)
Monocytes/µL	1,500 (1.5 × 10^9/L)
Eosinophils/µL	0 (0 × 10^9/L)
Basophils/µL	0 (0 × 10^9/L)
Toxic neutrophils	None
Platelets × 10³/µL	394 (0.394 × 10^{12}/L)
Coagulation tests	
↑ **Bleeding time (min)**	**>12**
PT (sec)	6.7/6.9
APTT (sec)	12.0/11.7
Factor VIII-related antigen (%)	80
Fibrinogen (mg/dL)	300 (3 g/L)
Plasma proteins (g/dL)	7.6 (76 g/L)

Table continued on following page

Serum Chemistry	
AST (SGOT) (IU/L)	54 (54 U/L)
ALT (SGPT) (IU/L)	58 (58 U/L)
ALP (IU/L)	63 (63 U/L)
Total protein (g/dL)	7.7 (77 g/L)
↑ **Albumin (g/dL)**	**4.5 (45 g/L)**
Globulin (g/dL)	3.2 (32 g/L)
Glucose (mg/dL)	125 (6.9 mmol/L)
Urea nitrogen (mg/dL)	28 (10 mmol/L)
Creatinine (mg/dL)	0.8 (70.7 μmol/L)
Calcium (mg/dL)	11.2 (2.8 mmol/L)
Phosphorus (mg/dL)	10.2 (3.3 mmol/L)
Sodium (mEq/L)	152 (152 mmol/L)
Potassium (mEq/L)	4.9 (4.9 mmol/L)
Na : K ratio	31
Chloride (mEq/L)	116 (116 mmol/L)
Total carbon dioxide (mEq/L)	18 (18 mmol/L)
Cholinesterase (IU/L)	1,332 (1,332 U/L)
Total resting T_3 (ng/dL)	174 (2.7 nm/L)
Total resting T_4 (μg/dL)	3.8 (48.9 nmol/L)

HEMOGRAM

Examination of the hemogram indicated a slight increase in the packed cell volume which may be caused by dehydration. The slight increase in serum albumin corroborates the presence of some dehydration.

The hemogram and biochemical profile are unusually unremarkable in a patient that has a history of bleeding diatheses. The platelet count and coagulation tests are normal as is the test for factor VIII-related antigen, which would rule out von Willebrand's disease. Platelet function is often abnormal in dogs with von Willebrand's disease. These findings would suggest a thrombasthenia, which is a platelet aggregation problem.

The bleeding diathesis was most likely secondary to a platelet function problem because the platelet count is normal, and there is no evidence of a coagulation factor deficiency even though bleeding began at an early age; therefore we must concentrate on more uncommon platelet function defects by conducting a platelet aggregation test.

Results of the platelet aggregation test were abnormal and the findings compatible with defective contact activation of platelets which has been reported in the basset hound.

DIAGNOSIS

Hereditary thrombocytopathy of basset hounds.

COMMENT

In patients with bleeding disorders, normal coagulation parameters, and normal platelet numbers the history should be examined for any drugs the patient may be taking, especially questions regarding any prostaglandin inhibitors such as aspirin.

Patient: Dog, Doberman pinscher, male, 3 years old.

Presenting Signs and Complaints: August 23, history of recurrent hemorrhages as evidenced by epistaxis and petechiation of the mucous membranes. On July 4, cut a foot and lost approximately a pint of blood before hemorrhage was controlled.

Physical Examination: Blood coming from nostrils; small hemorrhages on membranes and abdomen; laceration on left from footpad.

Problem List: 1. Epistaxis. 2. Petechiation of mucous membranes. 3. Lacerated footpad.

Hematology	July 4[a]	July 7	July 11
↓ RBC × 10⁶/μL	2.39 (2.39 × 10¹²/L)	↓ 2.4 (2.4 × 10¹²/L)	↓ 3.6 (3.6 × 10¹²/L)
↓ Hemoglobin (g/dL)	5.6 (3.47 mmol/L)	↓ 6.1 (3.79 mmol/L)	↓ 8.7 (5.4 mmol/L)
↓ PCV (%)	16 (0.16 volume fraction)	↓ 18.3 (0.18 volume fraction)	↓ 28.5 (0.29 volume fraction)
MCV (fL)	66.9	↑ 76.3	↑ 79.1
MCHC (g/dL)	35 (21.7 mmol/L)	33.3 (20.7 mmol/L)	↓ 30.5 (18.9 mmol/L)
↑ Reticulocytes (%)	2 (0.02 number fraction)	8 ↑ (0.08 number fraction)	↑ 8 (0.08 number fraction)
Corrected reticulocyte (%)	0.8 (0.008 number fraction)	↑ 3.2 (0.032 number fraction)	↑ 5.1 (0.051 number fraction)
Reticulocytes × 10³/μL	48 (48 × 10⁹/L)	↑ (216 × 10⁹/L)	↑ 288 (288 × 10⁹/L)
NRBC/100 WBC	0	0	0
Erythrocyte morphology	Normal		
Polychromasia	None	+	↑ 2+
Anisocytosis	None	+	↑ 2+
WBC × 10³/μL	13.8 (13.8 × 10⁹/L)	15.6 (15.6 × 10⁹/L)	
Myelocytes/μL	0 (0 × 10⁹/L)	0 (0 × 10⁹/L)	
Metamyelocytes/μL	0 (0 × 10⁹/L)	0 (0 × 10⁹/L)	
Band neutrophils/μL	276 (0.276 × 10⁹/L)	0 (0 × 10⁹/L)	
Segmented neutrophils/μL	9,800 (9.8 × 10⁹/L)	12,948 (12.9 × 10⁹/L)	
Lymphocytes/μL	3,724 (3.7 × 10⁹/L)	936 (0.94 × 10⁹/L)	
Monocytes/μL	0 (0 × 10⁹/L)	1,716 (1.72 × 10⁹/L)	
Eosinophils/μL	0 (0 × 10⁹/L)	0 (0 × 10⁹/L)	
Basophils/μL)	0 (0 × 10⁹/L)	0 (0 × 10⁹/L)	
Toxic neutrophils	None	None	
↓ Platelet × 10³/μL	7.0 (0.07 × 10¹²/L)	↓ 75[b] (0.075 × 10¹²/L)	425 (0.425 × 10¹²/L)
Coagulation tests			
PT	6.4		
APTT	15.7		
TCT	8.6		
Fibrinogen (mg/dL)	300 (3 g/L)	200 (2 g/L)	200 (2 g/L)
Plasma protein (g/dL)	5.8 (58 g/L)	5.1 (51 g/L)	5.8 (58 g/L)
von Willebrand factor (%)	126		
↑ Antiplatelet factor 3 antibody	Positive		

[a] Patient was treated with one dose of vincristine intravenously and oral corticosteroids.
[b] Large forms of platelets present.

HEMOGRAM

On admission there was a normocytic normochromic nonregenerative anemia that reflected the acute blood loss. The decreased plasma protein along with the low PCV supports blood loss. By July 11 the anemia was regenerative. A regenerative response to blood loss anemias is not as great as with hemolytic processes. There was a reticulocyte response by July 7 which persisted through July 11. Note that the corrected reticulocyte per cent and absolute reticulocyte count are better indicators of a regenerative response to anemia than the reticulocyte per cent alone.

The presence of antiplatelet antibodies supports an immune mediated thrombocytopenia. The platelet factor 3 release test is extremely difficult to complete, and because results are frequently equivocal it is seldom used today. An ELISA method for detecting antibodies to platelets have been developed and used successfully in research laboratories. Response to treatment is frequently used to support the diagnosis.

DIAGNOSIS

Immune mediated thrombocytopenia.

Patient: Dog Doberman pinscher, male, 2 years old.

Presenting Signs and Complaints: Owner reported that the dog was lethargic, drank a lot of water, had red colored urine, occasional dark colored stools, and a decreased appetite.

Physical Examination: Thin, yellow mucous membranes; dog passed red urine in examination room.

Problem List: 1. Icterus. 2. Hematuria. 3. Lethargy.

Hematology		Serum Chemistry	
RBC × 10⁶/μL	6.8 (6.8 × 10¹²/L)	AST (SGOT) (IU/L)	85 (85 U/L)
Hemoglobin (g/dL)	14.5 (8.99 mmol/L)	↑ ALT (SGPT) (IU/L)	149 (149 U/L)
PCV (%)	46 (0.46 volume fraction)	↑ ALP (IU/L)	2,043 (2,043 U/L)
MCV (fL)	67.6	↑ GGT (IU/L)	116 (116 U/L)
MCHC (g/dL)	31.5 (19.5 mmol/L)	↑ Total bilirubin (mg/dL)	5 (85.5 μmol/L)
Reticulocytes (%)	0.4 (0.04 number fraction)	↑ Conjugated bilirubin (mg/dL)	0.7 (12.0 μmol/L)
Reticulocytes/μL	27,200 (27.2 × 10⁹/L)	Total protein (g/dL)	6.6 (66 g/L)
RBC morphology	Normal	Albumin (g/dL)	3.1 (31 g/L)
WBC × 10³/μL	16.8 (16.8 × 10⁹/L)	Globulin (g/dL)	3.5 (35 g/L)
		Amylase (IU/L)	750 (750 U/L)
Myelocytes/μL	0 (0 × 10⁹/L)	Lipase (IU/L)	75 (75 U/L)
Metamyelocytes/μL	0 (0 × 10⁹/L)	Glucose (mg/dL)	118 (6.5 mmol/L)
↑ Band neutrophils/μL	504 (0.5 × 10⁹/L)	Urea nitrogen (mg/dL)	22 (7.9 mmol/L)
↑ Segmented neutrophils/μL	15,456 (15.5 × 10⁹/L)	Creatine (mg/dL)	1 (88.4 μmol/L)
↓ Lymphocyte × 10³/μL	504 (0.5 × 10⁹/L)	Calcium (mg/dL)	9.6 (2.4 mmol/L)
Monocytes × 10³/μL	336 (0.3 × 10⁹/L)	Phosphorus (mg/dL)	3.7 (1.2 mmol/L)
↓ Eosinophils × 10³/μL	0 (0 × 10⁹/L)	Sodium (mEq/L)	137 (137 mmol/L)
Basophils × 10³/μL	0 (0 × 10⁹/L)	Potassium (mEq/L)	5.3 (5.3 mmol/L)
Toxic neutrophils	None	Chloride (mEq/L)	106 (106 mmol/L)
Coagulation tests		Carbon dioxide (mEq/L)	21 (21 mmol/L)
PT (sec)	7.5	LDH (IU/L)	676 (676 U/L)
APTT (sec)	11.6	Creatine kinase (IU/L)	158 (158 U/L)
TCT	8.3	↓ Total T₃ (ng/dL)	50 (0.77 nmol/L)
Platelets × 10³μL	227 (0.227 × 10¹²/L)	↓ Total T₄ (mg/dL)	0.5 (6.44 nmol/L)
Fibrinogen (mg/dL)	400 (4 g/L)	↓ Free T₄ (ng/dL)	0.32 (25.3 pmol/L)
↓ Factor VIII-related antigen	<7%	↑ Cholesterol (mg/dL)	345 (8.97 mmol/L)
↑ Bleeding time (min)	9		
↑ Fecal occult blood	Positive		

Urinalysis (Cystocentesis)	
Appearance	Opaque, red
Specific gravity	1.063
pH	6.0
↑ Protein	3+
Glucose	Negative
Ketones	Negative
↑ Blood	4+
↑ Bilirubin	3+
Sediment	
↑ WBC/hpf	TNTC
↑ RBC/hpf	TNTC
Casts	None
↑ Bacteria	4+

HEMOGRAM

Neutrophilia with a left shift indicates an active inflammation. Lymphopenia and eosinopenia suggest the possibility of increased glucocorticoid activity.

URINALYSIS

The pyuria, hematuria, and bactiuria suggest infection and inflammation of the urinary tract. The type of infection is best determined by a pretreatment urine culture and antibiotic sensitivity (MIC) on urine collected by cystocentesis.

BIOCHEMICAL PROFILE

Patient has a severe (penetrant) form of the von Willebrand's disease gene and is either an affected (bleeder) or carrier (asymptomatic) heterozygote. There is platelet dysfunction in dogs with von Willebrand's disease although the platelet count is normal. This may be a contributing factor to the hematuria, intestinal hemorrhage, and prolonged bleeding time in this patient.

Hyperbilirubinemia with a normal packed cell volume indicates the presence of a hepatobiliary disorder. The marked increased serum activity of alkaline phosphatase and GGT with no history of steroid therapy and the hyperbilirubinemia denote a cholestatic disorder, either intrahepatic or extrahepatic. The slight increase in ALT indicates hepatocellular membrane leakage. Because of the severe hemostatic problems in this patient, noninvasive methods should be tried initially to differentiate the cause of the cholestasis. Ultrasonography of the hepatobiliary tree may help differentiate intrahepatic from extrahepatic cholestasis in some patients. Cholangitis/cholangiohepatitis should be considered especially in light of the inflammatory leukogram. A liver biopsy would be useful to confirm this suspicion. After a fresh blood transfusion (collected in plastic to preserve functional platelets) liver tissue may be obtained judiciously. The patient should be monitored carefully for postbiopsy hemorrhage complications. The decision to obtain liver tissue to direct therapy as well as indicate prognosis should be individualized for each patient. In some cases, including this one, the owner should be informed of the dangers, and the use of antibiotics for 2 to 3 weeks may be an appropriate alternative. Thyroid replacement during this period would also be important because the thyroid hormone does play a role in the hepatobiliary excretory process. This case is complicated further by the fact that the Doberman breed is predisposed to chronic liver disease. Because total bilirubin is increased there is no necessity to run a more sensitive liver function test such as BSP or bile acids.

Hypercholesterolemia and low total T_3 and T_4 with a concomitantly low free T_4 support hypothyroidism. Hypothyroidism occurs frequently in dogs with von Willebrand's disease. Platelet function is decreased in such dogs and is often corrected by the administration of thyroid to affected animals.

DIAGNOSIS

von Willebrand's disease with secondary platelet dysfunction and cholestatic liver disease.

COMMENT

The patient was treated with a broad spectrum antibiotic and thyroid supplementation. At the end of 2 weeks the bilirubin had returned to normal, and the alkaline phosphatase and GGT had decreased suggesting a response to therapy. At the end of a month the liver tests were normal, and the dog was clinically normal.

Patient: Dog, beagle, neutered male, 9 years old.

Presenting Signs and Complaints: Inappetent and listless.

Physical Examination: Thin; lethargic; enlarged prescapular and popliteal lymph nodes; abdomen distended, and liver seems large on palpation; skin dry; radiography revealed fluid in abdomen and an asymmetrically enlarged liver, the right lobe being the larger.

Ultrasonography: A mass with variable echogenecity with hypoechoic areas.

Problem List: 1. Lymphadenopathy. 2. Hepatomegaly. 3. Ascites. 4. Dry scaly skin. 5. Anorexia. 6. Lethargy.

Hematology		Serum Chemistry	
RBC × 10⁶/µL	5.45 (5.45 × 10¹²/L)	AST (SGOT) (IU/L)	42 (42 U/L)
Hemoglobin (g/dL)	13.9 (8.6 mmol/L)	↑ ALT (SGPT) (IU/L)	134 (134 U/L)
PCV (%)	38 (0.38 volume fraction)	↑ ALP (IU/L)	2,266 (2,266 U/L)
MCV (fL)	69	Total bilirubin (mg/dL)	0.5 (8.6 µmol/L)
MCHC (g/dL)	36 (22.3 mmol/L)	↑ Cholesterol (mg/dL)	387 (10.1 mmol/L)
Reticulocytes (%)	Not done	Total protein (g/dL)	8.1 (81 g/L)
NRBC/100 WBC	0	↓ Albumin (g/dL)	2.2 (22 g/L)
RBC morphology	Normal	Globulin (g/dL)	5.9 (59 g/L)
↑ WBC × 10³/µL	45.1 (45.1 × 10⁹/L)	Glucose (mg/dL)	111 (6.1 mmol/L)
Myelocytes/µL	0 (0 × 10⁹/L)	Urea nitrogen (mg/dL)	25 (8.9 mol/L)
Metamyelocytes/µL	0 (0 × 10⁹/L)	Creatinine (mg/dL)	1.0 (88.4 µmol/L)
↑ Band neutrophils/µL	1,353 (1.4 × 10⁹/L)	Calcium (mg/dL)	9.6 (2.4 mmol/L)
↑ Segmented neutrophils/µL	38,335 (38.3 × 10⁹/L)	Corrected calcium (mg/dL)	10.9 (2.7 mmol/L)
↓ Lymphocytes/µL	902 (0.9 × 10⁹/L)	Phosphorus (mg/dL)	5.2 (1.68 mmol/L)
↑ Monocytes/µL	4,059 (4.1 × 10⁹/L)	Sodium (mEq/L)	143 (143 mmol/L)
Eosinophils/µL	451 (0.45 × 10⁹/L)	Potassium (mEq/L)	4.3 (4.3 mmol/L)
Basophils/µL	0 (0 × 10⁹/L)	Na : K ratio	33.3
↑ Toxic neutrophils	2+	Chloride (mEq/L)	115 (115 mmol/L)
Platelet estimate	Adequate	↓ Carbon dioxide (mEq/L)	12 (12 mmol/L)
Fibrinogen (mg/dL)	300	LDH (IU/L)	171 (171 U/L)
Plasma proteins (g/dL)	8.3		
Coagulation tests	Patient/Control		
PT (sec)	8.2/8.5		
APTT (sec)	13.5/13.7		
TCT (sec)	7.2/7.3		

Urinalysis (Cystocentesis)	
Appearance	Clear, yellow
Specific gravity	1.047
pH	7.0
Protein	Negative
Glucose	Negative
Ketones	Negative
Blood	Negative

Table continued on following page

Urinalysis (Cystocentesis) *Continued*	
↑ **Bilirubin**	2+
Sediment	
WBC/hpf	0–1
RBC/hpf	0–1
Casts	None
Crystals	Occasional struvite
Bacteria	Negative

HEMOGRAM

The leukocytosis, which is comprised of a neutrophilia, and a left shift to bands, suggest an active inflammatory response. Toxic neutrophils further support an inflammatory response and imply a bacterial etiology. Fibrinogen is a reflection of an inflammatory response; however, in the carnivorous species the neutrophil response is a more sensitive reflection of a response to inflammation than is an increased in fibrinogen concentration (see the section on fibrinogen in Chapter 3). The lymphopenia and monocytosis are most likely associated with stress that accompanies the inflammatory process.

BIOCHEMICAL PROFILE

There is a slight increase in ALT, indicating hepatocellular membrane leakage. A marked increase in alkaline phosphatase is indicative of cholestasis or enzyme induction secondary to glucocorticoid increase. The liver tests taken together do not indicate whether there is a primary or secondary hepatic disorder. There is a hyperproteinemia with a hypoalbuminemia and hyperglobulinemia. The decrease in albumin concentration may be the result of down-regulation of albumin production by the liver secondary to hyperglobulinemia, although end-stage liver related to decreased albumin production cannot be ruled out. This is based on the fact that the patient does not have clinical evidence of a protein-losing enteropathy and no proteinuria. The hyperglobulinemia could be monoclonal or polyclonal. Because of the inflammatory picture presented on the leukogram, one can speculate that this is a polyclonal hyperglobulinemia associated with an inflammatory response.

Hyperbilirubinuria is suggestive of a cholestatic process attendant to the increased alkaline phosphatase activity. Bilirubin appears in the urine before there is an increase in the peripheral blood.

The overall picture is suggestive of an inflammatory process within the mass of the liver. Additional liver function tests are not indicated in this case because we know there is liver involvement. A surgical approach for diagnostic purposes is indicated.

DIAGNOSIS

Because coagulation tests were normal, surgery was done; liver biopsy revealed a hepatoma with small abscesses within the tumor mass.

Patient: Horse, Paso Fino, female, 6 years old.

Presenting Signs and Complaints: Diarrhea and lack of appetite. Two weeks prior to admission mare (7 months pregnant) was shipped from Dominican Republic. While in quarantine was noted to be anorectic and sore in all four limbs. Referring veterinarian diagnosed laminitis and treated animal with phenylbutazone. She developed a diarrhea and was treated with bismuth subsalicylate, mineral oil, and antibiotics with no improvement.

Physical Examination: Obese; walks hesitantly; has ridges on hoof walls of forefeet; profuse watery stool; 10% dehydration.

Problem List: 1. Diarrhea. 2. Overweight. 3. Moderately dehydrated. 4. Sore feet. 5. Prominent ridges on hoof walls of forefeet.

Hematology		Serum Chemistry[a]	
RBC × 10⁶/µL	6.94 (6.94 × 10¹²/L)	↑ AST (SGOT) (IU/L)	2,370 (2,370 U/L)
Hemoglobin (g/dL)	14.1 (8.75 mmol/L)	↑ ALP (IU/L)	1,380 (1,380 U/L)
PCV (%)	38 (0.38 volume fraction)	↑ GGT (IU/L)	29 (29 U/L)
MCV (fL)	55	↑Total bilirubin (mg/dL)	2.5 (42.8 µmol/L)
MCHC (g/dL)	37 (22.9 mmol/L)	↑ Conjugated bilirubin (mg/dL)	1.3 (22.2 µmol/L)
NRBC/100 WBC	0	Unconjugated bilirubin (mg/dL)	1.2 (20.6 µmol/L)
RBC morphology	Normal	↑ Triglycerides (mg/dL)	1,175 (12.93 µmol/L)
WBC × 10³/µL	17.2 (17.2 × 10⁹/L)	Total protein (g/dL)	6.0 (60 g/L)
		Albumin (g/dL)	2.7 (27 g/L)
Myelocytes/µL	0 (0 × 10⁹/L)	Globulin (g/dL)	3.3 (33 g/L)
Metamyelocytes/µL	0 (0 × 10⁹/L)	Glucose (mg/dL)	105 (5.8 mmol/L)
↑ Band neutrophils/µL	200 (0.2 × 10⁹/L)	↑ Urea nitrogen (mg/dL)	32 (11.4 mmol/L)
↑ Segmented neutro- phils/µL	11,300 (11.3 × 10⁹/L)	↑ Creatinine (mg/dL)	2.7 (238.7 µmol/L)
Lymphocytes/µL	4,700 (4.7 × 10⁹/L)	Calcium (mg/dL)	10.8 (2.7 mmol/L)
Monocytes/µL	800 (0.8 × 10⁹/L)	Phosphorus (mg/dL)	3.7 (1.2 mmol/L)
Eosinophils/µL	200 (0.2 × 10⁹/L)	↓ Sodium (mEq/L)	128 (128 mmol/L)
Basophils/µL	0 (0 × 10⁹/L)	↓ Potassium (mEq/L)	2.2 (2.2 mmol/L)
Toxic neutrophils	Doehle bodies	Na : K ratio	58.1
Platelets	Adequate	Chloride (mEq/L)	102 (102 mmol/L)
Plasma protein (g/dL)	6.9 (69 g/L)	Carbon dioxide (mEq/L)	18.4 (18.4 mmol/L)
↑ Fibrinogen (mg/dL)	800 (8 g/L)	Creatine kinase (IU/L)	250 (250 U/L)
Fecal culture	Salmonella (group B)		

[a] Turbid serum (lipemia).

Urinalysis (Catheter)	
Appearance	Cloudy, yellow
Specific gravity	1.031
pH	7.0
Protein	Negative
Glucose	Negative
Ketones	Negative
Blood	Negative

Table continued on following page

Urinalysis (Catheter) *Continued*	
↑ **Bilirubin**	3+
Sediment	
WBC/hpf	0–1
RBC/hpf	0–2
Casts	None seen
Crystals	Amorphous PO_4
Bacteria	None seen

HEMOGRAM

There is a mature neutrophilia with a slight left shift and a hyperfibrinogenemia denoting active inflammation. Hyperfibrinogenemia in the equine and ruminant species is a sensitive indicator of inflammation. These findings are consistent with inflammation. Döehle bodies in neutrophils are an indication of a systemic toxic process, either endotoxin or bacterial related. The inflammatory process is probably related to the *Salmonella* infection.

BIOCHEMICAL PROFILE

The hyperbilirubinemia and bilirubinuria along with a normal packed cell volume indicate a cholestatic process. The conjugated bilirubin is 52% of the total, and, in the equine, values greater than 25 to 30% suggest extrahepatic bile duct obstruction.

The increase in alkaline phosphatase and GGT activities also support a cholestatic process. In the equine, GGT may be increased secondary to enzyme leakage from the hepatobiliary system secondary to inflammation. The marked increase in AST activity with no increase in the creatinine kinase is consistent with enzyme leakage from hepatocytes. The increase in all liver enzymes confirms a hepatobiliary disorder.

Lipemia was accompanied by a marked increase in the triglyceride concentration, which was probably secondary to decreased hepatic lipoprotein synthesis and rapid fat mobilization from adipose tissue. The slight increase in urea nitrogen and creatinine is prerenal and related to the dehydration.

Electrolyte abnormalities (low potassium, low sodium) are probably a result of intestinal loss accompanying the diarrhea. Low sodium and potassium concentrations may also occur in lipemic patients if flame photometry is used for the assay.

The abnormal laboratory results support the presence of cholestasis, which may be either intrahepatic or extrahepatic. The history along with the presence of lipemia suggests the possibility of hepatic lipidosis, which can be confirmed by a liver biopsy. Coagulation parameters were assessed and found to be normal; a liver biopsy resulted in a histologic diagnosis of hepatic lipidosis. Had this been an extrahepatic process (as suggested by the bilirubins), the liver biopsy would have had findings suggestive of that process and appropriate diagnostic efforts could be pursued.

DIAGNOSIS

Hepatic lipidosis confirmed by liver biopsy.

Patient: Bovine, Holstein, female, 8 years old.

Presenting Signs and Complaints: Inappetent, and milk production decreased.

Physical Examination: Thin, yellow mucous membranes; poor rumen motility.

Problem List: 1. Rumen atony. 2. Icterus. 3. Weight loss.

Hematology		Serum Chemistry	
RBC × 10⁶/μL	8.8 (8.8 × 10¹²/L)	↑ **AST (SGOT) (IU/L)**	**525 (525 U/L)**
Hemoglobin (g/dL)	9.9 (6.14 mmol/L)	ALT (SGPT) (IU/L)	16.9 (16.9 U/L)
PCV (%)	27.5 (0.275 volume fraction)	ALP (IU/L)	36 (36 U/L)
MCV (fL)	45	↑ **GGT (IU/L)**	**25 (25 U/L)**
MCHC (g/dL)	37.4 (23.2 mmol/L)	↑ **Total bilirubin (mg/dL)**	**1.5 (25.6 μmol/L)**
NRBC/100 WBC	0	↑ **Conjugated bilirubin (mg/dL)**	**0.1 (1.7 μmol/L)**
Erythrocyte morphology	Normal	↑ **Unconjugated bilirubin (mg/dL)**	**1.4 (23.9 μmol/L)**
WBC × 10³/μL	8.8 (8.8 × 10⁹/L	↑ **Total protein (g/dL)**	**9.8 (98 g/L)**
Myelocytes/μL	0 (0 × 10⁹/L)	Albumin (g/dL)	3.7 (37 g/L)
Metamyelocytes/μL	0 (0 × 10⁹/L)	↑ **Globulin (g/dL)**	**6.1 (61 g/L)**
Band neutrophils/μL	0 (0 × 10⁹/L)	Cholesterol (mg/dL)	115 (2.99 mmol/L)
↑ **Segmented neutro-phils/μL**	**6,690 (6.69 × 10⁹/L)**	Urea nitrogen (mg/dL)	23 (8.2 mmol/L)
↓ **Lymphocytes/μL**	**1,760 (1.8 × 10⁹/L)**	Creatinine (mg/dL)	0.7 (61.9 μmol/L)
Monocytes/μL	0 (0 × 10⁹/L)	Glucose (mg/dL)	108 (5.94 mmol/L)
Eosinophils/μL	350 (0.35 × 10⁹/L)	Creatine kinase (IU/L)	55 (55 U/L)
Basophils/μL	0 (0 × 10⁹/L)	Sodium (mEq/L)	141 (141 mmol/L)
Toxic neutrophils	None seen	Potassium (mEq/L)	3.6 (3.6 mmol/L)
Platelet estimate	Adequate	Chloride (mEq/L)	111 (111 mmol/L)
↑ **Plasma protein (g/dL)**	**10.9 (109 g/L)**	Carbon dioxide (mEq/L)	18 (18 mmol/L)
↑ **Fibrinogen (mg/dL)**	**900 (9 g/L)**	Calcium (mg/dL)	9.8 (2.5 mmol/L)
		Phosphorus (mg/dL)	3.6 (1.16 mmol/L)

Urinalysis (Voided Sample)	
Appearance	Cloudy, yellow
↓ **Specific gravity**	**1.019**
pH	8.0
Protein	Negative
Glucose	Negative
Ketones	Negative
Blood	Negative
Bilirubin	Trace
Sediment	
↑ **WBC/hpf**	**10–15**
RBC/hpf	1–3
Casts	Negative
Crystals	Negative
↑ **Bacteria**	**3+**

HEMOGRAM

There is a neutrophilia, lymphopenia, and hyperfibrinogenemia indicative of an active inflammatory process. Fibrinogen is a sensitive indicator of inflammation in the bovine species.

BIOCHEMICAL PROFILE

Examination of the biochemical profile reveals increased AST suggestive of enzyme leakage from the liver or skeletal muscle. Hepatocellular damage is most likely the culprit as creatine kinase (a muscle enzyme) is normal. Because ALT concentration is low in the liver of ruminants it is of no value in assessing hepatocellular damage. The alkaline phosphatase is normal, however it has a low sensitivity for detecting liver disease in the ruminant. The GGT is increased. GGT is better than alkaline phosphatase as an indicator of cholestasis in ruminants. Hyperbilirubinemia, most of which is unconjugated, with a normal packed cell volume supports liver disease. There is little increase in conjugated bilirubin in the ruminant species in association with liver disease. The hyperproteinemia is caused by hyperglobulinemia which is probably the result of increased globulin production secondary to the inflammatory process and suggests chronicity.

The pyuria and bactiuria are probably caused by the collection method as opposed to bacterial cystitis since there is no hematuria or proteinuria.

DIAGNOSIS

Hepatic necrosis with multiple abscessation confirmed by laparotomy and histopathology of a liver biopsy.

Patient: Dog, Labrador, spayed female, 12 years old.

Presenting Signs and Complaints: Lack of appetite; dark colored urine for the last week; lethargic.

Physical Examination: Yellow mucous membranes.

Problem List: 1. Icterus. 2. Lethargy. 3. Anorexia.

Ultrasound: Markedly distended gallbladder with prominent intrahepatic biliary channels.

Hematology		Serum Chemistry	
RBC × 10⁶/μL	6.0 (6.0 × 10¹²/L)	AST (SGOT) (IU/L)	104 (104 U/L)
Hemoglobin (g/dL)	13 (8.1 mmol/L)	↑ ALT (SGPT) (IU/L)	**1,022 (1,022 U/L)**
PCV (%)	39 (0.39 volume fraction)	↑ Total bilirubin (mg/dL)	**13.3 (227.4 μmol/L)**
MCV (fL)	67	Urea nitrogen (mg/dL)	12 (4.28 mmol/L)
MCHC (g/dL)	33 (20.5 mmol/L)	Creatinine (mg/dL)	1.7 (150.3 μm/L)
RBC morphology	**Acanthocytes**	↑ Cholesterol (mg/dL)	**338 (8.8 mmol/L)**
WBC × 10³/μL	16.3 (16.3 × 10⁹/L)	↑ ALP (IU/L)	**1,214 (1,214 U/L)**
Myelocytes/μL	0 (0 × 10⁹/L)	Glucose (mg/dL)	101 (5.6 mmol/L)
Metamyelocytes/μL	0 (0 × 10⁹/L)	Amylase (IU/L)	750 (750 U/L)
↑ **Band neutrophils/μL**	**460 (0.46 × 10⁹/L)**	Lipase (IU/L)	15 (15 U/L)
↑ **Segmented neutrophils/μL**	**13,990 (13.99 × 10⁹/L)**	Phosphorus (mg/dL)	4.3 (1.39 mmol/L)
↓ **Lymphocytes/μL**	**690 (0.69 × 10⁹/L)**	Calcium (mg/dL)	10.2 (2.6 mmol/L)
Monocytes/μL	1,160 (1.1 × 10⁹/L)	Corrected calcium (mg/dL)	11.3 (2.8 mmol/L)
↓ **Eosinophils/μL**	**0 (0 × 10⁹/L)**	Total protein (g/dL)	7.5 (75 g/L)
Basophils/μL	0 (0 × 10⁹/L)	Albumin (g/dL)	2.4 (24 g/L)
Toxic neutrophils	None seen	Globulin (g/dL)	5.1 (51 g/L)
Platelets × 10³/μL	230 (0.23 × 10¹²/L)	Sodium (mEq/L)	149 (149 mmol/L)
Plasma protein (g/dL)	7.8 (78 g/L)	Potassium (mEq/L)	3.8 (3.8 mmol/L)
Fibrinogen (mg/dL)	300 (3 g/L)	Na : K ratio	39.2
		Chloride (mEq/L)	114 (114 mmol/L)
		Carbon dioxide (mEq/L)	22 (22 mmol/L)

Coagulation Tests	Day 1[a]	Day 5[a]
↑ **PT (sec)**	**17/11**	**12/10**
↑ **APTT (sec)**	**28/12**	**14/12**
TCT (sec)	7.8/8.0	7.6/7.8
Fibrin split products	Negative	

[a] Patient/control.

Urinalysis (Cystocentesis)	
Appearance	Clear, yellow
↓ **Specific gravity**	**1.021**
pH	7
Protein	+
Glucose	Negative
Ketones	Negative
Occult blood	Negative

Table continued on following page

Urinalysis (Cystocentesis) *Continued*	
↑ **Bilirubin**	**4+**
WBC/hpf	None
RBC/hpf	None
Casts/lpf	None
Bacteria	None

HEMOGRAM

Left shift with neutrophilia indicates active inflammation. Lymphopenia and eosinopenia suggest the possibility of increased glucocorticoid activity. Acanthocytes are associated more commonly with microangiopathic diseases such as hemangiosarcoma of the liver and spleen, certain liver disorders, and DIC.

URINALYSIS

Evaluation of the slightly low specific gravity depends upon knowing hydration state, water intake of patient, and serum urea, and creatinine levels. In this patient urea nitrogen and creatinine levels are normal, and there is no clinical evidence of renal disease.

BIOCHEMICAL PROFILE

Hyperbilirubinemia and increased serum alkaline phosphatase with a normal packed cell volume suggest a cholestatic disorder. The high ALT indicates altered membrane permeability of the hepatocytes; retained bile components can alter membrane components sufficiently to alter serum levels of ALT to this extent. The markedly increased cholesterol may also may reflect impaired bile flow as cholesterol is eliminated from the body in bile. The clinical chemistry values corroborate the ultrasonographic findings indicative of an extrahepatic cause of the impaired bile flow.

COAGULATION TESTS

Because of the presence of poikilocytes and abnormal coagulation parameters, fibrin split products were determined and found to be negative tending, supporting the absence of DIC and suggesting that the acanthocytosis is related to the liver disease.

Since the coagulation tests revealed abnormal clotting (patient time/control time = > 1.25), vitamin K was given subcutaneously, and the tests were repeated. After vitamin K therapy, the tests results returned toward normal. The existence of vitamin K-responsive coagulation aberrations substantiates further the presence of extrahepatic cholestasis. When there is impaired bile flow to the intestine because of bile duct obstruction, the fat-solubilizing bile acids cannot reach the intestines, and there is malabsorption of fat-soluble vitamins, in this case vitamin K. This causes a deficiency of the vitamin K-dependent coagulation factors. If vitamin K is then administered, the procoagulation components in the liver can be converted rapidly, in the presence of vitamin K, to active coagulation parameters. This is true with an obstructive lesion of the common bile duct. However, if cholestasis is due to liver failure such as cirrhosis or chronic hepatitis, the absence of vitamin K-dependent coagulation factors occurs because the liver cannot make the procoagulation factors. The parenteral administration of vitamin K does not alter the coagulation parameters because no active vitamin K-dependent factors are formed. Therefore the coagulation tests remain prolonged after administration of vitamin K in a patient with liver insufficiency secondary to chronic hepatitis/cirrhosis. These factors emphasize the need for preoperative preparation of any nonanemic icteric patient with regard to hemostasis.

DIAGNOSIS

Bile duct obstruction.

ADDITIONAL FINDINGS

Exploratory surgery revealed a tumor involving the duodenum, pancreas, and bile duct. Histologic diagnosis was pancreatic carcinoma. There is usually not an inflammatory component to this neoplastic growth in the pancreas, and therefore amylase and lipase values do not assist in the differential diagnosis of it. In some patients, 1 to 2 weeks after an attack of acute pancreatitis sufficient inflammatory/scar tissue will develop to cause obstruction of the common bile duct. In those patients amylase and lipase have also returned to normal by the time icterus develops, and the clinical presentation will mimic that of this patient. Histologic differentiation is required.

Patient: Dog, Labrador, spayed female, 4 years old.

Presenting Signs and Complaints: Suspected of cycad poisoning in February. Referring veterinarian removed 2 liters of serosanguinous abdominal fluid prior to referral.

Physical Examination: Abdomen distended; yellow mucous membranes; irregular heartbeat.

Problem List: 1. Ascites. 2. Icterus. 3. Cardiac arrhythmia.

Hematology	February 23	March 5	March 11
RBC × 10⁶/μL	6.1 (6.1 × 10¹²/L)	5.6 (5.6 × 10¹²/L)	5.65 (5.65 × 10¹²/L)
Hemoglobin (g/dL)	14.8 (9.18 mmol/L)	14.2 (8.81 mmol/L)	14.2 (8.81 mmol/L)
PCV (%)	42 (0.42 volume fraction)	37.6 (0.376 volume fraction)	38.5 (0.385 volume fraction)
MCV (fL)	68.8	67	68.2
MCHC (g/dL)	35.2 (21.8 mmol/L)	37.8 (22.7 mmol/L)	36.9 (22.1 mmol/L)
NRBC/100 WBC	0	2	0
RBC morphology	Normal	Normal	Normal
↑ WBC × 10³/μL	**17.5 (17.5 × 10⁹/L)**	15.96 (16 × 10⁹/L)	6.0 (6 × 10⁹/L)
Band neutrophils/μL	0 (0 × 10⁹/L)	0 (0 × 10⁹/L)	80 (0.08 × 10⁹/L)
↑ Segmented neutro-phils/μL	**14,875 (14.9 × 10⁹/L)**	↑ 14,400 (14.4 × 10⁹/L)	3,910 (3.9 × 10⁹/L)
↓ Lymphocytes/μL	**525 (0.53 × 10⁹/L)**	1,170 (1.2 × 10⁹/L)	1,000 (1.0 × 10⁹/L)
↑ Monocytes/μL	**2,100 (2.1 × 10⁹/L)**	330 (0.33 × 10⁹/L)	520 (0.52 × 10⁹/L)
↓ Eosinophils/μL	**0 (0 × 10⁹/L)**	↓ 60 (0.06 × 10⁹/L)	490 (0.49 × 10⁹/L)
Basophils/μL	0 (0 × 10⁹/L)	0 (0 × 10⁹/L)	0 (0 × 10⁹/L)
↑ Toxic neutrophils	+	None	None
Platelet estimate	**Adequate**	↓ Decreased	
Platelet × 10³/μL			↓ 77 (0.08 × 10¹²/L)

Coagulation Tests	March 5			March 11	
	Patient	Control		Patient	Control
↑ PT (sec)	13.8	9.8	↑ Fibrin degradation products + at 1:40		
↑ APTT (sec)	15.2	10.2	↑ PT (sec)	9.2	8.2
Fibrinogen (mg/dL)	400	<100	↑ APTT (sec)	12.1	10.2
	3/11		Fibrin split products	Negative	

Serum Chemistry	February 23	March 5	March 11	April 15
↑ AST (SGOT) (IU/L)	686 (686 U/L)	↑ 179 (179 U/L)	47 (47 U/L)	43 (43 U/L)
↑ ALT (SGPT) (IU/L)	3,800 (3,800 U/L)	↑ 202 (202 U/L)	↑ 160 (160 U/L)	79 (79 U/L)
↑ ALP (IU/L)	256 (256 U/L)	↑ 247 (247 U/L)	↑ 213 (213 U/L)	104 104 U/L)
GGT (IU/L)	8 (8 U/L)	↑ 28 (28 U/L)	↑ 20 (20 U/L)	1 (1 U/L)
Total bilirubin (mg/dL)	0.4 (6.8 μmol/L)	↑ 1.5 (25.7 μmol/L)	↑ 1.3 (22.2 μmol/L)	0.4 (6.8 μmol/L)
Conjugated bilirubin (mg/dL)	0.3 (5.1 μmol/L)	↑ 1.2 (20.5 μmol/L)	↑ 1.1 (19 μmol/L)	0.3 (5.1 μmol/L)
Unconjugated bilirubin (mg/dL)	0.1 (1.7 μmol/L)	0.3 (5.1 μmol/L)	0.2 (3.4 μmol/L)	0.1 (1.7 μmol/L)
Total protein (g/dL)	6.2 (62 g/L)	5.7 (57 g/L)	5.8 (58 g/L)	6.0 (60 g/L)
Albumin (g/dL)	2.9 (29 g/L)	2.5 (25 g/L)	2.7 (27 g/L)	2.9 (29 g/L)
Globulin (g/dL)	3.3 (3 g/L)	3.2 (32 g/L)	3.1 (31 g/L)	3.1 (31 g/L)
↑ Urea nitrogen (mg/dL)	42 (15 mmol/L)	12 (4.3 mmol/L)	8 (2.9 mmol/L)	12 (4.3 mmol/L)
↑ Creatinine (mg/dL)	2.3 (203 mm/L)	1.0 (88 μmol/L)	1.0 (88 μmol/L)	1.2 (106.1 μm/L)
Amylase (IU/L)	1,250 (1,250 U/L)			
Lipase (IU/L)	25 (25 U/L)			
Glucose (mg/dL)	86 (4.7 mmol/L)	72 (3.96 mmol/L)	107 (6 mmol/L)	96 (5.3 mmol/L)
Sodium (mEq/L)	149 (149 mmol/L)	147 (147 mmol/L)	148 (148 mmol/L)	146 (146 mmol/L)
Potassium (mEq/L)	4.4 (4.4 mmol/L)	3.9 (3.9 mmol/L)	4.0 (4 mmol/L)	4.2 (4.2 mmol/L)
Na : K ratio	33.8	38	37	34.7
Chloride (mEq/L)	101 (101 mmol/L)	105 (105 mmol/L)	125 (125 mmol/L)	110 (110 mmol/L)
Carbon dioxide (mEq/L)	22 (22 mmol/L)	23 (23 mmol/L)	17 (17 mmol/L)	18 (18 mmol/L)
Calcium (mg/dL)	9.8 (2.5 mmol/L)	9.5 (2.38 mmol/L)	10.1 (2.53 mmol/L)	9.9 (2.5 mmol/L)
Phosphorus (mg/dL)	4.2 (1.4 mmol/L)	3.7 (1.20 mmol/L)	4.2 (1.4 mmol/L)	4.3 (1.4 mmol/L)
Creatine kinase (IU/L)	135 (135 U/L)	95 (95 U/L)		
↑ Fasting bile acids (μmol/L)	38 (38 μmol/L)	↑ 55 (55 μmol/L)	↑ 90 (90 μmol/L)	↑ 28 (28 μmol/L)

Abdominocentesis	
Total protein (g/dL)	<2.5
RBC/μL	250,000
WBC/μL	1,600
Neutrophils	30%
Macrophages	70%

Urinalysis (Cystocentesis)	February 23	March 11
Appearance	Yellow	Medium yellow
Specific gravity	1.042	1.018
pH	7	6
Protein	Negative	Negative
Glucose	Negative	Negative
Ketones	Negative	Negative
Blood	Negative	Negative
Bilirubin	+	3+
Sediment		
WBC/hpf	0–2	2–3
RBC/hpf	0–1	None
Casts	2-4 hyaline	Negative
Crystals	Negative	Negative
Bacteria	Negative	Negative

HEMOGRAM (FEBRUARY 23)

The hemogram on February 23 was normal except for a glucocorticoid-stress differential leukocyte count.

BIOCHEMICAL PROFILE

The biochemical profile on February 23 revealed increased ALT and AST, the magnitudes of which imply a diffuse alteration of hepatocellular membranes. Because some AST is in the cytoplasm and some is bound to microsomal components, the marked increase in AST with a normal creatine kinase suggests an alteration of microsomal integrity within hepatocytes, suggesting a more severe insult to the liver (Figs. 5-1, 5-2). The relatively mild increase in alkaline phosphatase further support acute injury to the liver with minimal cholestasis. The urea nitrogen and creatinine increases along with the urine specific gravity denote a prerenal azotemia.

The fasting bile acid is abnormal and, although not essential for evaluation of this patient, indicates liver insufficiency. It was conducted to obtain a base line for future evaluation of the patient.

HEMOGRAM (MARCH 5)

The hemogram on March 5 revealed a decreased platelet count, and abnormal coagulation parameters were detected. The abnormal prothrombin and partial thromboplastin times with a positive test for fibrin split products and a decreased fibrinogen are suggestive of DIC.

BIOCHEMICAL PROFILE

The transaminases (AST, ALT) remain increased, indicating a continuation of damage to hepatocyte cell membranes and microsomes. The total bilirubin increase with a normal packed cell volume suggests a cholestatic process that is supported by a mild increase in alkaline phosphatase and GGT. The magnitudes of these increases are most compatible with an intrahepatic cholestatic problem. Differentiation between conjugated and unconjugated bilirubin does not contribute to further interpretation of the liver disorder. Fasting bile acids remain increased.

Abdominocentesis conducted on this day revealed a fluid compatible with a transudate with blood contamination. The transudate (total protein < 2.5 g/L suggests the presence of portal hypertension secondary to the diffuse nature of the liver disease.

HEMOGRAM (MARCH 11)

The hemogram on March 11 was normal except for a thrombocytopenia. The patient is receiving vitamin K_1 and heparin subcutaneously, and the coagulation values are returning to normal.

BIOCHEMICAL PROFILE (APRIL 15)

The biochemical profile on April 15 was normal except for the slightly increased fasting bile acids. Ultrasonography was performed; the gallbladder was full, but no other abnormalities were noted.

ADDITIONAL INFORMATION

A liver biopsy was performed on March 22. The biopsy was delayed to permit the coagulation values to return to normal subsequent to the use of vitamin K_1. The anatomic diagnosis was hepatitis, chronic/active, multifocal, moderate, in association with fibrosis, lipofuscin and hemosiderin accumulation periportal; evidence of hepatocellular regeneration. Histologic findings are compatible with hepatocellular collapse after an acute insult to the liver, the etiology of which is not apparent. Prognosis at this time remains guarded until the healing process is completed. A liver biopsy was not essential in this patient but was performed at the owner's request for prognostic purposes.

The reason for sequentially following bile acids in this patient becomes apparent when the liver enzymes have returned to normal. One notes that the fasting bile acids remain increased, indicating liver insufficiency. In some patients an acute insult may proceed to cirrhosis, in which case the fasting bile acids do not return to normal but plateau and gradually increase over time. If the healing process is complete with no cholestasis, fasting bile acids return to normal, a good prognostic sign.

A 6-month follow-up revealed a normal biochemical profile, normal bile acids, and the patient was clinically healthy.

DIAGNOSIS

Cycad poisoning with hepatic disease. Cycad toxicity is due to a group of azoxyglyciosides found in various quantities throughout the plant. This dog was known to have eaten seeds from *Zamia*. As few as two seeds have been known to cause poisoning.

Case 34

Patient: Dog, mixed breed, spayed, female, 10 years old.

Presenting Signs and Complaints: Intermittent inappetence for the past month; weak; seems to be drinking a lot of water.

Physical Examination: Weight loss, yellow discoloration of sclera, possible ascites.

Problem List: 1. Generalized weakness. 2. Icterus. 3. Abdominal radiographs revealed fluid.

Hematology		Serum Chemistry	
RBC × 10⁶/µL	6.63 (6.6 × 10¹²/L)	AST (SGOT) (IU/L)	134 (134 U/L)
Hemoglobin (g/dL)	15 (9.3 mol/L)	↑ **ATL (SGPT) (IU/L)**	**1,074 (1,074 U/L)**
PCV (%)	43.9 (0.44 volume fraction)	↑ **ALP (IU/L)**	**926 (926 U/L)**
MCV (fL)	66	↑ **GGT (IU/L)**	**23 (23 U/L)**
MCHC (g/dL)	34.1 (21.2 mmol/L)	Total bilirubin (mg/dL)	0.5 (8.6 µmol/L)
NRBC/100 WBC	0	Conjugated bilirubin (mg/dL)	0.4 (6.8 µmol/L)
RBC morphology	Normal	Total protein (g/dL)	6.6 (66 g/L)
WBC × 10³/µL	11.8 (11.8 × 10⁹/L)	↓ **Albumin (g/dL)**	**1.8 (18 g/L)**
		Globulin (g/dL)	4.8 (48 g/L)
Myelocytes/µL	0 (0 × 10⁹/L)	Amylase (IU/L)	2,129 (2,129 U/L)
Metamyelocytes/µL	0 (0 × 10⁹/L)	Lipase (IU/L)	50 (50 U/L)
Band neutrophils/µL	0 (0 × 10⁹/L)	↓ **Glucose (mg/dL)**	**38 (2.1 mmol/L)**
Segmented neutrophils/µL	8,296 (8.3 × 10⁹/L)	Urea nitrogen (mg/dL)	16 (5.71 mmol/L)
Lymphocytes/µL	1,592 (1.6 × 10⁹/L)	Creatinine (mg/dL)	0.6 (53 µmol/L)
Monocytes/µL	1,586 (1.6 × 10⁹/L)	Calcium (mg/dL)	10.4 (2.6 mmol/L)
Eosinophils/µL	366 (0.37 × 10⁹/L)	Phosphorus (mg/dL)	5.3 (1.71 mmol/L)
Basophils/µL	0 (0 × 10⁹/L)	Sodium (mEq/L)	150 (150 mmol/L)
Toxic neutrophils	None seen	Potassium (mEq/L)	5.0 (5 mmol/L)
Platelets × 10³/µL	Adequate	Chloride (mEq/L)	120 (120 mmol/L)
		Total carbon dioxide (mm/L)	21 (21 mmol/L)
Abdominal Fluid		↑ Fasting bile acids (µmol/L)	**256 (256 µmol/L)**
Specific gravity	1.011		
Protein (g/dL)	1.2 (12 g/L)		
Nucleated cells/µL	200 (0.2 × 10⁹/L)		
Lymphocytes (%)	5		
Macrophages (%)	95		

Urinalysis (Cystocentesis)	
Appearance	Light yellow
↓ **Specific gravity**	**1.008**
pH	6.5
Protein	Negative
Glucose	Negative
Ketones	Negative
Blood	Negative
Bilirubin	+
Sediment	
WBC/hpf	1–3
RBC/hpf	2–4
Casts	Negative
Crystals	Negative
Bacteria	Negative

BIOCHEMICAL PROFILE

The markedly increased ALT with a mild increase in AST indicates altered hepatocellular membrane integrity. Increased alkaline phosphatase and GGT are compatible with increased enzyme production reflecting cholestasis, or the enzymes can be induced by the administration of glucocorticoids. A review of the history for administration of such drugs should be made. Bilirubinuria and increases in alkaline phosphatase and GGT will precede hyperbilirubinemia secondary to a cholestatic process. Normal total protein and globulin levels with hypoalbuminemia and no other evidence of protein loss (diarrhea or proteinuria) leads one to suspect decreased liver production. Hypoglycemia may be related to increased insulin production or decreased production by the liver. When hypoglycemia is secondary to liver insufficiency it indicates a poor prognosis because of the tremendous reserve capacity of the liver for maintaining glucose homeostasis. Because of the liver enzyme abnormalities as well as suggestions of liver insufficiency reflected by the hypoalbuminemia and hypoglycemia, a fasting bile acids was run and found to be markedly increased, supporting liver insufficiency. Further biochemical efforts at diagnosis would not be useful at this time. Confirmation of the underlying pathology would require a liver biopsy.

If medications are used in an attempt to decrease the inflammatory component or delay further development of the fibrous component, fasting serum bile acids can be used as a guide to evaluate any improvement in liver function and can be periodically evaluated to see if there is progression of the cirrhotic process.

URINALYSIS

The low urine specific gravity is most likely a reflection of polydipsia/polyuria which may be related to the chronic liver insufficiency.

ABDOMINAL FLUID

Abdominal fluid with a low protein content and cell count is characteristic of a transudate. In this case it is probably a result of hepatic cirrhosis.

DIAGNOSIS

A liver biopsy was done, and histopathologic evaluation revealed cirrhosis with chronic active liver disease.

Patient: Dog, Skye terrier, male, 4 months old.

Presenting Signs and Complaints: Lethargic since purchased; diarrhea; sometimes weak in back legs and falls down.

Physical Examination: Very thin; little response to surroundings; incoordination when walking.

Problem List: 1. Lethargy. 2. Ataxia. 3. Thin.

Hematology		Serum Chemistry	
RBC × 10⁶/μL	4.82 (4.82 × 10¹²/L)	AST (SGOT) (IU/L)	55 (55 U/L)
Hemoglobin (g/dL)	8.5 (5.28 mmol/L)	ALT (SGPT) (IU/L)	59 (59 U/L)
PCV (%)	27 (0.27 volume fraction)	↑ **ALP (IU/L)**	**384 (384 U/L)**
↓ **MCV (fL)**	**58**	GGT (IU/L)	3 (3 U/L)
MCHC (g/dL)	32 (19.8 mmol/L)	Total bilirubin (mg/dL)	0.1 (1.7 μmol/L)
Reticulocytes (%)	0	Conjugated bilirubin (mg/dL)	0.0 (0 μmol/L)
NRBC/100 WBC	0	Unconjugated bilirubin (mg/dL)	0.1 (1.7 μmol/L)
RBC morphology	Normal	↑ **Total protein (g/dL)**	**4.0 (40 g/L)**
WBC × 10³/μL	15.2 (15.2 × 10⁹/L)	↓ **Albumin (g/dL)**	**2.1 (21 g/L)**
Myelocytes/μL	0 (0 × 10⁹/L)	Globulin (g/dL)	1.9 (19 g/L)
Metamyelocytes/μL	0 (0 × 10⁹/L)	↓ **Cholesterol (mg/dL)**	**68 (1.8 mmol/L)**
Band neutrophils/μL	0 (0 × 10⁹/L)	↓ **Urea nitrogen (mg/dL)**	**5 (1.8 mmol/L)**
Segmented neutrophils/μL	10,730 (10.7 × 10⁹/L)	Creatinine (mg/dL)	0.4 (35.4 μmol/L)
Lymphocytes/μLᵃ	2,430 (2.4 × 10⁹/L)	Glucose (mg/dL)	117 (6.44 mmol/L)
Monocytes/μL	1,740 (1.7 × 10⁹/L)	Sodium (mEq/L)	136 (136 mmol/L)
Eosinophils/μL	300 (0.3 × 10⁹/L)	Potassium (mEq/L)	4.2 (4.2 mmol/L)
Basophils/μL	0	Na : K ratio	32.3
Toxic neutrophils	None	Chloride (mEq/L)	111 (111 mmol/L)
Platelet estimate	Adequate	Carbon dioxide (mEq/L)	22 (22 mmol/L)
↓ **Plasma protein (g/dL)**	**4.3 (43 g/L)**	Calcium (mg/dL)	8.8 (2.2 mmol/L)
Fibrinogen (mg/dL)	300 (3 g/L)	Corrected calcium (mg/dL)	10.2 (2.6 mmol/L)
		Phosphorus (mg/dL)	8.6 (2.78 mmol/L)
		Iron (μg/dL)	112 (20.05 mm/L)
		↑ **Fasting bile acids (μmol/L)**	**182 (182 μmol/L)**
		↑ **Postmeal bile acids (μmol/L)**	**289 (289 μmol/L)**

ᵃ Few reactive lymphocytes.

Urinalysis (Cystocentesis)	
Appearance	Clear, yellow
Specific gravity	1.035
pH	6.8
Protein	Negative
Glucose	Negative
Ketones	Negative
Blood	Negative
Bilirubin	Negative
Sediment	
WBC/hpf	0–2
RBC/hpf	1–4
Casts	Negative
↑ **Crystals**	**Ammonium biurate 3+**
Bacteria	Negative

HEMOGRAM

The only abnormal hemogram finding is a decreased MCV. The most common cause for a decreased MCV is iron deficiency; in this case the serum iron is normal. However, in young animals showing neurologic signs a decreased MCV has been associated with congenital portosystemic vascular anomalies. PCV, RBC, and hemoglobin are normal for a puppy.

BIOCHEMICAL PROFILE

The increased serum alkaline phosphatase with a normal GGT in a growing animal most likely reflect alkaline phosphatase of bone origin since cholestasis would be expected to increase both enzymes. Hypoalbuminemia and low serum urea nitrogen are suggestive of liver insufficiency. Because of nondescript neurologic findings in a young animal with a decreased MCV, hypoalbuminemia, ammonium biurate crystals in the urine, and decreased serum urea nitrogen and cholesterol, a liver function test such as serum bile acids or ammonia measurement is appropriate. Ammonium biurate crystals are most commonly associated with portosystemic vascular anomalies.

The fasting bile acid is markedly increased. A postprandial bile acid is not necessary when the fasting bile acid is as markedly abnormal as in this case. However, to demonstrate the effect of gallbladder contraction and the intrahepatic circulation of bile acids a postprandial bile acid is shown in this case. Here it demonstrates the inability of the liver to extract bile acids.

DIAGNOSIS

A portal venogram confirmed the presence of a *portosystemic shunt*. The owners requested euthanasia. At necropsy the presence of portosystemic shunt was verified. Histologically there were vesicular polycavitational lesions at the junction of the gray/white matter in the CNS. Hyperammonia has been shown to produce similar lesions experimentally. The neurologic signs may have been a result of the degenerative process.

Patient: Cat, domestic shorthair, male, 4 months old.

Presenting Signs and Complaints: Attacked by neighbor's dog 2 days ago; since then it has been stiff and sore.

Physical Examination: Wounds on back; reluctant to move; generalized stiffness.

Problem List: 1. Muscle soreness. 2. Contusions.

Hematology		Serum Chemistry	
RBC × 10⁶/μL	5.86 (5.86 × 10¹²/L)	↑ **AST (SGOT) (IU/L)**	**562 (562 U/L)**
Hemoglobin (g/dL)	8.9 (5.52 mmol/L)	↑ **ALT (SGPT) (IU/L)**	**120 (120 U/L)**
PCV (%)	27 (0.27 volume fraction	ALP (IU/L)	41 (41 U/L)
MCV (fL)	46	GGT (IU/L)	3 (3 U/L)
MCHC (g/dL)	30.5 (18.9 mmol/L)	Total bilirubin (mg/dL)	0.1 (1.7 μmol/L)
NRBC/100 WBC	0	Conjugated bilirubin (mg/dL)	0.0 (0.0 μmol/L)
RBC morphology	Normal	Unconjugated bilirubin (mg/dL)	0.1 (1.7 μmol/L)
WBC × 10³/μL	11.6 (11.6 × 10⁹/L)	Total protein (g/dL)	6.0 (60 g/L)
Myelocytes/μL	0 (0 × 10⁹/L)	Albumin (g/dL)	3.2 (32 g/L)
Metamyelocytes/μL	0 (0 × 10⁹/L)	Globulins (g/dL)	2.8 (28 g/L)
Band neutrophils/μL	0 (0 × 10⁹/L)	Cholesterol (mg/dL)	127 (3.3 mmol/L)
Segmented neutrophils/μL	10,324 (10.3 × 10⁹/L)	Urea nitrogen (mg/dL)	32 (11.4 mmol/L)
↓ **Lymphocytes/μL**	**928 (0.93 × 10⁹/L)**	Creatinine (mg/dL)	1.9 (168.0 μmol/L)
Monocytes/μL	348 (0.35 × 10⁹/L)	Glucose (mg/dL)	120 (6.6 mmol/L)
Eosinophils/μL	0 (0 × 10⁹/L)	↓ **Creatine kinase (IU/L)**	**5,000 (5,000 U/L)**
Basophils/μL	0 (0 × 10⁹/L)	Sodium (mEq/L)	151 (151 mmol/L)
Toxic neutrophils	None seen	Potassium (mEq/L)	4.4 (4.4 mmol/L)
Platelet estimate	Adequate	Na : K ratio	34.3
Plasma protein (g/dL)	6.3 (63 g/L)	Chloride (mEq/L)	116 (116 mmol/L)
Fibrinogen (mg/dL)	300 (3 g/L)	Carbon dioxide (mEq/L)	16 (16 mmol/L)
		Calcium (mg/dL)	10.4 (2.6 mmol/L)
		Phosphorus (mg/dL)	5.6 (1.81 mmol/L)
		↑ **LDH (IU/L)**	**1,789 (1,789 U/L)**

HEMOGRAM

Lymphopenia and eosinopenia support increased glucocorticoid activity.

BIOCHEMICAL PROFILE

Slightly increased ALT and marked increase in AST indicate enzyme leakage from both liver and skeletal muscle. However, the marked increase in AST compared with ALT suggests that injury to skeletal muscle is the predominant organ system affected. The increased creatinine kinase confirms skeletal muscle injury. The concentration of creatinine kinase in the muscle tissue of the cat is one third to one fourth less than other species. Therefore the magnitude of creatine kinase increase in the cat must be evaluated more critically from a clinical standpoint.

LDH is present in all cells of the body. An elevation in serum LDH activity indicates tissue damage or alteration in cell membrane permeability. In this case the increase is most likely associated with the damaged tissues.

DIAGNOSIS

Muscle and liver injury.

Patient: Horse, thoroughbred, male, 2 years old.

Presenting Signs and Complaints: Growth removed surgically 2 days ago; today animal is reluctant to move.

Physical Examination: Sutured wound on right neck; animal appears to be weak and stiff.

Problem List: 1. Generalized muscle soreness. 2. Weak.

Serum Chemistry	Day 1	Day 3
↑ **AST (SGOT) IU/L**	**3,210 (3,210 U/L)**	**13,200 (3,200 U/L)**
ALT (SGPT) (IU/L)	68 (68 U/L)	72 (72 U/L)
ALP (IU/L)	273 (273 U/L)	266 (266 U/L)
SD (mU/ml)	12 (12 U/L)	
Total protein (g/dL)	6.1 (61 g/L)	5.5 (5.5 g/L)
Albumin (g/dL)	3.5 (35 g/L)	3.1 (32 g/L)
Globulin (g/dL)	2.6 (2.6 g/L)	2.4 (24 g/L)
Glucose (mg/dL)	84 (4.62 mmol/L)	88 (4.84 mmol/L)
Urea nitrogen (mg/dL)	28 (10 mmol/L)	19 (6.78 mmol/L)
Creatinine mg/dL	2 (176.8 μmol/L)	1.4 (123.7 μmol/L)
Calcium (mg/dL)	10.1 (2.5 mmol/L)	9.7 (2.43 mmol/L)
Phosphorus (mg/dL)	3.1 (1.0 mmol/L)	4.1 (1.32 mmol/L)
Sodium (mEq/L)	138 (138 mmol/L)	148 (148 mmol/L)
Potassium (mEq/L)	2.6 (2.6 mmol/L)	4.0 (4.0 mmol/L)
Chloride (mEq/L)	99 (99 mmol/L)	100 (100 mmol/L)
Total carbon dioxide (mEq/L)	26 (26 mmol/L)	30 (30 mmol/L)
↑ **Creatine kinase (IU/L)**	**15,111 (15,111 U/L)**	**15,200 (15,200 U/L)**

BIOCHEMICAL PROFILE

There is a marked increase in AST which can be a reflection of either hepatocellular leakage or skeletal muscle cell leakage. In the equine species, the ALT does not help differentiate between the liver and skeletal muscle because ALT has poor sensitivity for hepatocellular enzyme leakage. One can do a creatine kinase and, as shown in this case in which it is increased markedly, assume that the AST is of skeletal muscle origin as well. Sorbitol dehydrogenase (SD) is a liver-specific enzyme, and evaluation of the SD serum concentration can be used as measurement of enzyme leakage from hepatocytes. The SD would be increased if there was liver injury.

DIAGNOSIS

Skeletal muscle damage.

Patient: Cat, Persian, spayed female, 5 years old.

Presenting Signs and Complaints: Recurrent fever; on two previous occasions has responded to antibiotics, now fever has persisted despite three different antibiotics. Lethargic

Physical Examination: Temperature 105° F; thin; radiographs indicated a mild increase in abdominal fluid.

Problem List: 1. Pyrexia. 2. Weight loss. 3. Lethargy. 4. Ascites.

Hematology		Serum Chemistry	
RBC × 10⁶/µL	6.1 (6.1 × 10¹²/L)	AST (SGOT) (IU/L)	26 (26 U/L)
Hemoglobin (g/dL)	11.9 (7.38 mmol/L)	ALT (SGPT) (IU/L)	41 (41 U/L)
PCV (%)	36 (0.36 volume fraction)	ALP (IU/L)	6 (6 U/L)
MCV (fL)	44	GGT (IU/L)	1 (1 U/L)
MCHC (g/dL)	33 (20.5 mmol/L)	Total bilirubin (mg/dL)	0.2 (3.4 µmol/L)
NRBC/100 WBC	0	↑ **Total protein (g/dL)**[a]	**8.8 (88 g/L)**[a]
RBC morphology	Normal	Albumin (g/dL)	2.2 (22 g/L)
WBC × 10³/µL	10.7 (10.7 × 10⁹/L)	↑ **Globulin (g/dL)**	**6.6 (66 g/L)**
Myelocytes/µL	0 (0 × 10⁹/L)	Cholesterol (mg/dL)	162 (4.21 mmol/L)
Metamyelocytes/µL	0 (0 × 10⁹/L)	Glucose (mg/dL)	24 (1.32 mmol/L)
Band neutrophils/µL	107 (0.11 × 10⁹/L)	Amylase (IU/L)	586 (586 U/L)
Segmented neutrophils/µL	9,844 (9.8 × 10⁹/L)	Lipase (IU/L)	35 (35 U/L)
↓ **Lymphocytes/µL**	**535 (0.54 × 10⁹/L)**	Urea nitrogen (mg/dL)	15 (5.4 mmol/L)
Monocytes/µL	214 (0.2 × 10⁹/L)	Creatinine (mg/dL)	1 (88.4 µmol/L)
↓ **Eosinophils/µL**	**0 (0 × 10⁹/L)**	Phosphorus (mg/dL)	5.1 (1.65 mmol/L)
Basophils/µL	0 (0 × 10⁹/L)	Calcium (mg/dL)	8.8 (2.2 mmol/L)
Toxic neutrophils	None	Corrected calcium (mg/dL)	10.1 (2.53 mmol/L)
Platelets × 10³/µL	230 (0.23 × 10¹²/L)	Sodium (mEq/L)	152 (152 mmol/L)
Blood parasites	None seen	Potassium (mEq/L)	4.3 (4.3 mmol/L)
Plasma protein (g/dL)	7.6 (76 g/L)	Na : K ratio	29.8
Fibrinogen (mg/dL)	100	Chloride (mEq/L)	102 (102 mmol/L)
		Carbon dioxide (mEq/L)	20 (20 mmol/L)
		Creatine kinase (IU/L)	45 (45 U/L)

[a] Protein electrophoresis = polyclonal gammopathy.

Urinalysis (Cystocentesis)	
Appearance	Clear, yellow
Specific gravity	1.036
pH	7
Protein	Negative
Glucose	Negative
Ketones	Negative
Occult blood	Negative
Bilirubin	Negative
WBC/hpf	Negative
RBC/hpf	Negative
Casts/lpf	+ Hyaline
Crystals	Negative
Bacteria	Negative

Abdominocentesis	
Gross appearance	Light yellow, slightly hazy, sticky
↑ Total protein (g/dL)	**5.7 (57 g/L)**
RBC/μL	1,200 (0.12 × 10^{12}/L)
↑ WBC/μL	**4,200 (4.2 × 10^9/μL)**
Segmented neutrophils	42% (nondegenerate)
Macrophages	43% (large foamy)
Lymphocytes	5%
Bacteria	No bacteria seen

HEMOGRAM

Lymphopenia and eosinopenia support increased glucocorticoid activity.

BIOCHEMICAL PROFILE

The notable finding in the biochemical profile is the hyperproteinemia which is the result of hyperglobulinemia. There is a mild hypoalbuminemia which is most likely a reflection of the increased globulin that has down-regulated albumin production by the liver. This is supported by the fact that the cat does not have evidence of a protein-losing enteropathy clinically, nor is there protein loss in the urine.

Hyperglobulinemia may be monoclonal or polyclonal and can be differentiated by serum protein electrophoresis. Serum electrophoresis was completed, and the polyclonal gammopathy suggested prolonged anitigen stimulation.

Several drops of abdominal fluid were obtained for evaluation with the results reported above. The effusion had a high total protein with a mild increase in cells. This effusion is best classified as an exudate as it has a protein content greater than 2.5 g/dL and neutrophils are present. The normal morphology of the neutrophils and the absence of bacteria support a nonseptic exudative effusion. An effusion with a remarkable increased protein and a polyclonal hyperglobulinemia

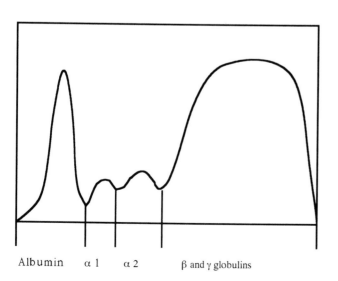

CASE 38. Serum electrophoresis with polyclonal gammopathy. Note the marked increase in the β–γ globulin peak.

Albumin   α 1   α 2   β and γ globulins

of serum are characteristic of feline infectious peritonitis (FIP). FIP titers are variable and difficult to interpret as they are frequently negative in cats with the infection.

An albumin to globulin ratio of less than 0.8 in the effusion, determined by a protein electrophoresis of the fluid, in cats is highly predictive for supporting a diagnosis of FIP.

DIAGNOSIS

The patient continued to do poorly for the next month and was euthanized; FIP was confirmed histologically.

Patient: Dog, fox terrier, female, 4 years old.

Presenting Signs and Complaints: Drinks a lot of water; frequently urinates large volumes; will not eat.

Physical Examination: No other clinical abnormalities.

Problem List: 1. Polyuria/polydipsia. 2. Anorexia.

Hematology	
RBC × 10⁶/μL	4.79 (4.79 × 10¹²/L)
Hemoglobin (g/dL)	11.8 (7.32 mmol/L)
PCV (%)	32.9 (33 volume fraction)
MCV (fL)	69
MCHC (g/dL)	35.8 (22.2 mmol/L)
NRBC/100 WBC	0
RBC morphology	Normal
WBC × 10³/μL	11.7 (11.7 × 10⁹/L)
Myelocytes/μL	0 (0 × 10⁹/L)
Metamyelocytes/μL	0 (0 × 10⁹/L)
Band neutrophils/μL	0 (0 × 10⁹/L)
Segmented neutrophils/μL	10,060 (10.1 × 10⁹/L)
↓ **Lymphocytes/μL**	**700 (0.70 × 10⁹/L)**
Monocytes/μL	470 (0.47 × 10⁹/L)
Eosinophils/μL	470 (0.47 × 10⁹/L)
Basophils/μL	0 (0 × 10⁹/L)
Toxic neutrophils	None seen
Platelet estimate	Adequate

Serum Chemistry	
AST (SGOT) (IU/L)	36 (36 U/L)
ALT (SGPT) (IU/L)	54 (54 U/L)
ALP (IU/L)	52 (52 U/L)
GGT (IU/L)	1 (1 U/L)
Total bilirubin (mg/dL)	0.1 (1.7 μmol/L)
Direct bilirubin (mg/dL)	0 (0 μmol/L)
Indirect bilirubin (mg/dL)	0.1 (1.7 μmol/L)
Total protein (g/dL)	6.0 (60 g/L)
Albumin (g/dL)	2.6 (26 g/L)
Globulin (g/dL)	3.4 (34 g/L)
↑ **Cholesterol (mg/dL)**	**372 (9.7 mmol/L)**
↑ **Urea nitrogen (mg/dL)**	**150 (53.6 mmol/L)**
↑ **Creatinine (mg/dL)**	**4.2 (371.3 μmol/L)**
Glucose (mg/dL)	102 (5.6 mmol/L)
↑ **Amylase (IU/L)**	**2,870 (2,870 U/L)**
Lipase (IU/L)	601 (301 U/L)
Sodium (mEq/L)	150 (150 mmol/L)
Potassium (mEq/L)	4.8 (4.8 mmol/L)
Na : K ratio	31.3
Chloride (mEq/L)	106 (106 mmol/L)
Carbon dioxide (mEq/L)	22 (22 mmol/L)
Calcium (mg/dL)	11.2 (2.80 mmol/L)
↑ **Corrected calcium (mg/dL)**	**12.1 (3.03 mmol/L)**
↑ **Phosphorus (mg/dL)**	**12.6 (4.07 mmol/L)**
Creatine kinase (IU/L)	100 (100 U/L)
LDH (IU/L)	150 (150 U/L)
Total resting T₄ (μg/dL)	2.1 (27.03 nmol/L)

Urinalysis (Cystocentesis)	
Appearance	Clear, pale yellow
↓ **Specific gravity**	**1.011**
pH	6.5
↓ **Protein**	**4+**
Glucose	Negative
Ketones	Negative
Occult blood	Negative
Bilirubin	Negative
WBC/hpf	2–4
RBC/hpf	1–3
Casts/lpf	None
Crystals	None
Bacteria	Negative
Urine protein (mg/dL)	200
Urine creatinine (mg/dL)	54
↑ **Urine protein/creatine ratio**	**3.7**

HEMOGRAM

Lymphopenia suggests increased glucocorticoid activity. The erythrocytes are normocytic normochromic. The low RBC parameters with no evidence of polychromasia suggest a nonregenerative or poorly regenerative anemia.

BIOCHEMICAL PROFILE AND URINALYSIS

The proteinuria, increased urea nitrogen, and creatinine associated with an inappropriate (low) urine specific gravity and hyperphosphatemia all support primary renal insufficiency and a protein-losing nephropathy. The urine protein/urine creatinine ratio of 3.7 quantifies the marked proteinuria.

The presence of hypercalcemia may be related to the kidney disease. However, one cannot absolutely rule out the possibility that the renal disease is caused by renal calcinosis, in which case the hypercalcemia may have preceded the renal disease.

The biochemical profile and urinalysis indicate a primary renal insufficiency which may be responsible for the poorly regenerative anemia because of the lack of erythropoietin. The hypercholesterolemia may be the result of altered lipid metabolism, the mechanism of which is poorly understood, which sometimes occurs with chronic renal failure. In this case hyperamylasemia is undoubtedly a result of decreased renal function. Values for amylase greater than three- to fourfold support acute pancreatitis when there is concurrent renal insufficiency.

DIAGNOSIS

Primary renal insufficiency. Histologic examination of renal tissue would be necessary to define the cause of the kidney disease further.

COMMENT

The patient was euthanized at the owner's request, and at necropsy both kidneys were small, shrunken, and fibrous, compatible with end-stage kidney. No etiology was determined.

Patient: Horse, quarterhorse, female, 20 years old.

Presenting Complaints: Frequent voluminous urination; increased water intake; weight loss.

Physical Examination: Thin; slightly (5%) dehydrated.

Problem List: 1. Polyuria and polydipsia. 2. Thin. 3. Dehydration.

Hematology		Serum Chemistry	
↓ RBC × 10⁶/µL	6.66 (6.66 × 10¹²/L)	AST (SGOT) (IU/L)	233 (233 U/L)
↓ Hemoglobin (g/dL)	10.7 (6.6 mmol/L)	ALP (IU/L)	249 (249 U/L)
↓ PCV (%)	27 (0.27 volume fraction)	GGT (IU/L)	1 (1 U/L)
MCV (fL)	40.5	Total bilirubin (mg/dL)	0.6 (10.3 µmol/L)
MCHC (g/dL)	39.6 (24.6 mmol/L)	Conjugated bilirubin (mg/dL)	0.1 (1.7 µmol/L)
RDW (%)	18.2 (0.182 volume fraction)	Unconjugated bilirubin (mg/dL)	0.5 (8.6 µmol/L)
RBC morphology	Normal	Total protein (g/dL)	8.4 (84 g/L)
↑ WBC × 10³/µL	20.9 (20.9 × 10⁹/L)	Albumin (g/dL)	3.0 (30 g/L)
Metamyelocytes/µL	0 (0 × 10⁹/L)	Globulin (g/dL)	5.4 (54 g/L)
Band neutrophils/µL	0 (0 × 10⁹/L)	Cholesterol (mg/dL)	96 (2.5 mmol/L)
↑ Segmented	18,884 (18.9 × 10⁹/L)	↑ Urea nitrogen (mg/dL)	86 (30.7 mmol/L)
neutrophils/µL			
Lymphocytes/µL	1,526 (1.5 × 10⁹/L)	↑ Creatinine (mg/dL)	6.9 (610.0 µmol/L)
Monocytes/µL	218 (0.22 × 10⁹/L)	Glucose (mg/dL)	116 (6.38 mmol/L)
Eosinophils/µL	218 (0.22 × 10⁹/L)	Sodium (mEq/L)	145 (145 mmol/L)
Basophils/µL	54 (0.05 × 10⁹/L)	Potassium (mEq/L)	4.8 (4.8 mmol/L)
Toxic neutrophils	None seen	Chloride (mEq/L)	92 (92 mmol/L)
Platelet estimate	Adequate	Carbon dioxide (mEq/L)	35 (35 mmol/L)
		↑ Calcium (mg/dL)	16.2 (4.1 mmol/L)
		↓ Phosphorus (mg/dL)	2.0 (0.65 mmol/L)

Urinalysis (Catheter)	
Appearance	Cloudy, yellow
↓ Specific gravity	1.010
pH	8
↑ Protein	3+
Glucose	Negative
Ketones	Negative
↑ Blood	+
Bilirubin	Negative
Sediment	
↑ WBC/hpf	10–30
↑ RBC/hpf	40–50
Casts	None
Bacteria	Negative

HEMOGRAM

There is a mild normocytic normochromic anemia. In the horse erythrocyte parameters indicating erythrogenesis are very insensitive. Since horses do not respond to anemia with reticulocytosis the best method to determine the regenerative status of an anemia is by doing a reticulocyte count on bone marrow. The leukocytosis and mature neutrophilia are suggestive of inflammation or stress.

BIOCHEMICAL PROFILE

The profile is remarkable for a marked azotemia (increased urea nitrogen and creatinine), hypercalcemia, and hypophosphatemia associated with inappropriate (low) urine specific gravity. In the horse the kidney is involved in calcium balance, and hypercalcemia frequently develops with renal failure. The increased number of erythrocytes and leukocytes in the urine could be associated with obtaining the specimen, but an inflammatory process involving the kidneys remains a possibility in this case. The proteinuria could reflect the inflammatory process, or if the cells are contaminants from the catheterization, the proteinuria would reflect glomerular damage. Further differentiation with the clinicopathologic parameters expressed at this point is not possible.

DIAGNOSIS

Primary renal insufficiency with secondary anemia and hypercalcemia.

Patient: Dog, Great Dane, male, 4 years old.

Presenting Complaints: Swollen leg with incomplete response to antibiotics the past 6 months.

Physical Examination: Right hind leg swollen; several fistular tracts present; thin; slightly dehydrated.

Problem List: 1. Chronic osteomyelitis. 2. Dehydration.

Hematology		Serum Chemistry	
RBC × 10⁶/µL	7.02 (7.02 × 10¹²/L)	AST (SGOT) (IU/L)	7 (7 U/L)
Hemoglobin (g/dL)	17.5 (10.9 mmol/L)	ALT (SGPT) (IU/L)	1 (1 U/L)
PCV (%)	49.1 (0.49 volume fraction)	ALP (IU/L)	17 (17 U/L)
MCV (fL)	70	Total bilirubin (mg/dL)	0.2 (3.4 µmol/L)
MCHC (g/dL)	35.6 (22.1 mmol/L)	Total protein (g/dL)	7.2 (72 g/L)
NRBC/100 WBC	0	↓ Albumin (g/dL)	1.4 (14 g/L)
RBC morphology	Normal	↑ Globulin (g/dL)	5.8 (58 g/L)
WBC × 10³/µL	20.1 (20.1 × 10⁹/L)	↑ Cholesterol (mg/dL)	609 (15.8 mmol/L)
Myelocytes/µL	0 (0 × 10⁹/L)	↑ Urea nitrogen (mg/dL)	49 (17.5 mmol/L)
Metamyelocytes/µL	0 (0 × 10⁹/L)	↑ Creatinine (mg/dL)	2.8 (247.5 µmol/L)
Band neutrophils/µL	201 (0.2 × 10⁹/L)	Glucose (mg/dL)	76 (4.18 mmol/L)
↑ Segmented neutrophils/µL	17,085 (17.1 × 10⁹/L)	Sodium (mEq/L)	138 (138 mmol/L)
↓ Lymphocytes/µL	603 (0.6 × 10⁹/L)	Potassium (mEq/L)	4 (4.0 mmol/L)
↑ Monocytes/µL	1,608 (1.6 × 10⁹/L)	Na : K ratio	4.5
Eosinophils/µL	603 (0.6 × 10⁹/L)	Chloride (mEq/L)	113 (113 mmol/L)
Basophils/µL	0 (0 × 10⁹/L)	↓ Carbon dioxide (mEq/L)	12 (12 mmol/L)
Platelets × 10³/µL	245 (0.245 × 10¹²/L)	Calcium (mg/dL)	8.9 (2.23 mmol/L)
Plasma protein (g/dL)	8.0 (80 g/L)	Corrected calcium (mg/dL)	11.0 (2.75 mmol/L)
↑ Fibrinogen (mg/dL)	800 (8.0 g/L)	Phosphorus (mg/dL)	7.7 (2.49 mmol/L)

Urinalysis (Cystocentesis)	
Appearance	Pale yellow
↓ Specific gravity	1.020
pH	6
↑ Protein	4+
Glucose	Negative
Ketones	Negative
Occult blood	Negative
Bilirubin	Negative
WBC/hpf	0–1
RBC/hpf	0–2
↑ Casts/lpf	2–5 granular
Crystals	None seen
Bacteria	Negative
Urine protein (mg/dL)	600
Urine creatinine (mg/dL)	79
↑ Urine protein/creatine ratio	7.59

HEMOGRAM

There is a slight increase in total leukocyte count with a mature neutrophilia, monocytosis, lymphopenia, and eosinopenia compatible with stress with excessive glucocorticoid production or, pertinent to this case, a response to an inflammatory process, presumably chronic based on the history. The hyperfibrinogemia further supports an inflammatory process.

BIOCHEMICAL PROFILE AND URINALYSIS

Significant alterations in the biochemical profile include increased urea nitrogen and creatinine (azotemia). This, along with the inappropriate (low) urine specific gravity suggest primary renal disease, which is also supported by the marked proteinuria and the presence of granular casts, indicating renal tubular degeneration. Hypoalbuminemia is marked and probably represents urine loss whereas the hyperglobulinemia is most likely a result of the chronic inflammatory process. The decreased total CO_2 is suggestive of a metabolic acidosis often associated with renal insufficiency. This may be caused in part, by phosphate and sulfate retention resulting from decreased renal function. Hyperphosphatemia occurs when there is a decrease in the glomerular filtration rate. Hypercholesterolemia may also be associated with chronic renal insufficiency and is one component of the nephrotic syndrome which is apparent in this patient. The reason for hypercholesterolemia in the nephrotic syndrome is not known. Hyperfibrinogenemia may be related to the inflammation but also occurs with the nephrotic syndrome by an unknown mechanism.

DIAGNOSIS

Nephrotic syndrome.

COMMENT

The patient was managed medically for 3 months but continued to lose weight, developed inappetance, and the renal parameters became more abnormal. The owners requested euthanasia. Histologically *renal amyloidosis*, most probably secondary to the chronic infectious process, was diagnosed.

Patient: Cow, Hereford, 5 years old.

Presenting Signs and Complaints: Passing red urine with clumps of red; lost weight; inappetence.

Problem List: 1. Hematuria. 2. Thin. 3. Anorexia.

Hematology		Serum Chemistry	
RBC × 10⁶/μL	5.8 (5.8 × 10¹²/L)	AST (SGOT) (IU/L)	82 (82 U/L)
Hemoglobin (g/dL)	8.7 (5.39 mmol/L)	ALT (SGPT) (IU/L)	28 (28 U/L)
PCV (%)	26 (0.26 volume fraction)	ALP (IU/L)	100 (100 U/L)
MCV (fL)	44.8	GGT (IU/L)	3 (3 U/L)
MCHC (g/dL)	33.4 (20.7 mmol/L)	Total bilirubin (mg/dL)	0.1 (1.7 μmol/L)
NRBC/100 WBC	0	Conjugated bilirubin (mg/dL)	0.1 (1.7 μmol/L)
RBC morphology		Unconjugated bilirubin (mg/dL)	0 (0.0 μmol/L)
Polychromasia	None	Cholesterol (mg/dL)	124 (3.2 mmol/L)
Anisocytosis	**2+**	Total protein (g/dL)	6.5 (65 g/L)
Poikilocytosis	None	Albumin (g/dL)	3.0 (30 g/L)
↑ **WBC × 10³/μL**	**16.0 (16 × 10⁹/L)**	Globulin (g/dL)	3.5 (35 g/L)
		Glucose (mg/dL)	52 (2.9 mmol/L)
Myelocytes/μL	0 (0 × 10⁹/L)	Urea nitrogen (mg/dL)	20 (7.1 mmol/L)
Metamyelocytes/μL	0 (0 × 10⁹/L)	↑ **Creatinine (mg/dL)**	**3.2 (282.9 μmol/L)**
↑ **Band neutrophils/μL**	**1,600 (1.6 × 10⁹/L)**	Calcium (mg/dL)	10.2 (2.6 mmol/L)
↑ **Neutrophils/μL**	**11,200 (11.2 × 10⁹/L)**	Phosphorus (mg/dL)	5.9 (1.9 mmol/L)
↓ **Lymphocytes/μL**	**2,400 (2.4 × 10⁹/L)**	Sodium (mEq/L)	143 (143 mmol/L)
Monocytes/μL	800 (0.8 × 10⁹/L)	Potassium (mEq/L)	4.8 (4.8 mmol/L)
↓ **Eosinophils/μL**	**0 (0 × 10⁹/L)**	Na : K ratio	29.8
Basophils/μL	0 (0 × 10⁹/L)	Chloride (mEq/L)	108 (108 mmol/L)
↑ **Toxic neutrophils**	**Present**	Carbon dioxide (mEq/L)	31 (31 mmol/L)
Platelets	Adequate		
↑ **Fibrinogen (mg/dL)**	**800 (8 g/L)**		
Plasma protein (g/dL)	7.3 (73 g/L)		

Urinalysis (Catheter)	
Appearance	Cloudy, red
Specific gravity	1.053
pH	8.5
↑ **Protein**	**3+**
Glucose	Negative
Ketones	Negative
↑ **Blood**	**3+**
Bilirubin	Negative
Sediment	
↑ **WBC/hpf**	**TNTC**
↑ **RBC/hpf**	**TNTC**
↑ **Casts**	**Rare WBC**
Crystals	None
↑ **Bacteria**	**Many coccobacillary Gram + rods**
Urine culture	***Corynebacterium renale***

HEMOGRAM

The hemogram is characterized by a leukocytosis, neutrophilia, left shift, lympho-penia, and eosinopenia supportive of an inflammatory response which is appar-ently severe. The presence of inflammation is further supported by the hyperfi-brinogenemia (see Chapter 3 for an additional discussion). The underlying bacterial etiology is implied by the toxic neutrophils.

BIOCHEMICAL PROFILE

The creatinine is increased with a normal urea nitrogen. In the ruminant increased creatinine is an indication of renal insufficiency. Because of rumen metabolism, urea nitrogen is of low sensitivity as a renal function test. The inflammatory hemogram along with the renal insufficiency and the presence of a bacterial infec-tion in the lower urinary tract support pyelonephritis. Renal tubular function is adequate as reflected by the high urine specific gravity.

DIAGNOSIS

Bacterial pyelonephritis with renal insufficiency.

Patient: Dog, German shepherd, male, 1 year old.

Presenting Signs and Complaints: Vomited twice yesterday; has gotten progressively weaker; collapsed this morning.

Physical Examination: Unable to rise; not responsive; depressed spinal reflexes; normal TPR; referred to neurologic service.

Problem List: 1. Weakness. 2. Almost comatose.

Hematology			Serum Chemistry	
RBC × 10⁶/µL	8.7	(8.7 × 10¹²/L)	**AST (SGOT) (IU/L)**	**125 (125 U/L)**
Hemoglobin (g/dL)	18.0	(11.2 mmol/L)	**ALT (SGPT) (IU/L)**	**258 (258 U/L)**
PCV (%)	55	(0.55 volume fraction)	ALP (IU/L)	32 (32 U/L)
MCV (fL)	63.2		GGT (IU/L)	1 (1 U/L)
MCHC (g/dL)	32.7	(20.3 mmol/L)	Total bilirubin (mg/dL)	0.2 (3.4 µmol/L)
NRBC/100 WBC	None		Conjugated bilirubin (mg/dL)	0.1 (1.7 µmol/L)
RBC morphology	Normal		Total protein (g/dL)	7.1 (71 g/L)
WBC × 10³/µL	18.7	(18.7 × 10⁹/L)	Albumin (g/dL)	3.6 (36 g/L)
			Globulin (g/dL)	3.5 (35 g/L)
Myelocytes/µL	0	(0 × 10⁹/L)	Amylase (IU/L)	850 (850 U/L)
Metamyelocytes/µL	0	(0 × 10⁹/L)	Lipase (IU/L)	125 (125 U/L)
Band neutrophils/µL	185	(0.19 × 10⁹/L)	↑ **Glucose (mg/dL)**	**169 (9.3 mmol/L)**
Neutrophils/µL	**15,725 ↑ (15.7 × 10⁹/L)**		↑ **Urea nitrogen (mg/dL)**	**67 (24 mmol/L)**
Lymphocytes/µL	**925 ↓ (0.9 × 10⁹/L)**		↑ **Creatinine (mg/dL)**	**3.2 (282.9 µmol/L)**
Monocytes/µL	**1,850 ↑ (1.9 × 10⁹/L)**		↓ **Calcium (mg/dL)**	**7.6 (1.9 mmol/L)**
Eosinophils/µL	**0 ↓ (0 × 10⁹/L)**		↑ **Phosphorus (mg/dL)**	**9.9 (3.2 mmol/L)**
Basophils/µL	0	(0 × 10⁹/L)	Sodium (mEq/L)	149 (149 mmol/L)
Toxic neutrophils	None seen		Potassium (mEq/L)	5.0 (5.0 mmol/L)
Platelets × 10³/µL	225	(0.225 × 10¹²/L)	Chloride (mEq/L)	95 (95 mmol/L)
			↓ **Carbon dioxide (mEq/L)**	**13.9 (13.9 mmol/L)**
↑ **Anion gap (Na + K)−**	**45.1**		LDH (IU/L)	1,535 (1535 U/L)
(Cl + TCO₂)[a]				
↑ **Serum osmolality (mOS/kg)**[b]	**350**		CK (IU/L)	250 (250 U/L)
↑ **Base excess (mEq/L)**	**−11.8**		Cholinesterase (IU/L)	1,027 (1027 U/L)
			↓ **Blood pH**	**7.267**
			↓ **PaCO₂ (mmHg)**	**30.2 (4.02 kPa)**
			PaO₂ (mmHg)	41.2 (5.48 kPa)
			↓ **HCO₃ (mEq/L)**	**13.0 (13 mmol/L)**

[a] Normal anion gap = 12–16.
[b] Normal serum osmolality = 280–310.

Urinalysis (Cystocentesis)	
Appearance	Dark yellow
Specific gravity	1.035
pH	6.5
Protein	+
Glucose	Negative
Blood	Negative
Bilirubin	Negative
Sediment	
WBC/hpf	1–3
RBC/hpf	1.5
Casts	+Hyaline
↑ **Crystals**	**2+ Calcium oxalate monohydrate**
Bacteria	Negative

HEMOGRAM

The leukogram (leukocytosis, neutrophilia, lymphopenia, eosinopenia, and mono-cytosis) is compatible with stress.

BIOCHEMICAL PROFILE

The mildly increased AST and ALT suggest enzyme leakage from hepatocytes. Azotemia and hyperphosphatemia indicate renal insufficiency. The urine specific gravity is inappropriate to the magnitude of the creatinine and urea nitrogen concentrations. This is probably an acute process because the tubules can still concentrate to a moderate degree.

The total CO_2 is decreased, suggesting metabolic acidosis. The anion gap of 45.1 is high, indicating the presence of increased unmeasured anions such as those associated with renal insufficiency (see Chapter 6, Table 6-5). Serum osmolality is increased, indicating the presence of osmotically active substances.

Hyperglycemia frequently accompanies ethylene glycol toxicity (see the discussion in Chapter 7).

The presence of calcium oxalate monohydrate crystals is indicative of ethylene glycol toxicity. Hypocalcemia results from excess formation of calcium oxalate crystals. These crystals are important to recognize because they strongly support a clinical diagnosis of ethylene glycol toxicosis. They appear similar to hippuric acid crystals.

The presence of ethylene glycol will increase serum osmolality.

DIAGNOSIS

Primary renal insufficiency secondary to ethylene glycol toxicosis.

COMMENTS

The mild increase in transaminases is unexplained but may reflect altered membrane permeability as a result of metabolic acidosis and/or altered hepatic blood flow.

Patient: Cat, domestic shorthair, neutered male, mature.

Presenting Signs and Complaints: Straining to urinate.

Physical Examination: On palpation the urinary bladder was markedly distended, and urine could not be expressed manually; 5% dehydration.

Problem List: 1. Distended urinary bladder. 2. Painful abdomen. 3. Dehydration.

Hematology		Serum Chemistry	
RBC × 10⁶/µL	8.9 (8.9 × 10¹²/L)	AST (SGOT) (IU/L)	44 (44 U/L)
Hemoglobin (g/dL)	13.8 (8.6 mmol/L)	ALT (SGPT) (IU/L)	59 (59 U/L)
PCV (%)	46 (0.46 volume fraction)	ALP (IU/L)	35 (35 U/L)
MCV (fL)	51.7	Total protein (g/dL)	7.1 (71 g/L)
MCHC (g/dL)	33.3 (20.6 mmol/L)	Albumin (g/dL)	3.7 (37 g/L)
NRBC/100 WBC	0	Globulin (g/dL)	3.4 (34 g/L)
RBC morphology	Normal	↑ Glucose (mg/dL)	282 (15.5 mmol/L)
↑ WBC × 10³/µL	22.0 (22 × 10⁹/L)	↑ Urea nitrogen (mg/dL)	144 (51.4 mmol/L)
		↑ Creatinine (mg/dL)	8.3 (733.7 µmol/L)
Myelocytes/µL	0 (0 × 10⁹/L)	Calcium (mg/dL)	7.2 (1.8 mmol/L)
Metamyelocytes/µL	0 (0 × 10⁹/L)	↑ Phosphorus (mg/dL)	7.9 (2.55 mmol/L)
Band neutrophils/µL	0 (0 × 10⁹/L)	Sodium (mEq/L)	144 (144 mmol/L)
↑ Segmented	20,020 (20 × 10⁹/L)	↑ Potassium (mEq/L)	8.1 (8.1 mmol/L)
neutrophils/µL			
↓ Lymphocytes/µL	660 (0.66 × 10⁹/L)	↓ Na : K ratio	17.8
↑ Monocytes/µL	1,320 (1.3 ×10⁹/L)	Chloride (mEq/L)	110 (110 mmol/L)
↓ Eosinophils/µL	0 (0 × 10⁹/L)	↓ Carbon dioxide (mEq/L)	9 (9 mmol/L)
Basophils/µL	0 (0 × 10⁹/L)		
↑ Toxic neutrophils	+		
Platelets	Adequate		

Urinalysis (Cystocentesis)	
Appearance	Cloudy, red
Specific gravity	1.048
pH	7.0
↑ **Protein**	3+
Glucose	Negative
Ketones	Negative
↑ **Blood**	3+
Bilirubin	Negative
Sediment	
↑ **WBC/hpf**	50–75
↑ **RBC/hpf**	TNTC
Casts	Negative
Crystals	Negative
Bacteria	None seen

HEMOGRAM

Leukocytosis, neutrophilia, monocytosis, lymphopenia and eosinopenia are compatible with a stress/inflammatory pattern.

BIOCHEMICAL PROFILE

The increased blood glucose is compatible with stress-induced gluconeogenesis. The markedly increased urea nitrogen, creatinine, phosphorus, and potassium indicate renal insufficiency, the result of lower urinary tract obstruction. The physical examination that indicated urinary obstruction suggests that the renal insufficiency is a secondary problem. The markedly decreased total CO_2 indicates metabolic acidosis. The acidosis may also be responsible for some of the hyperkalemia as potassium enters the plasma and hydrogen enters cells in acidotic animals.

URINALYSIS

The presence of blood, leukocytes, and protein indicates inflammation. The absence of bacteria suggests that this is a sterile cystitis.

DIAGNOSIS

Renal insufficiency secondary to urinary outflow obstruction.

Patient: Colt, thoroughbred, female, 6 hours old.

Presenting Complaints: Labored respirations, rapid and shallow.

Physical Examination: Scleral injection; 3-cm swelling on ventral abdomen; unable to stand. Radiographs: air bronchograms and diffuse interstitial infiltrates compatible with bacterial pneumonia.

Problem List: 1. Extreme weakness. 2. Dyspnea.

Hematology		Serum Chemistry	
PCV (%)	43 (0.43 volume fraction)	Urea nitrogen (mg/dL)	30 (10.71 mmol/L)
NRBC/100 WBC	0	Creatinine (mg/dL)	1.8 (159.1 μmol/L)
RBC morphology	Normal	Glucose (mg/dL)	49 (40.5 mmol/L)
↑ **WBC × 10³/μL**	**48.5 (48.5 × 10¹²/L)**	Sodium (mEq/L)	147 (147 mmol/L)
Metamyelocytes/μL	0 (0 × 10⁹/L)	Potassium (mEq/L)	3.4 (3.4 mmol/L)
↑ **Band neutrophils/μL**	**1,455 (1.46 × 10⁹/L)**	Na : K ratio	43.2
↑ **Segmented neutrophils/** **μL**	**44,135 (44.1 × 10⁹/L)**	Chloride (mEq/L)	105 (105 mmol/L)
↓ **Lymphocytes/μL**	**970 (0.97 × 10⁹/L)**	Arterial blood gas	
Monocytes/μL	1,940 (1.9 × 10⁹/L)	pH	7.377
↓ **Eosinophils/μL**	**0 (0 × 10⁹/L)**	P_{CO_2} (mmHg)	40 (5.32 pKa)
Basophils/μL	0 (0 × 10⁹/L)	P_{O_2} (mmHg)	63 (8.379 pKa)
Toxic neutrophils	None seen	HCO_3 (mEq/L)	23 (23 mmol/L)
Platelet × 10³/μL	195 (0.195 × 10¹²/L)	**Zn precipitation test for**	**<200 mg (<2 g/L)**
↓ **Plasma protein (g/dL)**	**2.5 (25 g/L)**	**IgG**	
↑ **Fibrinogen (mg/dL)**	**700 (7 g/L)**		

Abdominocentesis[a]	
Specific gravity	1.015
Protein (g/dL)	<2.5 (<25 g/L)
RBC/μL	2,000 (0.002 × 10¹²/L)
WBC/μL	28,000 (28 × 10⁹/L)
92% nondegenerate, segmented neutrophils	
8% macrophages	
↑ **Creatinine (mg/dL)**	**3.5 (309.4 μmol/L)**

[a] Taken 18 hours after entering. Foal is stronger but has not urinated since arrival.

Serum Values at This time	
Creatinine (mg/dL)	1.0 (88.4 μmol/L)
Sodium (mEq/L)	136 (136 mmol/L)
Potassium (mEq/L)	4.2 (4.2 mmol/L)
Chloride (mEq/L)	100 (100 mmol/L)

HEMOGRAM

The marked leukocytosis with neutrophilia and left shift represents an acute inflammatory response. A bacterial etiology should be considered. Inflammation is supported by the hyperfibrinogenemia.

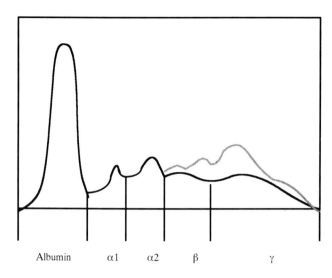

CASE 45. Protein electrophoretic tracing showing a very low β–γ concentration. The *dotted line* represents a normal β–γ peak.

Albumin   α1   α2   β   γ

BIOCHEMICAL PROFILE

There is a hypoproteinemia which, in part, is caused by the failure of colostral transfer as indicated by the low zinc precipitation test. Hypoglobulinemia was confirmed by protein electrophoresis.

ABDOMINOCENTESIS

The abdominal fluid has a normal protein concentration but is high in nondegenerate neutrophils. This is a modified transudate resulting from a sterile inflammation.

The increased creatinine concentration in the abdominal fluid contrasted with a normal serum creatinine supports uroperitoneum. The creatinine concentration in the abdominal fluid is normally less than or equal to that of serum.

DIAGNOSIS

Ruptured urinary bladder.

COMMENT

The ruptured urinary bladder was confirmed and repaired at laparotomy. Urine has higher potassium and lower sodium concentrations than interstitial fluid; therefore hyponatremia and hyperkalemia are also frequent findings in patients with uroperitoneum. In this patient the duration was apparently short enough that these electrolyte disturbances did not develop.

Patient: Dog, Great Dane, female, 4 months old.

Presenting Signs and Complaints: Red urine; strains to urinate.

Physical Examination: Blood in urine.

Problem List: 1. Hematuria. 2. Stranguria.

Hematology		Serum Chemistry	
RBC × 10⁶/μL	5.3 (5.3 × 10¹²/L)	AST (SGOT) (IU/L)	25 (25 U/L)
Hemoglobin (g/dL)	12.1 (7.50 mmol/L)	ALT (SGPT) (IU/L)	24 (24 U/L)
PCV (%)	36.5 (0.365 volume fraction)	↑ **ALP (IU/L)**	**140 (140 U/L)**
MCV (fL)	70	GGT (IU/L)	11
MCHC (g/dL)	36.5 (22.6 mmol/L)	Total bilirubin (mg/dL)	0.2 (3.4 μmol/L)
NRBC/100 WBC	0	Conjugated bilirubin (mg/dL)	0.1 (1.7 μmol/L)
RBC morphology	Normal	Unconjugated bilirubin (mg/dL)	0.21 (1.7 μmol/L)
WBC × 10³/μL	12.0 (12.0 × 10⁹/L)	Total protein (g/dL)	5.7 (57 g/L)
Myelocytes/μL	0 (0 × 10⁹/L)	Albumin (g/dL)	3.1 (31 g/L)
Metamyelocytes/μL	0 (0 × 10⁹/L)	Globulin (g/dL)	2.6 (26 g/L)
Band neutrophils/μL	0 (0 × 10⁹/L)	Cholesterol (mg/dL)	121 (3.15 mmol/L)
Segmented neutrophils/μL	8,610 (8.6 × 10⁹/L)	Urea nitrogen (mg/dL)	19 (6.78 mmol/L)
Lymphocytes/μL	2,830 (2.8 × 10⁹/L)	Creatinine (mg/dL)	1.6 (141.4 μm/L)
Monocytes/μL	350 (0.35 × 10⁹/L)	Glucose (mg/dL)	131 (7.21 mmol/L)
Eosinophils/μL	110 (0.11 × 10⁹/L)	Amylase (IU/L)	350 (350 U/L)
Basophils/μL	110 (0.11 × 10⁹/L)	Lipase (IU/L)	22 (22 U/L)
Toxic neutrophils	None	Sodium (mEq/L)	152 (152 mmol/L)
Platelet estimate	Adequate	Potassium (mEq/L)	4.5 (4.5 mmol/L)
		Na : K ratio	33.7
		Chloride (mEq/L)	110 (110 mmol/L)
		Carbon dioxide (mEq/L)	25 (25 mmol/L)
		Calcium (mg/dL)	9.9 (2.48 mmol/L)
		Corrected calcium (mg/dL)	10.32.58 mmol/L)
		↑ **Phosphorus (mg/dL)**	**7.7 (2.5 mmol/L)**

Urinalysis (Catheter)	
Appearance	**Cloudy, reddish yellow**
Specific gravity	1.032
↑ **pH**	**8.0**
↑ **Protein**	**3+**
Glucose	Negative
Ketones	Negative
↑ **Blood**	**3+**
Bilirubin	Negative
Sediment	
↑ **WBC/hpf**	**TNTC**
↑ **RBC/hpf**	**25–50**
Casts	Negative
Crystals	Negative
↑ **Bacteria**	**3+ Gram-negative rods**
Urine culture	**Heavy growth *Escherichia coli***

URINALYSIS AND BIOCHEMICAL PROFILE

The pyuria, hematuria, and bacteriuria support the presence of a lower urinary tract infection and inflammation. Alkaline urine in this patient is probably due to metabolism of urea by *E. coli*.

BIOCHEMICAL PROFILE

The serum alkaline phosphatase and phosphorus are higher than normal for an adult animal but are normal for a growing animal.

DIAGNOSIS

Urinary bladder cystitis.

Patient: Dog, Boston terrier, spayed female, 3 years old.

Presenting Signs and Complaints: Diarrhea with increased frequency; weight loss for 3 months; appetite varies between normal to increased; has been to several veterinarians; multiple antidiarrheal drugs administered with partial response.

Physical Examination: Stool is soft, to liquid; thin.

Problem List: 1. Chronic diarrhea. 2. Weight loss.

Hematology		Serum Chemistry	
RBC × 10⁶/μL	5.3 (5.3 × 10¹²/L)	AST (SGOT) (IU/L)	83 (83 U/L)
Hemoglobin (g/dL)	13.3 (8.25 mmol/L)	ALT (SGPT) (IU/L)	14 (14 U/L)
PCV (%)	37.9 (0.38 volume fraction)	ALP (IU/L)	25 (25 U/L)
MCV (fL)	71	GGT (IU/L)	2 (2 U/L)
MCHC (g/dL)	35.2 (21.8 mmol/L)	Total bilirubin (mg/dL)	0.1 (1.7 μmol/L)
Reticulocytes (%)	1.7 (0.017 number fraction)	Conjugated bilirubin (mg/dL)	0.0 (0.0 μmol/L)
Reticulocytes × 10³/μL	9.0 (9 × 10⁹/L)	Unconjugated bilirubin (mg/dL)	0.1 (1.7 μmol/L)
NRBC/100 WBC	1	↓ Total protein (g/dL)	**3.1 (31 g/L)**
RBC morphology	Normal	↓ Albumin (g/dL)	**1.6 (16 g/L)**
WBC × 10³/μL	11.3 (11.3 × 10⁹/L)	↓ Globulin (g/dL)	**1.5 (15 g/L)**
Myelocytes/μL	0 (0 × 10⁹/L)	↓ Cholesterol (mg/dL)	**86 (2.2 mmol/L)**
↑ **Metamyelocytes/μL**	**110 (0.11 × 10⁹/L)**	Urea nitrogen (mg/dL)	14 (4.99 mmol/L)
↑ **Band neutrophils/μL**	**330 (0.33 × 10⁹/L)**	Creatinine (mg/dL)	0.6 (53.0 μmol/L)
Segmented neutrophils/μL	10,390 (10.39 × 10⁹/L)	Glucose (mg/dL)	120 (6.6 mmol/L)
↓ **Lymphocytes/μL**	**330 (0.33 × 10⁹/L)**	Amylase (IU/L)	2,100 (2,100 U/L)
Monocytes/μL	110 (0.11 × 10⁹/L)	Lipase (IU/L)	75 (75 U/L)
↓ **Eosinophils/μL**	**0 (0 × 10⁹/L)**	Sodium (mEq/L)	144 (144 mmol/L)
Basophils/μL	0 (0 × 10⁹/L)	Potassium (mEq/L)	4.6 (4.6 mmol/L)
Toxic neutrophils	None seen	Na : K ratio	31.3
Platelet estimate	**Increased**	Chloride (mEq/L)	119 (119 mmol/L)
↑ **Platelet × 10³μL**	**1,100 (1.1 × 10¹²/L)**	Carbon dioxide (mEq/L)	21 (21 mmol/L)
↓ **Plasma protein (g/dL)**	**3.4 (34 g/L)**	↓ **Calcium (mg/dL)**	**6.4 (1.6 mmol/L)**
Fibrinogen (mg/dL)	300 (3 g/L)	Corrected calcium (mg/dL)	8.3 (2.08 mmol/L)
		Phosphorus (mg/dL)	2.8 (0.90 mmol/L)
		↓ **TLI (μg/L)**	**0.8**
		↑ **Folate (μg/L)**	**80**
		Cobalamin (ng/L)	**400**

Urinalysis (midstream collect)	
Appearance	**Cloudy, yellow**
Specific gravity	1.024
pH	6.5
↑ **Protein**	**3+**
Glucose	Negative
Ketones	Negative
↑ **Blood**	**2+**
Bilirubin	Negative
Sediment	
↑ **WBC/hpf**	**TNTC**
↑ **RBC/hpf**	**TNTC**
Casts	None
Crystals	None
↑ **Bacteria**	**3+**

HEMOGRAM

Left shift indicates active inflammation, and the magnitude of the shift suggests an acute severe response with increased peripheral utilization of neutrophils. Lymphopenia and eosinopenia indicate increased glucocorticoid activity. In this case it is probably a part of a stress response to the inflammation. Platelet increases may occur in association with iron deficiency for reasons that are poorly understood. Serum iron was not determined in this patient, and the cause of the thrombocytosis remains unexplained.

URINALYSIS

Proteinuria, pyuria, hematuria, and bacteriuria support inflammatory renal or urinary tract disease. Because this is a midstream collection by the owner one must consider the possibility of posturinary tract contamination. The urinalysis should be repeated on a sample collected by cystocentesis.

BIOCHEMICAL PROFILE

Hypoproteinemia is a result of hypoalbuminemia and hypoglobulinemia. A parallel decrease in albumin and globulin is commonly associated with a protein-losing enteropathy, and there is historic support for that diagnosis. Hypocholesterolemia may be a reflection of malabsorption. The decreased TLI concentration is indicative of exocrine pancreatic insufficiency. The increased serum folate concentration with a normal serum cobalamin is most compatible with bacterial overgrowth, a common complication of a number of intestinal disorders. The working clinical diagnosis at this point is exocrine pancreatic insufficiency with secondary intestinal bacterial overgrowth. The marked decrease in proteins is unusual in these conditions and suggests that an underlying protein-losing enteropathy may also be present.

The owners elected to try a course of antibiotics for several weeks and pancreatic enzyme replacement for 2 months before additional tests were done. At the end of 2 months the stool characteristic had improved although the patient had not gained weight, and the lymphopenia and hypoproteinemia persisted. Biopsy of the small intestine indicated severe lymphangectasia. Biopsy of the pancreas indicated atrophy and fibrosis.

DIAGNOSIS

Exocrine pancreatic insufficiency, lymphangectasia with bacterial overgrowth.

COMMENT

Persistent lymphopenia with chronic diarrhea is common in patients with lymphangectasia. Lymphopenia is caused by cell loss through dilated lymphatics into the lumen of the intestine.

Patient: Dog, terrier, male, 8 years old.

Presenting Signs and Complaints: Depressed; inappetent; vomited three times last night.

Physical Examination: Supple abdomen with intestinal gas and fluid on palpation; nonresponsive.

Problem List: 1. Depression. 2. Inappetence. 3. Vomiting.

Hematology		Serum Chemistry[a]	
RBC × 10⁶/µL	6.6 (6.6 × 10¹²/L)	↑ AST (SGOT) (IU/L)	**210 (210 U/L)**
Hemoglobin (g/dL)	Too lipemic	↑ ALT (SGPT) (IU/L)	**180 (180 U/L)**
PCV (%)	43.4 (0.434 volume fraction)	↑ ALP (IU/L)	**327 (327 U/L)**
MCV (fL)	66	↑ GGT (IU/L)	**28 (28 U/L)**
MCHC (g/dL)	Too lipemic	↑ Total bilirubin (mg/dL)	**3.2 (54.7 µmol/L)**
NRBC/100 WBC	0	↑ Conjugated bilirubin (mg/dL)	**2.9 (49.6 µmol/L)**
RBC morphology	Normal	Unconjugated bilirubin (mg/dL)	0.3
↑ WBC × 10³/µL	**24.7 (24.7 × 10⁹/L)**	Total protein (g/dL)	7.2 (72 g/L)
Myelocytes/µL	0 (0 × 10⁹/L)	↑ Albumin (g/dL)	**4.5 (45g/L)**
Metamyelocytes/µL	0 (0 × 10⁹/L)	Globulin (g/dL)	2.7 (27 g/L)
Band neutrophils/µL	0 (0 × 10⁹/L)	↑ Cholesterol (mg/dL)	**369 (9.59 mmol/L)**
↑ Segmented neutrophils/µL	**22,971 (23 × 10⁹/L)**	Urea nitrogen (mg/dL)	12 (4.28 mmol/L)
↓ Lymphocytes/µL	**247 (0.25 × 10⁹/L)**	Creatinine (mg/dL)	1.2 (106.1 µmol/L)
Monocytes/µL	988 (0.99 × 10⁹/L)	Glucose (mg/dL)	72 (3.96 mmol/L)
Eosinophils/µL	494 (0.49 × 10⁹/L)	↑ Amylase (IU/L)	**>5,000 (5,000 U/L)**
Basophils/µL	0 (0 × 10⁹/L)	↑ Lipase (IU/L)	**1,270 (1,270 U/L)**
Toxic neutrophils	None seen	↓ Sodium (mEq/L)	**139 (139 mmol/L)**
Platelet estimate	Adequate	Potassium (mEq/L)	3.2 (3.2 mmol/L)
Plasma protein (g/dL)	7.6 (76 g/L)	↓ Chloride (mEq/L)	**86 (86 mmol/L)**
Fibrinogen (mg/dL)	400 (4 g/L)	↑ Carbon dioxide (mEq/L)	**28 (28 mmol/L)**
		↓ Calcium (mg/dL)	**7.2 (1.8 mmol/L)**
		↓ Corrected calcium (mg/dL)	**6.2 (1.55 mmol/L)**
		Phosphorus (mg/dL)	5.4 (1.74 mmol/L)
		↑ LDH (IU/L)	**755 (755 U/L)**

[a] Serum is lipemic.

Urinalysis (catheter)	
Appearance	Clear, yellow
Specific gravity	1.048
pH	6.5
Protein	Negative
Glucose	Negative
Ketones	Negative
Blood	Negative
↑ Bilirubin	+
Sediment	
WBC/hpf	1–2
RBC/hpf	0–1
Casts	Negative
Crystals	Negative
Bacteria	Negative

HEMOGRAM

Leukocytosis with a mature neutrophilia and lymphopenia may be indicative of glucocorticoid activity associated with stress or may reflect the presence of inflammation.

BIOCHEMICAL PROFILE

Increased ALT and AST support enzyme leakage resulting from increased cell membrane permeability associated with hepatocellular damage. Since the AST increase is greater than the ALT, leakage from skeletal muscle must also be considered. The alkaline phosphatase and GGT are increased, indicating increased enzyme production secondary to cholestasis or enzyme-inducing drugs. Hyperbilirubinemia is also supportive of cholestasis, however the + bilirubin in the urine is inappropriate for the magnitude of the hyperbilirubinemia. When the serum bilirubin is greater than 1.0 mg/dL a 3+ or 4 + bilirubinuria will be present. The inappropriate relationship in this case suggests that the hyperbilirubinemia is an artifact. Lipemia will falsely increase the serum bilirubin value.

The marked increases in amylase and lipase are indicative of acute pancreatic injury. An increase in liver enzymes is frequent in dogs with acute pancreatitis (Fig. 7–5).

The corrected calcium is low. Hypocalcemia can occur in association with acute pancreatitis. Hyperalbuminemia with normal globulin and normal total protein suggests mild dehydration. Albumin is often artificially increased in lipemic samples.

Hypochloridemia, hypokalemia, hyponatremia, and alkalosis (high CO_2) are secondary to vomiting.

LDH is present in all cells of the body. An elevation in serum LDH activity indicates tissue damage or alteration in cell membrane permeability.

DIAGNOSIS

Acute pancreatitis with secondary liver disease.

COMMENT

The liver tests will return to normal after successful symptomatic management of the acute pancreatitis. If there is a secondary complication to the pancreatitis such as a diffuse inflammatory process causing extrahepatic obstruction, the cholestatic enzymes will increase, and the bilirubin will increase within 7 to 10 days.

Patient: Horse, standardbred, female, 15 years old.

Presenting Complaints: Not eating; weight loss; firm dark colored stools.

Physical Examination: Very thin; firm stool black in color; pale, yellow mucous membranes; increased pulse and respiratory rates.

Problem List: 1. Anorexia. 2. Weight loss. 3. Anemia. 4. Dark colored feces. 5. Icterus.

Hematology		Serum Chemistry	
↓ RBC × 10⁶/μL	5.3 (5.3 × 10¹²/L)	↑ AST (SGOT) (IU/L)	435 (435 U/L)
↓ Hemoglobin (g/dL)	5.5 (3.41 mmol/L)	ALT (SGPT) (IU/L)	10 (10 U/L)
↓ PCV (%)	17.5 (0.175 volume fraction)	ALP (IU/L)	35 (35 U/L)
↓ MCV (fL)	38	GGT (IU/L)	1 (1 U/L)
↓ MCHC (g/dL)	30 (18.6 mmol/L)	↑ Total bilirubin (mg/dL)	5.5 (94.1 μmol/L)
↑ RDW (%)ᵃ	24.2 (0.24 volume fraction)	↓ Total protein (g/dL)	4.3 (43 g/L)
Reticulocytes/μL	0	↓ Albumin (g/dL)	2.0 (10 g/L)
NRBC/100 WBC	0	↓ Globulin (g/dL)	2.3 (23 g/L)
RBC morphology		Glucose (mg/dL)	87 (4.9 mmol/L)
Polychromasia	0	Urea nitrogen (mg/dL)	12 (4.28 mmol/L)
↑ Anisocytosis	2 +	Creatinine (mg/dL)	0.6 (53.0 μmol/L)
Poikilocytosis	0	Calcium (mg/dL)	9.8 (2.45 mmol/L)
↑ WBC × 10³/μL	16.3 (16.3 × 10⁹/L)	Phosphorus (mg/dL)	3.5 (1.13 mmol/L)
		Sodium (mEq/L)	150 (150 mmol/L)
Myelocytes/μL	0 (0 × 10⁹/L)	Potassium (mEq/L)	4.5 (4.5 mmol/L)
Metamyelocytes/μL	0 (0 × 10⁹/L)	Chloride (mEq/L)	102 (102 mmol/L)
↑ Band neutrophils/μL	326 (0.33 × 10⁹/L)	Carbon dioxide (mEq/L)	24 (24 mmol/L)
↑ Segmented neutrophils/μL	13,203 (13.2 × 10⁹/L)	LDH (IU/L)	236 (236 U/L)
Lymphocytes/μL	2,445 (2.4 × 10⁹/L)	↓ Serum iron (μg/dL)	38 (6.8 mm/L)
Monocytes/μL	163 (0.16 × 10⁹/L)	↑ Fecal occult blood	Positive
Eosinophils/μL	163 (0.16 × 10⁹/L)		
Basophils/μL	0 (0 × 10⁹/L)		
Toxic neutrophils	None		
Platelet estimate	Adequate		
↓ Plasma protein (g/dL)	4.5 (45 g/L)		
Fibrinogen (mg/dL)	200 (2 g/L)		

ᵃ Red cell distribution width.

HEMOGRAM

There is an anemia that is difficult to classify in the horse since reticulocytes are not released from the bone marrow. However, the increased RDW (indicating the presence of a subpopulation of erythrocytes, either microcytes or macrocytes) along with the low normal MCV support iron deficiency, confirmed by the low serum iron. The decreased plasma protein (both albumin and globulin) supports blood loss. The leukocytosis with a mild left shift indicates an inflammatory response.

BIOCHEMICAL PROFILE

There is a mild increase in AST suggestive of enzyme leakage from hepatocytes or skeletal muscle. The hypoproteinemia is a result of decreases in both albumin and globulins, most compatiable with blood loss. The low serum ions aids in confirming the iron deficiency.

The positive test for fecal blood suggests hemorrhage into the gastrointestinal tract.

Hyperbilirubinemia may be associated with hepatic disease or the result of inanition.

COMMENTS

A gastric lavage was performed. It was positive for blood, and cytologically inflammatory cells and carcinoma cells were present. At necropsy an ulcerated gastric neoplasm was noted which was histologically described as a squamous cell carcinoma.

DIAGNOSIS

Squamous cell carcinoma of stomach.

Patient: Dog, Akita, male, 3 years old.

Presenting Signs and Complaints: Diarrhea, small amounts, increased frequency; occasional vomiting, 6 weeks duration; no weight loss; appetite normal.

Physical Examination: No abnormal findings.

Problem List: 1. Diarrhea.

Hematology		Serum Chemistry (Slightly Hemolyzed)	
RBC × 10⁶/μL	7.41 (7.41 × 10¹²/L)	AST (SGOT) (IU/L)	43 (43 U/L)
Hemoglobin (g/dL)	15.9 (9.9 mmol/L)	ALT (SGPT) (IU/L)	20 (20 U/L)
PCV (%)	43 (0.43 volume fraction)	ALP (IU/L)	50 (50 U/L)
↓ MCV (fL)	58	↓ Total protein (g/dL)	5.3 (53 g/L)
MCHC (g/dL)	37 (22.9 mmol/L)	↓ Albumin (g/dL)	1.5 (15 g/L)
NRBC/100 WBC	0	↑ Globulin (g/dL)	3.8 (38 g/L)
RBC morphology	Normal	Glucose (mg/dL)	92 (5.1 mmol/L)
↑ WBC × 10³/μL	22.6 (22.6 × 10⁹/L	Urea nitrogen (mg/dL)	12 (4.28 mmol/L)
		Creatinine (mg/dL)	1.6 (141.4 μmol/L)
Myelocytes/μL	0 (0 × 10⁹/L)	Calcium (mg/dL)	8.3 (2.1 mmol/L)
Metamyelocytes/μL	0 (0 × 10⁹/L)	Corrected calcium (mg/dL)	10.3 (2.6 mmol/L)
Band neutrophils/μL	0 (0 × 10⁹/L)	Phosphorus (mg/dL)	3.6 (1.16 mmol/L)
Segmented neutrophils/μL	6,780 (6.8 × 10⁹/L)	Sodium (mEq/L)	148 (148 mmol/L)
Lymphocytes/μL	3,729 (3.7 × 10⁹/L)	↑ Potassium (mEq/L)	8.5 (8.5 mmol/L)
Monocytes/μL	339 (0.34 × 10⁹/L)	↓ Na : K ratio	17.4
↑ Eosinophils/μL	11,413 (11.4 × 10⁹/L)	Chloride (mEq/L)	119 (119 mmol/L)
↑ Basophils/μL	339 (0.34 × 10⁹/L)	Carbon dioxide (mEq/L)	21 (21 mmol/L)
Platelet estimate	Adequate	TLI (μg/L)	11.6 (11.6 μg/L)
Fibrinogen (mg/dL)	200 (2 g/L)	Cobalamin (ng/L)	426 (426 ng/L)
Plasma protein (g/dL)	5.6 (56 g/L)	Folate (μg/L)	10.8 (10.8 μg/L)

Fecal Examination: fecal parasites negative on several samples.

Urinalysis (Catheter)	
Appearance	Light yellow
↑ Specific gravity	1.018
↑ pH	7.5
Protein	Negative
Glucose	Negative
Ketones	Negative
Blood	Negative
Bilirubin	Negative
Sediment	
↑ WBC/hpf	50
RBC/hpf	Rare
Casts	Negative
Crystals	Triple phosphate
↑ Bacteria	Many Cocci

HEMOGRAM

The erythrocytes are microcytic. This may be normal in the Akita breed. Other considerations should include iron deficiency, or it may be associated with congenital portosystemic vascular anomalies.

There is a leukocytosis that is characterized by a marked eosinophilia.

BIOCHEMICAL PROFILE

The hypoalbuminemia with a negative urine protein is suggestive of decreased hepatic production.

The hyperkalemia and resulting low Na : K ratio is because Akita dogs have a high concentration of potassium in their erythrocytes, and hemolysis causes a factitious hyperkalemia.

A direct fecal examination for leukocytes was made, and some neutrophils were present indicating an inflammatory process. Colonic endoscopy was performed with scrapings for cytology which indicated numerous eosinophils. Biopsies were also obtained and supported eosinophilic colitis. Occasionally fecal examination for leukocytes will be positive for eosinophils, supporting the clinical diagnosis and obviating the need for a biopsy.

Because of the hypoalbuminemia, fasting serum bile acids were completed. The fasting serum bile acids was 56 μmol/L, supportive of liver insufficiency. Ultrasound examination of the abdomen was compatible for a portosystemic vascular anomaly.

DIAGNOSIS

Eosinophilic colitis, liver insufficiency.

COMMENT

In this patient the clinical presentation and diagnostics were for eosinophilic colitits. Serendipitously the hypoalbuminemia led us to do a fasting serum bile acids, and we uncovered a portosystemic vascular anomaly most likely congenital in origin. The owners declined additional diagnostic tests until the patient was successfully managed for the colitis. Cirrhosis could not be ruled out in this patient, however, with the normal liver enzymes and the age of the animal a congenital problem was most likely.

Case 51

Patient: Dog, poodle, female, 11 years old.

Presenting Signs and Complaints: Lethargic for 2 to 3 weeks; not eating; vomited once or twice; soft scant stools.

Physical Examination: Lethargy; weak; weight loss; resists abdominal palpation, but ascites is suspected; dark.

Problem List: 1. Anorexia. 2. Ascites. 3. Mild dehydration.

Hematology		Serum Chemistry	
↓ RBC × 10⁶/μL	4.56 (4.56 × 10¹²/L)	↑ AST (SGOT) (IU/L)	126 (126 U/L)
↓ Hemoglobin (g/dL)	11.8 (7.32 mmol/L)	ALT (SGPT) (IU/L)	50 (50 U/L)
↓ PCV (%)	30.5 (0.305 volume fraction)	↑ ALP (IU/L)	262 (262 U/L)
MCV (fL)	67	GGT (IU/L)	1 (1 U/L)
MCHC (g/dL)	38.6 (23.9 mmol/L)	Total bilirubin (mg/dL)	0.6 (10.3 μmol/L)
NRBC/100 WBC	0	Conjugated bilirubin (mg/dL)	0.2 (3.4 μmol/L)
RBC morphology	Normal	Unconjugated bilirubin (mg/dL)	0.4 (6.9 μmol/L)
↑ WBC × 10³/μL	68.1 (68.1 × 10⁹/L)	↑ Total protein (g/dL)	7.9 (79 g/L)
↑ Myelocytes/μL	681 (0.68 × 10⁹/L)	↓ Albumin (g/dL)	2.2 (22 g/L)
↑ Metamyelocytes/μL	2724 (2.7 × 10⁹/L)	↑ Globulin (g/dL)	7.0 (70 g/L)
↑ Band neutrophils/μL	4086 (4.1 × 10⁹/L)	Cholesterol (mg/dL)	196 (5.1 mmol/L)
↑ Segmented neutrophils/μL	42,903 (42.9 × 10⁹/L)	↑ Urea nitrogen (mg/dL)	56 (20 mmol/L)
↑ Lymphocytes/μL[a]	12,258 (12.1 × 10⁹/L)	↑ Creatinine (mg/dL)	2.0 (176.8 μmol/L)
↑ Monocytes/μL	5448 (5.4 × 10⁹/L)	Glucose (mg/dL)	97 (5.34 mmol/L)
↓ Eosinophils/μL	0 (0 × 10⁹/L)	Amylase (IU/L)	610 (610 U/L)
Basophils/μL	0 (0 × 10⁹/L)	Lipase (IU/L)	25 (25 U/L)
↑ Toxic neutrophils	2+	Creatinine kinase (IU/L)	168 (168 U/L)
Platelet estimate	Adequate	Sodium (mEq/L)	140 (140 mmol/L)
Fecal occult blood	Positive	Potassium (mEq/L)	4.1 (4.1 mmol/L)
		Chloride (mEq/L)	104 (104 mmol/L)
		↓ Carbon dioxide (mEq/L)	13 (13 mmol/L)
		Calcium (mg/dL)	8 (2.0 mmol/L)
		Corrected calcium (mg/dL)	9.3 (2.33 mmol/L)
		Phosphorus (mg/dL)	5.1 (1.65 mmol/L)
		↑ LDH (IU/L)	1272 (1272 U/L)

[a] Most lymphocytes large and immature.

Abdominal Fluid[a]	
Appearance	Hazy, red
Specific gravity	1.024
↑ Protein (g/dL)	4.5 (45 g/L)
↑ WBC/μL	63,360 (63.4 × 10⁹/L)
↑ RBC/μL	30,000 (0.003 × 10¹²/L)

[a] Abdominal fluid cytology: many degenerate neutrophils; bacterial rods are numerous; supports septic infection.

Urinalysis (Cystocentesis)	
Appearance	Clear, yellow
Specific gravity	1.040
pH	6.5
Protein	Negative
Glucose	Negative
Ketones	Negative
Blood	Negative
↑ **Bilirubin**	3+
Sediment	
WBC/hpf	1–2
RBC/hpf	2–3
Casts	Rare hyaline
Crystals	Negative
Bacteria	Negative

HEMOGRAM

Leukocytosis, neutrophilia with a severe left shift to myelocytes, indicates an acute severe inflammatory response. The marked neutrophilia with a marked left shift are suggestive of a leukeimoid pattern (see Chapter 3). Toxic neutrophils often occur with bacterial infections, and the abdominal fluid findings support sepsis. Lymphocytosis of this magnitude with immature morphology supports the presence of a neoplastic process.

The anemia is nonregenerative and probably secondary to chronic disease.

BIOCHEMICAL PROFILE

Since the serum urea nitrogen is increased inappropriately in relation to the creatinine one should consider hemorrhage into the gastrointestinal tract as the cause of the urea nitrogen increase. The positive fecal occult blood supports hemorrhage into the intestinal tract.

Mild increase of serum ALP may be associated with stress or early cholestasis and is frequently abnormal in patients with sepsis. The high normal bilirubin with a bilirubinuria is also compatible with early cholestasis and has been reported as a reflection of cholestasis associated with sepsis.

The mild increase in AST with normal ALT indicates that the AST is probably not of liver origin but from a nonspecific tissue source, which is further supported by the LDH increase, also implying nonspecific tissue necrosis. If the AST originated from muscle the creatine kinase would be increased.

The hypoalbuminemia may represent gastrointestinal loss, maldigestion, or there may be a compensatory decrease as a result of the high globulin. The increased globulin may be monoclonal, a paraprotein associated with lymphosarcoma, or polyclonal, associated with inflammation.

ABDOMINOCENTESIS

The findings indicate a septic exudate.

DIAGNOSIS

Ruptured intestine secondary to lymphosarcoma.

COMMENT

At the request of the owners to determine if the neoplastic process could be resected, the patient was stabilized, and a laparotomy was performed. Thickened loops of intestine with an ulcer in the jejunal section were noted. A fine needle aspirate of the intestinal wall was done, and an intraoperative diagnosis of lymphosarcoma was made. The neoplastic process was considered too extensive for resection. For academic purposes, the serum was electrophoresed and there was a monoclonal gammopathy.

Patient: Dog, Labrador X, Female, 7 years old.

Presenting Signs and Complaints: Increased water consumption and urination for the past 3 or 4 weeks.

Physical Examination: Unremarkable.

Problem List: Polyuria/polydipsia.

Hematology		Serum Chemistry	
RBC × 10⁶/μL	7.87 (7.87 × 10¹²/L)	AST (SGOT) (IU/L)	19 (19 U/L)
Hemoglobin (g/dL)	18.8 (11.7 mmol/L)	ALT (SGPT) (IU/L)	50 (50 U/L)
PCV (%)	51.4 (0.514 volume fraction)	ALP (IU/L)	87 (87 U/L)
MCV (fL)	65	GGT (IU/L)	1 (1 U/L)
MCHC (g/dL)	36.6 (22.7 mmol/L)	Total bilirubin (mg/dL)	1 (17.1 μmol/L)
NRBC/100 WBC	0	Conjugated bilirubin (mg/dL)	0 (0 μmol/L)
RBC morphology	Normal	Unconjugated bilirubin (mg/dL)	1 (17.1 μmol/L)
WBC × 103/μL	11.3 (11.3 × 10⁹/L)	Total protein (g/dL)	7 (70 g/L)
Band neutrophils/μL	0 (0 × 10⁹/L)	Albumin (g/dL)	2.8 (28 g/L)
Segmented neutrophils/μL	7571 (7.6 × 10⁹/L)	Globulin (g/dL)	4.2 (42 g/L)
Lymphocytes/μL	3503 (3.5 × 10⁹/L)	Cholesterol (mg/dL)	288 (7.49 mmol/L)
Monocytes/μL	226 (0.23 × 10⁹/L)	Urea nitrogen (mg/dL)	19 (6.78 mmol/L)
Eosinophils/μL	**0 (0 × 10⁹/L)**	Creatinine (mg/dL)	1.2 (106.1 μm/L)
Basophils/μL	0 (0 × 10⁹/L)	Glucose (mg/dL)	113 (6.22 mmol/L)
Toxic neutrophils	None	Sodium (mEq/L)	41 (41 mmol/L)
		Potassium (mEq/L)	4.4 (4.4 mmol/L)
		Na : K ratio	2.1
		Chloride (mEq/L)	110 (110 mmol/L)
		Carbon dioxide (mEq/L)	24 (24 mmol/L)
		↑ **Calcium (mg/dL)**	**12.7 (3.2 mmol/L)**
		↑ **Corrected calcium (mg/dL)**	**13.4 (3.4 mmol/L)**
		↓ **Phosphorus (mg/dL)**	**1.7 (0.55 mmol/L)**
		Creatine kinase (IU/L)	630 (630 U/L)
		T₄ (μg/dL)	2.1 (27.03 nmol/L)
		↑ **Parathormone (pg/ml)**[a]	**65**

[a] Normal = 10–33 (pg/ml)

Urinalysis (Cystocentesis)	
Appearance	Clear, light yellow
Specific gravity	1.015
pH	6.5
Protein	Negative
Glucose	Negative
Ketones	Negative
Blood	Negative
Bilirubin	Negative
Sediment	
WBC/hpf	0–1
RBC/hpf	1–2
Casts	Negative
Crystals	Negative
Bacteria	Negative

BIOCHEMICAL PROFILE

Hypercalcemia and hypophosphatemia are suggestive of hyperparathyroidism. The high parathormone confirms hyperparathyroidism.

    The hypercalcemia caused renal tubular toxicity impairing the resorptive capacity and precipitating the clinical signs of polyuria/polydipsia.

DIAGNOSIS

An enlarged parathyroid was removed on exploratory surgery. Biopsy supported parathyroid neoplasia.

Patient: Dog, miniature schnauzer, spayed female, 10 years old.

Presenting Signs and Complaints: Inappetence; occasional vomiting; weight loss; polydipsia and polyuria for past 2 to 3 months.

Physical Examination: Thin.

Problem List: 1. Vomiting. 2. Weight loss. 3. Polyuria and polydipsia.

Hematology		Serum Chemistry	
RBC × 10⁶/μL	5.6 (5.6 × 10¹²/L)	AST (SGOT) (IU/L)	Lipemia
↑ Hemoglobin (g/dL)	26.4 (16.4 mmol/L)	↑ ALT (SGPT) (IU/L)	1544 (1544 U/L)
PCV (%)	38 (0.38 volume fraction)	ALP (IU/L)	Lipemia
MCV (fL)	67.9	GGT (IU/L)	Lipemia
↑ MCHC (g/dL)	69.5 (43.1 mmol/L)	Total bilirubin (mg/dL)	3.4 (58.1 μmol/L)
↑ NRBC/100 WBC	8	Conjugated bilirubin (mg/dL)	3.0 (51.3 μmol/L)
RBC morphology	Normal	Unconjugated bilirubin (mg/dL)	0.4 (6.8 μmol/L)
WBC × 10³/μL	16.5 (16.5 × 10⁹/L)	Total protein (g/dL)	6.3 (63 g/L)
Myelocytes/μL	0 (0 × 10⁹/L)	Albumin (g/dL)	3.2 (32 g/L)
Metamyelocytes/μL	0 (0 × 10⁹/L)	Globulin (g/dL)	3.1 (31 g/L)
Band neutrophils/μL	160 (0.16 × 10⁹/L)	↑ Cholesterol (mg/dL)	680 (17.7 mmol/L)
↑ Segmented neutrophils/ μL	13,200 (13.2 × 10⁹/L)	Urea nitrogen (mg/dL)	21 (7.5 mmol/L)
Lymphocytes/μL	1630 (16 × 10⁹/L)	Creatinine (mg/dL)	0.9 (79.6 μmol/L)
Monocytes/μL	810 (0.81 × 10⁹/L)	↑ Glucose (mg/dL)	399 (22 mmol/L)
Eosinophils/μL	650 (0.65 × 10⁹/L)	Amylase (IU/L)	250 (250 U/L)
Basophils/μL	0 (0 × 10⁹/L)	Lipase (IU/L)	10 (10 U/L)
Toxic neutrophils	None seen	↓ Sodium (mEq/L)	122 (122 mmol/L)
Platelet estimate	Adequate	Potassium (mEq/L)	3.6 (3.6 mmol/L)
		Na : K ratio	33.8
		Chloride (mEq/L)	109 (109 mmol/L)
		↓ Carbon dioxide (mEq/L)	8 (8 mmol/L)
		Calcium (mg/dL)	9.1 (2.28 mmol/L)
		Corrected calcium (mg/dL)	9.4 (2.35 mmol/L)
		Phosphorus (mg/dL)	5.5 (1.78 mmol/L)
		↓ Blood pH	7.2
		Pco₂ (mm/L)	29.6
		↓ HCO₃ (mEq/L)	12.4 (12.4 mmol/L)
		↓ Base excess (mEq/L)	−12.8 (−12.8 mmol/L)
		↑ Anion gap (mEq/L)	29.6 (29.6 mmol/L)

Urinalysis (Cystocentesis)	
Appearance	Cloudy, yellow
Specific gravity	1.017
↓ pH	5.5
Protein	Trace
↑ Glucose	4+
↑ Ketones	3+
Blood	Negative
Bilirubin	Negative
Sediment	
WBC/hpf	0–3
RBC/hpf	None
Casts	None
Crystals	None
Bacteria	None

HEMATOLOGY

There is a normocytic anemia. An increased MCHC is physiologically impossible and always reflects an artifact. In this case it is secondary to lipemia.

There are no significant alterations in total leukocyte count. There is a mature neutrophilia that could be secondary to stress or may represent an occult inflammation. The eosinopenia suggests the possibility of increased glucocorticoid activity. Finding eight NRBC may have been incidental, but NRBC may be present in considerable numbers in healthy miniature schnauzers for unknown reasons.

BIOCHEMICAL PROFILE

Hyperglycemia with glucosuria and ketonuria supports the diagnosis of diabetes mellitus. The high cholesterol is probably associated with abnormal lipid metabolism attendant to the metabolic disturbance.

The marked increase in serum ALT activity indicates enzyme leakage through altered hepatocellular membranes; in this case hepatic lipidosis which often accompanies diabetes mellitus is probably the cause.

The low serum carbon dioxide, low blood pH, and negative base excess indicate acidosis. The anion gap of approximately 30 supports increased nonvolatile metabolic acids. In this case it is probably a result of the presence of ketones.

Hyponatremia may be secondary to the hyperosmolar diuresis accompanying hyperglycemia or may be an artifact of lipemia if flame photometry was used for electrolyte determination.

LIPIDEMIA

Lipidemia in this patient probably is associated with diabetes mellitus. The hyperlipidemia associated with diabetes mellitus is in part a reflection of insufficient insulin to activate the lipoprotein lipase within the circulation. Consequently there is a build-up in very low density lipoproteins and chylomicrons resulting in hyperlipidemia and hypercholesterolemia.

URINALYSIS

Glucosuria has induced polydipsia/polyuria resulting in an osmotic diuresis.

DIAGNOSIS

Diabetes mellitus with ketoacidosis.

Patient: Dog, beagle, female, 10 years old.

Presenting Signs and Complaints: Frequent fainting episodes, especially when excited; recovers in a few minutes; increasing frequency; seems weak all the time.

Physical Examination: Very weak, almost in a coma, pale mucous membranes; dry skin; many fleas.

Problem List: 1. Weakness. 2. Anemia. 3. Fleas.

Hematology		Serum Chemistry	
↓ **RBC × 10⁶/μL**	**5.4 (5.4 × 10¹²/L)**	AST (SGOT) (IU/L)	82 (82 U/L)
↓ **Hemoglobin (g/dL)**	**9.9 (6.1 mmol/L)**	ALT (SGPT) (IU/L)	76 (76 U/L)
↓ **PCV (%)**	**30 (0.30 volume fraction)**	ALP (IU/L)	85 (85 U/L)
↓ **MCV (fL)**	**56**	GGT (IU/L)	1 (1 U/L)
MCHC (g/dL)	33 (20.5 mmol/L)	Total bilirubin (mg/dL)	0.1 (1.7 μmol/L)
Reticulocytes (%)	0.2 (0.002 number fraction)	Conjugated bilirubin (mg/dL)	0.1 (1.7 μmol/L)
Reticulocytes/μL	10,800 (10.8 × 10⁹/L)	Total protein (g/dL)	7.9 (79 g/L)
RBC morphology	Normal	Albumin (g/dL)	3.8 (38 g/L)
WBC × 10³/μL	17.8 (17.8 × 10⁹/L)	Globulin (g/dL)	4.1 (41 g/L)
		↑ **Cholesterol (mg/dL)**	**380 (9.9 mmol/L)**
Myelocytes/μL	0 (0 × 10⁹/L)	Urea nitrogen (mg/dL)	20 (7.1 mmol/L)
Metamyelocytes/μL	0 (0 × 10⁹/L)	Creatinine (mg/dL)	1.2 (106.1 μmol/L)
Band neutrophils/μL	0 (0 × 10⁹/L)	↓ **Glucose (mg/dL)**	**36 (2.0 mmol/L)**
↑ **Segmented neutrophils/μL**	**16,910 (16.9 × 10⁹/L)**	Amylase (IU/L)	350 (350 U/L)
↓ **Lymphocytes/μL**	**712 (0.71 × 10⁹/L)**	Lipase (IU/L)	67 (67 U/L)
Monocytes/μL	178 (0.18 × 10⁹/L)	Sodium (mEq/L)	151 (151 mmol/L)
Eosinophils/μL	0 (0 × 10⁹/L)	Potassium (mEq/L)	4.9 (4.9 mmol/L)
Basophils/μL	0	Chloride (mEq/L)	98 (98 mmol/L)
Toxic neutrophils	None	Carbon dioxide (mEq/L)	21 (21 mmol/L)
Platelets × 10³/μL	325	Calcium (mg/dL)	8.5 (2.13 mmol/L)
		Phosphorus (mg/dL)	5.3 (1.7 mmol/L)
		↑ **Insulin (μU/μL)**	**60 (431 pmol/L)**
		↑ **AIGR**	**1000**
		↓ **Serum iron (μg/dL)**	**44 (7.88 μmol/L)**

Urinalysis (Cystocentesis)	
Appearance	Clear, yellow
Specific gravity	1.043
pH	6.5
Protein	Negative
Glucose	Negative
Ketones	Negative
Blood	Negative
Bilirubin	Negative
Sediment	
WBC/hpf	0–1
RBC/hpf	2–4
Casts	Negative
Crystals	Negative
Bacteria	Negative

HEMOGRAM

The leukocytosis, mature neutrophilia, lymphopenia, and eosinopenia support increased glucocorticoid activity, probably as a result of stress. There is a microcytic normochromic nonregenerative anemia. This type of anemia is most compatible with iron deficiency which is supported by the decreased serum iron concentration. Iron deficiency in this dog is probably caused by the blood loss associated with the flea infestation.

BIOCHEMICAL PROFILE

There is a hypoglycemia. Hypoglycemia commonly is an artifact if serum is not separated from RBC soon after the clot forms (for additional information see Chapter 7 and Table 7–2).

In this case the high insulin ($N = 5$ to 22 mU/μL) together with hypoglycemia is consistent with an insulin-producing neoplasm of pancreatic islet cells. This was confirmed by histopathology.

DIAGNOSIS

Insulin-producing neoplasia of the islets of Langerhans.

Patient: Bovine, Holstein, female, 6 years old.

Presenting Signs and Complaints: Calved 4 days ago; has diarrhea, and has difficulty rising.

Physical Examination: Increased pulse and respiratory rates; ping on left posterior thorax and flank; no rumen activity detected; temperature 103.6° F.

Problem List: 1. Accelerated pulse and respiratory rates. 2. Pyrexia. 3. Rumen atony. 4. Ping on left posterior thorax and flank.

Hematology		Serum Chemistry	
RBC × 10⁶/µL	5.59 (5.6 × 10¹²/L)	AST (SGOT) (IU/L)	158 (158 U/L)
Hemoglobin (g/dL)	9.8 (6.08 mmol/L)	ALP (IU/L)	28 (28 U/L)
PCV (%)	27 (0.27 volume fraction)	Total bilirubin (mg/dL)	0.2 (3.4 µmol/L)
MCV (fL)	48.3	Conjugated bilirubin (mg/dL)	0.1 (1.7 µmol/L)
MCHC (g/dL)	36.3 (22.5 mmol/L)	Unconjugated bilirubin (mg/dL)	0.1 (1.7 µmol/L)
Reticulocytes (%)	0	Total protein (g/dL)	7.8 (78 g/L)
NRBC/100 WBC	0	Albumin (g/dL)	3.2 (32 g/L)
RBC morphology	Normal	Globulin (g/dL)	4.6 (46 g/L)
WBC × 10³/µL	11,670 (11.7 × 10⁹/L)	Urea nitrogen (mg/dL)	13 (4.6 mmol/L)
Band neutrophils/µL	0 (0 × 10⁹/L)	Creatinine (mg/dL)	0.5 (44.2 mmol/L)
Segmented neutrophils/µL	2801 (2.8 × 10⁹/L)	↑ **Glucose (mg/dL)**	**105 (5.8 mmol/L)**
Lymphocytes/µL	7702[a] (7.7 × 10⁹/L)	Sodium (mEq/L)	132 (132 mmol/L)
Monocytes/µL	1050 (1.1 × 10⁹/L)	↓ **Potassium (mEq/L)**	**2.5 (2.5 mmol/L)**
Eosinophils/µL	117 (0.12 × 10⁹/L)	↓ **Chloride (mEq/L)**	**88 (88 mmol/L)**
Basophils/µL	0 (0 × 10⁹/L)	↑ **Carbon dioxide (mEq/L)**	**39 (39 mmol/L)**
Platelet estimate	Adequate	Calcium (mg/dL)	3.2 (30 mmol/L)
Plasma protein (g/dL)	6.1 (61 g/L)	Phosphorus (mg/dL)	7.8 (2.52 mmol/L)
Fibrinogen (mg/dL)	300 (3 g/L)		

[a] Some lymphocytes have characteristics of blasts.

Urinalysis (Voided)	
Appearance	Slightly cloudy, yellow
Specific gravity	1.032
↓ **pH**	**6.0**
Protein	Negative
Glucose	Negative
Ketones	Negative
Occult blood	Negative
Bilirubin	Negative
↑ **WBC/hpf**	**18–25**
↑ **RBC/hpf**	**10–15**
Casts/lpf	None
↑ **Bacteria**	**3+**

HEMOGRAM

The hemogram is unremarkable; however, it is unusual not to have lymphopenia in a ruminant that is clinically stressed. Lymphocytosis in stressed cattle is suggestive of lymphoid neoplasia, and the presence of immature forms of lymphocytes is additional evidence of lymphosarcoma.

BIOCHEMICAL PROFILE

There is a hyperglycemia; most increases in serum glucose in cattle are secondary to stress and are transient once the underlying condition is corrected. Hypochloridemia, hypokalemia, and metabolic alkalosis with a paradoxical aciduria are present. In ruminants the sequestration of gastric fluid in a third space such as a displaced abomasum causes a loss of hydrogen and chloride to the outside of the body. The loss of chloride necessitates that the kidney reabsorb bicarbonate as the alternative anion contributing to the alkalosis. The loss of the hydrogen ion necessitates that the kidney exchange potassium for sodium in maintaining fluid balance/electrolyte neutrality contributing to the hypokalemia. The preferential renal resorption of bicarbonate instead of chloride also results in acid urine in a patient with systemic alkalosis (paradoxic aciduria).

DIAGNOSIS

Lymphosarcoma and displacement of abomasum to the right. This was confirmed by laparotomy and corrected surgically. Four days later the biochemical profile was normal.

Patient: Dog, mixed, female, 7 years old.

Presenting Signs and Complaints: No bowel movements for 3 days; owner obtained Fleet enemas from a practitioner and gave three the same day; dog seizured several times.

Physical Examination: Not responsive.

Problem List: 1. Semi-comatosed.

Hematology		Serum Chemistry	
RBC × 10⁶/μL	7.5 (7.5 × 10¹²/L)	AST (SGOT) (U/L)	51 (51 U/L)
Hemoglobin (g/dL)	16.8 (10.4 mmol/L)	ALT (SGPT) (IU/L)	64 (64 U/L)
PCV (%)	50 (0.50 volume fraction)	ALP (IU/L)	147 (147 U/L)
MCV (fL)	66.7	↑ Cholesterol (mg/dL)	242 (6.3 mmol/L)
MCHC (g/dL)	33.6 (20.8 mmol/L)	Total protein (g/dL)	6.0 (60 g/L)
NRBC/100 WBC	0	Albumin (g/dL)	3.1 (31 g/L)
RBC morphology	Normal	Globulin (g/dL)	2.9 (29 g/L)
WBC × 10³/μL	14.0 (14 × 10⁹/L)	↑ Glucose (mg/dL)	212 (11.7 mmol/L)
		↑ Urea nitrogen (mg/dL)	84 (30 mmol/L)
Band neutrophils/μL	0 (0 × 10⁹/L)	↑ Creatinine (mg/dL)	6.7 (592.3 μmol/L)
Segmented			
neutrophils/μL	11,760 (11.8 × 10⁹/L)	↓ Calcium (mg/dL)	4.1 (1.0 mmol/L)
Lymphocytes/μL	1,120 (1.1 × 10⁹/L)	↓ Corrected calcium (mg/dL)	4.5 (1.1 mmol/L)
Monocytes/μL	980 (0.98 × 10⁹/L)	↑ Phosphorus (mg/dL)	11.4 (3.7 mmol/L)
Eosinophils/μL	140 (0.14 × 10⁹/L)	↑ Sodium (mEq/L)	166 (166 mmol/L)
Basophils/μL	0 (0 × 10⁹/L)	↓ Potassium (mEq/L)	3.3 (3.3 mmol/L)
Toxic neutrophils	None	Na : K ratio	37.9
Platelet estimate	Adequate	↓ Chloride (mEq/L)	98 (98 mmol/L)
		Carbon dioxide (mEq/L)	20 (20 mmol/L)
		Cholinesterase (IU/L)	3,326 (3,326 U/L)

Urinalysis (Cystocentesis)

Appearance	Clear yellow
Specific gravity	1.048
pH	7
Protein	Negative
Glucose	Negative
Ketones	Negative
Blood	Negative
Bilirubin	Negative
Sediment	
WBC/hpf	0–1
RBC/hpf	0–2
Casts	Negative
Crystals	Negative
Bacteria	Negative

HEMOGRAM

No significant abnormalities.

BIOCHEMICAL PROFILE

Hyperglycemia, hypocalcemia, hyperphosphatemia, hypernatremia, and hypokalemia are present. The clinical signs are most likely attributed to the hypernatremia causing the obtundation, and the seizure-like activity is probably related to the hypocalcemia. Hyperglycemia may be an indication of diabetes mellitus or associated with stress accompanying the underlying disorder; if caused by stress the glucose will return to normal with management of the underlying condition. Hypernatremia and hyperphosphatemia are associated with the absorption of the ions from the large bowel associated with the hypertonic solution (Fleet enema). The mechanism for the hyperphosphatemic related hypocalcemia is not clear. The hypokalemia may be related to preexisting vomiting which was not noted or through potassium exchange for sodium via the colon. The hypochloridemia may have been related to a transcolonic exchange with phosphate.

The increased urea nitrogen and creatinine with a concentrated urine specific gravity indicate prerenal azotemia secondary to dehydration.

DIAGNOSIS

Hypertonic enema-associated electrolyte disturbances. Patient was managed aggressively with appropriate electrolyte solutions and returned to normal within 24 hours.

Patient: Dog, spaniel, male, 8 years old.

Presenting Signs and Complaints: Losing weight for several weeks; lethargic; appetite remains good; drinking large quantities of water and increased urination.

Physical Examination: Pale membranes; thin; small hemorrhages on membranes.

Problem List: 1. Anemia. 2. Weight loss. 3. Petechiae on mucous membranes. 4. Polyuria and polydipsia.

Hematology		Clinical Chemistry	
↓ **RBC × 10⁶/μL**	**2.37 (2.37 × 10¹²/L)**	AST (SGOT) (IU/L)	25 (25 U/L)
↓ **Hemoglobin (g/dL)**	**5.3 (3.29 mmol/L)**	ALT (SGPT) (IU/L)	20 (20 U/L)
↓ **PCV (%)**	**16.2 (0.16 volume fraction)**	ALP (IU/L)	75 (75 U/L)
MCV (fL)	68	GGT (IU/L)	3 (3 U/L)
MCHC (g/dL)	32.9 (20.3 mmol/L)	Total bilirubin (mg/dL)	0.2 (3.4 μmol/L)
↑ **Reticulocytes (%)**	**4.1 (0.041 number fraction)**	Conjugated bilirubin (mg/dL)	0.1 (1.7 μmol/L)
Corrected reticulocytes (%)	1.5 (0.015 number fraction)	Unconjugated bilirubin (mg/dL)	0.1 (1.7 μmol/L)
↑ **Reticulocytes/μL**	**97,170 (97.17 × 10⁹/L)**	Total protein (g/dL)	7.2 (72 g/L)
↑ **NRBC/100 WBC**	**25**	Albumin (g/dL)	3.9 (39 g/L)
RBC morphology		Globulins (g/dL)	3.3 (33 g/L)
Spherocytes	None	Cholesterol (mg/dL)	156 (4.06 mmol/L)
Polychromasia	+	Urea nitrogen (mg/dL)	12 (4.28 mmol/L)
↑ **Anisocytosis**	**2+**	Creatinine (mg/dL)	1.0 (88.4 μmol/L)
Poikilocytosis	None	Glucose (mg/dL)	89 (80.5 mmol/L)
↓ **WBC × 10³/μL**	**4.5 (4.5 × 10⁹/L)**	Amylase (IU/L)	250 (250 U/L)
Myelocytes/μL	0 (0 × 10⁹/L)	Lipase (IU/L)	25 (25 U/L)
Metamyelocytes/μL	0 (0 × 10⁹/L)	Creatine kinase (IU/L)	225 (225 U/L)
Band neutrophils/μL	90 (0.09 × 10⁹/L)	Sodium (mEq/L)	145 (145 mmol/L)
↓ **Segmented neutrophils/μL**	**2,115 (2.12 × 10⁹/L)**	Potassium (mEq/L)	4.2 (4.2 mmol/L)
Lymphocytes/μL[a]	1,395 (1.4 × 10⁹/L)	Na : K ratio	34.5
Monocytes/μL	900 (0.9 × 10⁹/L)	Chloride (mEq/L)	1021 (02 mmol/L)
↓ **Eosinophils/μL**	**0 (0 × 10⁹/L)**	Carbon dioxide (mEq/L)	21 (21 mmol/L)
Basophils/μL	0 (0 × 10⁹/L)	↑ **Calcium (mg/dL)**	**13.7 (3.4 mmol/L)**
↓ **Platelets × 10³/μL**	**33 (0.03 × 10¹²/L)**	↑ **Corrected calcium (mg/dL)**	**13.3 (3.3 mmol/L)**
		Phosphorus (mg/dL)	5.3 (1.71 mmol/L)

[a] Lymphocyte morphology is normal.

Urinalysis (Cystocentesis)	
Appearance	Clear, light yellow
↓ **Specific gravity**	**1.014**
pH	6.5
All chemistry tests	Negative

HEMOGRAM

There is a leukopenia secondary to the neutropenia. Thrombocytopenia is present. The anemia is poorly regenerative with a corrected reticulocyte count of only 1.5% and an absolute reticulocyte count of 97,170. Inappropriate numbers of NRBCs can be a reflection of myelophthisis, endotoxemia, or hemangiosarcoma. The neutropenia, thombocytopenia, and nonregenerative anemia are indications for examination of the bone marrow. Furthermore, the presence of a paraneoplastic process in the marrow might be suspected because of the otherwise unexplained hypercalcemia.

BIOCHEMICAL PROFILE

There is a hypercalcemia which, in the dog and cat, is the most commonly associated with lymphosarcoma. However, in this age patient, hyperparathyroidism should also be kept in the differential diagnosis.

URINALYSIS

The low urine specific gravity of 1.014 with no azotemia reflects impaired tubular reabsorption ability that is often associated with hypercalcemia, which is toxic to the renal tubule epithelial cells resulting in the clinical signs of polyuria/polydipsia.

BONE MARROW EXAMINATION

Cytologic examination of a bone marrow aspirate revealed a hypercellular preparation. No megakaryocytes were noted. Occasional myeloid and erythroid components were present. The majority of the cells are immature lymphocytes indicating lymphosarcoma invasion of the bone marrow.

COMMENT

Proliferation of lymphocytes in the bone marrow disrupts the microenvironment, displacing normal cellular elements and allows for the abnormal release of the few remaining nucleated erythrocytes that are noted in the peripheral blood. Some patients may have leukemic cells in the peripheral blood whereas others, as in this case, do not. Reasons for such differences are poorly understood.

DIAGNOSIS

Lymphosarcoma of the bone marrow with secondary hypercalcemia and renal tubular nephropathy.

Patient: Dog, pointer, male, 12 years old.

Presenting Signs and Complaints: Dog is kept in outdoor kennel; lethargic for several months; can not hunt for more than 15 or 20 minutes until becoming lame; seems to have trouble eating anything other than soft canned dog food; face looks distorted.

Physical Examination: Marked peridontal disease and plaque formation; facial bones deformed and seem soft; lame in front legs, slightly dehydrated; pale mucous membranes; purulent skin lesions in axilla; thin.

Problem List: 1. Facial deformity. 2. Lameness. 3. Pyoderma in axilla. 4. Anemia. 5. Thin. 6. Dehydration.

Hematology			Serum Chemistry	
↓ **RBC × 10⁶/μL**	**3.5**	**(3.5 × 10¹²/L)**	AST (SGOT) (IU/L)	68 (68 U/L)
↓ **Hemoglobin (g/dL)**	**7.1**	**(4.4 mmol/L)**	ALT (SGPT) (IU/L)	85 (85 U/L)
↓ **PCV (%)**	**22**	**(0.22 volume fraction)**	↑ **ALP (IU/L)**	**285 (285 U/L)**
MCV (fL)	62.9		GGT (IU/L)	12 (12 U/L)
MCHC (g/dL)	32.3	(20 mmol/L)	Total bilirubin (mg/dL)	0.2 (3.4 μmol/L)
Reticulocytes (%)	0		Conjugated bilirubin (mg/dL)	0.1 (1.7 μmol/L)
NRBC/100 WBC	0		Total protein (g/dL)	7.2 (72 g/L)
RBC morphology	Normal		Albumin (g/dL)	3.2 (32 g/L)
WBC × 10³/μL	**34.2** ↑	**(34.2 × 10⁹/L)**	Globulin (g/dL)	4.0 (40 g/L)
			↑ **Urea nitrogen (mg/dL)**	**184 (65.7 mmol/L)**
Myelocytes/μL	0	(0 × 10⁹/L)	↑ **Creatinine (mg/dL)**	**6.1 (539.2 μmol/L)**
Metamyelocytes/μL	0	(0 × 10⁹/L)	↑ **Glucose (mg/dL)**	**180 (9.9 mmol/L)**
↑ **Band neutrophils/μL**	**1,026**	**(1.03 × 10⁹/L)**	Amylase (IU/L)	1,200 (1,200 U/L)
↑ **Segmented**				
neutrophils/μL	**30,780**	**(30.8 × 10⁹/L)**	Lipase (IU/L)	180 (180 U/L)
↓ **Lymphocyte/μL**	**342**	**(0.34 × 10⁹/L)**	Sodium (mEq/L)	143 (143 mmol/L)
↑ **Monocytes/μL**	**2,052**	**(2.1 × 10⁹/L)**	↑ **Potassium (mEq/L)**	**6.1 (6.1 mmol/L)**
↓ **Eosinophils/μL**	**0**	**(0 × 10⁹/L)**	↓ **Na : K ratio**	**23.4**
Basophils/μL	0	(0 × 10⁹/L)	Chloride (mEq/L)	98 (98 mmol/L)
Toxic neutrophils	None		↓ **Total carbon dioxide (mm/L)**	**7.0 (7 mmol/L)**
Platelet estimate	Adequate		↓ **Calcium (mg/dL)**	**6.4 (1.6 mmol/L)**
			↓ **Corrected calcium (mg/dL)**	**6.7 (1.7 mmol/L)**
			↑ **Phosphorus (mg/dL)**	**21 (6.8 mmol/L)**
			↑ **LDH (IU/L)**	**876 (876 U/L)**
			↑ **CK (IU/L)**	**3,200 (3,200 U/L)**

Urinalysis (Cystocentesis)	
↓ **Specific gravity**	**1.010**
pH	6
↑ **Protein**	**3+**
Glucose	Negative
Ketones	Negative
↑ **Blood**	**3+**
Bilirubin	Negative
Sediment	
WBC/hpf	0–1
RBC/hpf	None seen
Casts	None
Crystals	None
Bacteria	None

HEMOGRAM

Leukocytosis, neutrophilia, and left shift are compatible with an acute inflammatory response. Lymphopenia, eosinopenia, and monocytosis are probably stress induced.

There is a normocytic normochromic nonregenerative anemia.

BIOCHEMICAL PROFILE AND URINALYSIS

The azotemia (increased serum urea nitrogen and creatinine) and hyperphosphatemia along with an inappropriately low specific gravity in a dog that is dehydrated confirm primary renal failure. The presence of occult blood in the urine with no RBCs suggests hemoglobinuria, myoglobinuria, or hematuria with RBC lysis in the hypotonic urine. In this case it is suspected that blood contaminated the specimen during cystocentesis and subsequently lysed in the hypotonic urine.

Proteinuria without evidence of inflammation indicates glomerular pathology. The significance of the proteinuria can be determined by quantitative measurement of urine protein and creatinine concentrations and calculation of a urine protein to urine creatinine ratio.

The anemia is most likely associated with the uremic syndrome and inadequate erythropoietin production by the kidneys.

Hyperglycemia with no urine glucose suggests that the urine was formed prior to the hyperglycemia or that the urine glucose result is a false negative caused by the presence of ascorbic acid or use of an outdated glucose test strip. Glucose intolerance occurs secondary to chronic renal failure.

The corrected serum calcium is low. Hypocalcemia, renal failure, and bone disease suggest secondary hyperparathyroidism.

The low total carbon dioxide is compatible with metabolic acidosis. The anion gap is 44.1 mEq/L (N = 12 to 16). Unmeasured anions are retained in chronic renal failure.

The moderate increase in alkaline phosphatase is probably related to metabolic bone disease.

DIAGNOSIS

Chronic renal failure with secondary hyperparathyroidism and metabolic bone disease.

Patient: Dog, sharpei, male, 4 years old.

Presenting Signs and Complaints: Inappetence and lethargy for the past 4 to 6 weeks; vomiting occasionally for last 2 weeks.

Physical Examination: Thin; 5% dehydration.

Problem List: 1. Vomiting. 2. Weight loss. 3. Inappetence. 4. Lethargy. 5. Dehydration.

Hematology			Serum Chemistry	
RBC × 10⁶/μL	6.51	(6.5 × 10¹²/L)	AST (SGOT) (IU/L)	24 (24 U/L)
Hemoblogin (g/dL)	13.5	(8.37 mmol/L)	ALT (SGPT) (IU/L)	28 (28 U/L)
PCV (%)	40	(0.40 volume fraction)	ALP (IU/L)	21 (21 U/L)
MCV (fL)	62		GGT (IU/L)	2 (2 U/L)
MCHC (g/dL)	34	(21.1 mmol/L)	Cholesterol (mg/dL)	198 (5.14 mmol/L)
NRBC/100 WBC	0		↑ Total protein (g/dL)	8.0 (80 g/L)
RBC morphology	Normal		↑ Albumin (g/dL)	4.9 (49 g/L)
↑ WBC × 10³/μL	26.8	(26.8 × 10⁹/L)	Globulin (g/dL)	3.1 (31 g/L)
			Glucose (mg/dL)	114 (6.3 mmol/L)
Myelocytes/μL	0	(0 × 10⁹/L)	↑ Urea nitrogen (mg/dL)	69 (25 mmol/L)
Metamyelocytes/μL	0	(0 × 10⁹/L)	↑ Creatinine (mg/dL)	2.1 (185.6 μmol/L)
Band neutrophils/μL	0	(0 × 10⁹/L)	Calcium (mg/dL)	10.7 (2.7 mmol/L)
↑ Segmented				
neutrophils/μL	21,708	(21.7 × 10⁹/L)	Corrected calcium (mg/dL)	11.1 (2.8 mmol/L)
Lymphocytes/μL	1,876	(1.9 × 10⁹/L)	Phosphorus (mg/dL)	7.0 (2.3 mmol/L)
↑ Monocytes/μL	2,680	(2.7 × 10⁹/L)	↓ Sodium (mEq/L)	123 (123 mmol/L)
Eosinophils/μL	536	(0.54 × 10⁹/L)	↑ Potassium (mEq/L)	6.4 (6.4 mmol/L)
Basophils/μL	0	(0 × 10⁹/L)	↓ Na : K ratio	19.2
Toxic neutrophils	None		↓ Chloride (mEq/L)	91 (91 mmol/L)
Platelets	Adequate		↓ Carbon dioxide (mEq/L)	14 (14 mmol/L)
Plasma protein (g/dL)	8.3 ↑ (83 g/L)		Resting cortisol (μg/dL)	0.8 (22.1 nmol/L)
Fibrinogen (mg/dL)	200	(2 g/L)	↓ Post-ACTH cortisol (μg/dL)	0.9 (24.8 nmol/L)

Urinalysis (Cystocentesis)	
Appearance	Light yellow
Specific gravity	1.016
pH	5.5
Protein	Negative
Glucose	Negative
Ketones	Negative
Blood	Negative
Bilirubin	Trace
Sediment	
WBC/hpf	Negative
RBC/hpf	Negative
Casts	Negative
Crystals	Negative
Bacteria[a]	Negative

[a] Contaminated sample, many fungal spores.

HEMOGRAM

There is a leukocytosis comprised predominantly of a mature neutrophilia, which may reflect a response to inflammation or stress. The presence of eosinophils in a stressed animal showing a neutrophilia and monocytosis is inappropriate, and one should consider the absence of glucocorticoids. There is also an increase in plasma proteins suggestive of dehydration or hyperglobulinemia.

BIOCHEMICAL PROFILE

There is an azotemia (serum urea nitrogen and creatinine increased) and hyperphosphatemia indicative of renal insufficiency. Because the urine specific gravity is low, a primary renal insufficiency is suggested. There is a remarkable decrease in sodium with a moderate increase in potassium and a sodium to potassium ratio (19.2) compatible with hypoadrenocorticism. The total carbon dioxide is decreased, indicating metabolic acidosis. There is a hypochloridemia. The patient was treated for renal insufficiency and Addison's disease while cortisols were pending. The resting and post-ACTH stimulation cortisols are diagnostic for hypoadrenocorticism. Dogs with hypoadrenocorticism usually have a mild metabolic acidosis which corrects when the condition is managed.

DIAGNOSIS

Hypoadrenocorticism with secondary renal insufficiency.

COMMENTS

In general, hypovolemia-induced prerenal azotemia is recognized by an increased urine specific gravity. In this case that rule of thumb does not apply. Some dogs with hypoadrenocorticism have an impaired ability to concentrate urine because chronic sodium loss depletes renal medullary sodium. This causes loss of the normal medullary concentrating gradient thereby impairing water reabsorption by the renal collecting tubules. In this patient the azotemia with a specific gravity in or near the fixed range caused the referring veterinarian to miss a diagnosis of hypoadrenocorticism. One should be cognizant of the age as well as the sodium to potassium ratio when evaluating these patients. If there is any doubt, cortisols should be determined before and after administration of ACTH.

Patient: Dog, terrier cross, female, 7 years old.

Presenting Signs and Complaints: Losing weight; increased food and water intake.

Physical Examination: Thin dry skin; bilateral alopecia over back and sides; pendulous abdomen.

Problem List: 1. Polyuria/polydipsia. 2. Polyphagia. 3. Alopecia. 4. Pendulous abdomen.

Hematology		Serum Chemistry	
RBC × 10⁶/µL	6.49 (6.5 × 10¹²/L)	AST (SGOT) (IU/L)	51 (51 U/L)
Hemoglobin (g/dL)	17.2 (10.7 mmol/L)	↑ ALT (SGPT) (IU/L)	606 (606 U/L)
PCV (%)	46.1 (0.46 volume fraction)	↑ ALP (IU/L)	2,032 (2,032 U/L)
MCV (fL)	71	↑ GGT (IU/L)	247 (247 U/L)
MCHC (g/dL)	37.4 (22.2 mmol/L)	Total bilirubin (mg/dL)	0.1 (1.7 µmol/L)
NRBC/100 WBC	0	Conjugated bilirubin (mg/dL)	0 (0 µmol/L)
RBC morphology	Normal	Unconjugated bilirubin (mg/dL)	0.1 (1.7 µmol/L)
WBC × 10³/µL	10.9 (10.9 × 10⁹/L)	Total protein (g/dL)	6.5 (65 g/L)
Myelocytes/µL	0 (0 × 10⁹/L)	Albumin (g/dL)	4.0 (40 g/L)
Metamyelocytes/µL	0 (0 × 10⁹/L)	Globulin (g/dL)	2.5 (25 g/L)
Band neutrophils/µL	0 (0 × 10⁹/L)	↑ Cholesterol (mg/dL)	299 (7.8 mmol/L)
Segmented			
neutrophils/µL	10,246 (10.2 × 10⁹/L)	Urea nitrogen (mg/dL)	8 (2.9 mmol/L)
↓ Lymphocytes/µL	109 (0.11 × 10⁹/L)	Creatinine (mg/dL)	1.1 (97.2 µm/L)
Monocytes/µL	545 (0.55 × 10⁹/L)	Glucose (mg/dL)	92 (5.1 mmol/L)
↓ Eosinophils/µL	0 (0 × 10⁹/L)	Amylase (IU/L)	334 (334 U/L)
Basophils/µL	0	Lipase (IU/L)	133 (122 U/L)
Toxic neutrophils	None	Sodium (mEq/L)	145 (145 mmol/L)
Platelet estimate	Adequate	Potassium (mEq/L)	4.1 (4.1 mmol/L)
		Na:K ratio	35.4
		Chloride (mEq/L)	108 (108 mmol/L)
		Carbon dioxide (mEq/L)	21 (21 mmol/L)
		Calcium (mg/dL)	10 (2.5 mmol/L)
		Phosphorus (mg/dL)	3.4 (1.1 mmol/L)
		LDH (IU/L)	198 (198 U/L)
		Total T₃ (ng/dL)	180 (2.8 nmol/L)
		↓ Total T₄ (µg/dL)	0.6 (7.7 nmol/L)
		Total free T₄ (ng/dL)	0.71 (56.1 pmol/L)

Cortisol Tests	
↑ Resting cortisol (µg/dL)	9.9 (273 nmol/L)
↑ Post-ACTH cortisol (µg/dL)	50 (1,380 nmol/L)
Dexamethasone suppression	
↑ Base cortisol (µg/dL)	13.9 (383.6 nmol/L)
↑ Low dose dexamethasone after 6 hours cortisol (µg/dL)	6.0 (165.6 nmol/L)
↑ Low dose dexamethasone after 8 hours cortisol (µg/dL)	6.1 (168.4 nmol/L)
↑ Base cortisol (µg/dL)	12.7 (350.5 nmol/L)
↑ High dose dexamethasone after 8 hours cortisol (µg/dL)	4.6 (127.0 nmol/L)

Urinalysis (Cystocentesis)	
Appearance	Clear, pale yellow
↓ **Specific gravity**	**1.005**
pH	6.5
Protein	Negative
Glucose	Negative
Ketones	Negative
Blood	Negative
Bilirubin	Negative
Sediment	
WBC/hpf	0–1
RBC/hpf	Negative
Casts	Negative
Crystals	Negative
Bacteria	Negative

HEMOGRAM

The lymphopenia and eosinopenia are consistent with increased glucocorticoid activity.

BIOCHEMICAL PROFILE

The high pre- and post-ACTH cortisols strongly indicated the presence of hyperadrenocorticism. After this finding the owner was given the choice of assuming that the dog had pituitary-dependent hyperadrenocorticism or electing to complete dexamethasone suppression tests in hope of a more precise diagnosis. The latter route was chosen. The lack of a decreased cortisol after a low dose of dexamethasone supported hyperadrenocorticism. The response to high dose dexamethasone in which the postdexamethasone cortisol was less than half the pretest value suggested that the condition was pituitary dependent hyperadrenocorticism.

The increased ALT (SGPT) indicates enzyme leakage from the hepatocytes. The ALT is more commonly increased than is the AST in patients with corticosteroid-induced hepatopathy. The AST usually remains within the normal range in such patients. The reasons for aminotransferase leakage in association with glucocorticoid hepatopathy are not clear, but it is suspected that there is altered membrane permeability secondary to the metabolic aberration in the liver. In patients with corticosteroid-induced hepatopathy the alkaline phosphatase activity is disproportionately increased in relation to the ALT. This pattern of liver test abnormalities in the presence of a normal serum bilirubin should lead one to consider a glucocorticoid-induced hepatopathy.

The alkaline phosphatase and GGT increases are most likely secondary to drug-stimulated enzyme induction as opposed to being a cholestatic phenomenon. The canine liver is profoundly sensitive to corticosteroids. Liver function tests (BSP retention, fasting bile acids) may also be abnormal in patients with glucocorticoid hepatopathy and are not helpful in further biochemical differential diagnosis. An increase in cholesterol is occasionally observed in patients with hyperadrenocorticism. Liver-related parameters usually return to normal after successful treatment of the condition.

A decrease in T_4 often accompanies hypercortisolemia.

DIAGNOSIS

The owner elected not to treat the animal. Histopathology after necropsy revealed pituitary chromophobe adenoma, bilateral adrenal hyperplasia, and diffuse severe vacuolar degeneration in liver compatible with the presence of excess cortico-steroids.

Patient: Dog, Doberman, spayed female, 8 years old.

Presenting Signs and Complaints: Has had an allergic skin condition for 2 years. Has been treated with corticosteroids continually for last year. Now urinates large quantities frequently and drinks a lot of water. Skin not itching now but is very dry. Owner thinks abdomen is swollen. The patient was seen at another veterinary hospital, and abnormal liver tests were noted on the biochemical profile; the patient was referred for further evaluation for chronic active liver disease which does occur in the Doberman breed.

Physical Examination: Thin dry skin; hair loss over back; obese; enlarged liver on palpation.

Problem List: 1. Polyuria/polydipsia. 2. Bilateral alopecia. 3. Hepatomegaly.

Hematology	Day 1	Day 21
RBC × 10⁶/μL	7.1 (7.1 × 10¹²/L)	6.8 (6.8 × 10¹²/L)
Hemoglobin (g/dL)	14.0 (8.69 mmol/L)	13.9 (8.63 mmol/L)
PCV (%)	42 (42 volume fraction)	41 (41 volume fraction)
MCV (fL)	59.1	60.3
MCHC (g/dL)	33.3 (20.6 mmol/L)	33.9 (20.3 mmol/L)
NRBC/100 WBC	0	0
RBC morphology	Normal	Normal
↑ WBC × 10³/μL	**19,500 (19.5 × 10⁹/L)**	14,000 (14 × 10⁹/L)
Myelocytes/μL	0 (0 × 10⁹/L)	0 (0 × 10⁹/L)
Metamyelocytes/μL	0 (0 × 10⁹/L)	0 (0 × 10⁹/L)
Band neutrophils/μL	195 (0.2 × 10⁹/L)	140 (0.14 × 10⁹/L)
↑ Segmented neutrophils/μL	**18,135 (18.1 × 10⁹/L)**	10,500 (10.5 × 10⁹/L)
↓ Lymphocytes/μL	**585 (0.59 × 10⁹/L)**	2,620 (2.6 × 10⁹/L)
Monocytes/μL	585 (0.59 × 10⁹/L)	420 (0.42 × 10⁹/L)
↓ Eosinophils/μL	**0 (0 × 10⁹/L)**	420 (0.42 × 10⁹/L)
Basophils/μL	0 (0 × 10⁹/L)	0 (0 × 10⁹/L)
Toxic neutrophils	None	None
Platelet estimate	Adequate	Adequate

Serum Chemistry	Day 1	Day 21
↑ AST (SGOT) (IU/L)	**101 (101 U/L)**	86 (86 U/L)
↑ ALT (SGPT) (IU/L)	**435 (435 U/L)**	120 (120 U/L)
↑ ALP (IU/L)	**7,350 (7,350 U/L)**	↑ 5,350 (5,350 U/L)
↑ GGT (IU/L)	**27 (27 U/L)**	↑ 20 (20 U/L)
Total bilirubin (mg/dL)	0.4 (6.8 μmol/L)	0.5 (8.5 μmol/L)
Conjugated bilirubin (mg/dL)	0.2 (3.4 μmol/L)	0.4 (6.8 μmol/L)
Unconjugated bilirubin (mg/dL)	0.2 (3.4 μmol/L)	0.1 (1.7 μmol/L)
Total protein (g/dL)	6.3 (63 g/L)	6.5 (65 g/L)
Albumin (g/dL)	3.2 (32 g/L)	3.4 (34 g/L)
Globulin (g/dL)	3.1 (31 g/L)	3.1 (31 g/L)
↑ Cholesterol (mg/dL)	**687 (17.9 mmol/L)**	↑ 589 (15.3 mmol/L)
Urea nitrogen (mg/dL)	12 (4.3 mmol/L)	15 (5.4 mmol/L)

Table continued on following page

Serum Chemistry	Day 1	Day 21
Creatinine (mg/dL)	0.8 (70.7 μmol/L)	0.9 (79.6 μmol/L)
Glucose (mg/dL)	103 (5.7 mmol/L)	98 (5.4 mmol/L)
Amylase (IU/L)	325 (325 U/L)	305 (305 U/L)
Lipase (IU/L)	75 (75 U/L)	25 (25 U/L)
Sodium (mEq/L)	154 (154 mmol/L)	148 (148 mmol/L)
Potassium (mEq/L)	4.6 (4.6 mmol/L)	4.8 (4.8 mmol/L)
Na : K ratio	33.4	30.8
Chloride (mEq/L)	101 (101 mmol/L)	98 (98 mmol/L)
Carbon dioxide (mEq/L)	22 (22 mmol/L)	21 (21 mmol/L)
Calcium (mg/dL)	8.2 (2.05 mmol/L)	8.4 (2.1 mmol/L)
Phosphorus (mg/dL)	4.3 (1.4 mmol/L)	4.1 (1.3 mmol/L)
↑ **Fasting bile acids (μmol/L)**	**51 (51 μmol/L)**	10 (10 μmol/L)
↓ **Resting cortisol (μg/dL)**	**0.5 (13.8 nmol/L)**	2.1 (58 nmol/L)
↑ **Post-ACTH cortisol (μg/dL)**	**0.4 (11.0 nmol/L)**	7.5 (207 nmol/L)
T_3 (ng/dL)	185 (2.85 nmol/L)	
T_4 (μg/dL)	3.6 (46.3 nmol/L)	

Urinalysis (Cystocentesis)	Day 1	Day 21
Appearance	Clear, light yellow	Clear, yellow
↓ **Specific gravity**	**1.004**	**1.035**
pH	6.5	6.0
Protein	Negative	Negative
Glucose	Negative	Negative
Ketones	Negative	Negative
Blood	Negative	Negative
Bilirubin	Negative	Negative
Sediment		
WBC/hpf	0–1	0–3
RBC/hpf	Negative	1–2
Casts	Negative	Negative
Crystals	Negative	Negative
Bacteria	Negative	Negative

Ultrasonic examination of the liver demonstrated a diffusely enlarged liver and a full gallbladder. No abnormalities were noted.

HEMOGRAM (DAY 1)

The leukocytosis and differential count are compatible with stress (excess corticosteroids) or inflammation.

BIOCHEMICAL PROFILE (DAY 1)

There is a mild to moderate increase in transaminases implying enzyme leakage through hepatocellular membranes. The reason for aminotransferases to leak in association with glucocorticoid hepatopathy is not clear, but it is suspected that there is altered membrane permeability as a result of the metabolic derangement in the liver. If there is a leakage enzyme increase in glucocorticoid-induced hepatopathy it is usually the ALT without a concurrent increase in AST. When both aminotransferases are increased one should have a higher index of suspicion that there may be a concurrent inflammatory disorder within the liver and follow the liver tests after the underlying metabolic condition has been managed successfully. Histologic examination of the liver in some patients with severe glucocorticoid hepatopathy indicates that the vacuolar change can be severe enoiugh to cause small focal areas of suppurative hepatitis. This may also be an explanation for both aminotransferases to be increased. The practitioner should be aware of this potential histologic finding and not be misled into considering a bacterial component to the liver disorder. The vacuolar change will be diffuse and severe and will be the predominant finding on a biopsy; this should guide the practitioner in the interpretation of the biopsy.

A fasting bile acids was done for academic purposes to demonstrate their lack of value in further differentiating certain liver disorders biochemically. The fasting bile acids is moderately increased (normal is less than 12 μmol/L).

The marked increases in alkaline phosphatases and GGT with no hyperbilirubinemia support drug-induced enzyme production. Hypercholesterolemia could be associated with excessive glucocorticoids or hypothyroidism. The normal T_3 and T_4 rule out hypothyroidism. The cortisol tests are suppressed by exogenous cortisol and coroborate the presence of iatrogenic Cushing's syndrome.

A needle biopsy of the liver was done; diffuse severe vacuolar degeneration was found and focal suppurative hepatitis noted. These findings are compatible with glucocorticoid-induced hepatopathy and are not compatible with chronic active liver disease of the Doberman breed.

MANAGEMENT

After reviewing the initial laboratory data and liver biopsy, no further medication was indicated, and the patient was reevaluated 3 weeks later.

HEMOGRAM (DAY 21)

The hemogram has returned to normal.

BIOCHEMICAL PROFILE (DAY 14)

The serum liver leakage enzymes (ALT and AST) and fasting bile acids have returned toward normal, and the adrenal glands now responds to ACTH. If a chronic active liver disease was present but masked by the glucocorticoid hepatopathy it is likely that the fasting serum bile acids would remain abnormal on subsequent examinations; this would suggest the need for a wedge biopsy in some patients. Alkaline phsophatase and GGT are still increased and may take weeks to months to return to normal for several reasons. First, the patient received an injectable long-acting glucocorticoid that may still be having endogenous glucticoid effects. Second, once the liver is stimulated to produce these enzymes it takes a period of time for those factories to decrease their *de novo* protein synthesis of them. Third, the serum half-life of alkaline phosphatase in the dog is approximately 3 days and from a kinetic viewpoint will take a period of time to return to normal.

DIAGNOSIS

Iatrogenic hyperadrenocorticism with glucocorticoid-induced hepatopathy.

Patient: Dog, Dachshund, male, 3 years old.

Presenting Signs and Complaints: Does not seem to have any energy, skin is dry and flaky, has gained weight recently in spite of being on a low-calorie specialty diet.

Physical Examination: Obese, dry scaly skin, hair loss over back and hind legs.

Problem List: 1. Obesity. 2. Lethargy. 3. Alopecia. 4. Dry hair coat.

Hematology		Serum Chemistry	
↓ **RBC × 10⁶/μL**	**4.5 (4.5 × 10¹²/L)**	AST (SGOT) (IU/L)	24 (24 U/L)
↓ **Hemoglobin (g/dL)**	**9.8 (6.08 mmol/L)**	ALT (SGPT) (IU/L)	32 (32 U/L)
↓ **PCV (%)**	**28 (0.28 volume fraction)**	ALP (IU/L)	57 (57 U/L)
Plasma protien (g/dL)	6.7 (67 g/L)		
MCV (fL)	62.2	GGT (IU/L)	1 (1 U/L)
MCHC (g/dL)	35 (21.70 mmol/L)	Total bilirubin (mg/dL)	0.1 (1.7 μmol/L)
Reticulocytes (%)	0.9 (0.009 number fraction)	Conjugated bilirubin (mg/dL)	0.1 (1.7 μmol/L)
Corrected reticulocyte (%)	0.5 (0.005 number fraction)	Unconjugated bilirubin (mg/dL)	0 (0 μmol/L)
Reticulocytes/μL	40,500 (40.5 × 10⁹/L)	Total protein (g/dL)	7.1 (71 g/L)
NRBC/100 WBC	3	Albumin (g/dL)	3.7 (37 g/L)
RBC morphology	Normal	Globulin (g/dL)	3.4 (34 g/L)
WBC × 10³/μL	10.5 (10.5 × 10⁹/L)	↑ **Cholesterol (mg/dL)**	**580 (15 mmol/L)**
Myelocytes/μL	0 (0 × 10⁹/L)	Urea nitrogen (mg/dL)	15 (5.4 mmol/L)
Metamyelocytes/μL	0 (0 × 10⁹/L)	Creatinine (mg/dL)	0.7 (61.9 μmol/L)
Band neutrophils/μL	0 (0 × 10⁹/L)	Glucose (mg/dL)	105 (5.8 mmol/L)
Segmented neutrophils/μL	7560 (7.6 × 10⁹/L)	Sodium (mEq/L)	148 (148 mmol/L)
Lymphocytes/μL	2310 (2.3 × 10⁹/L)	Potassium (mEq/L)	4.2 (4.2 mmol/L)
Monocytes/μL	315 (0.32 × 10⁹/L)	Na : K ratio	35.2
Eosinophils/μL	315 (0.32 × 10⁹/L)	Chloride (mEq/L)	103 (103 mmol/L)
Basophils/μL	0 (0 × 10⁹/L)	Carbon dioxide (mEq/L)	24 (24 mmol/L)
Toxic neutrophils	None	Calcium (mg/dL)	8.7 (2.05 mmol/L)
Platelet estimate	Adequate	Inorganic phosphate (mg/dL)	3.5 (1.13 mmol/L)
Platelets × 10³/μL	250 (0.25 × 10¹²/L)	↑ **Creatine kinase (IU/L)**	**775 (775 U/L)**
		↑ **Total T₃ (ng/dL)**	**750 (11.6 nmol)**
		Total T₄ (μg/dL)	1.3 (16.7 nmol/L)

Urinalysis (Cystocentesis)	
Appearance	Clear, yellow
Specific gravity	1.043
pH	6
Protein	Negative
Glucose	Negative
Ketones	Negative
Blood	Negative
Bilirubin	Negative
Sediment	
WBC/hpf	0–1
RBC/hpf	0–3
Casts	Negative
Crystals	Negative
Bacteria	Negative

HEMOGRAM

There is a nonregenerative normocytic normochromic anemia.

BIOCHEMICAL PROFILE

The T_3 is increased. Patients with T_3 concentrations this high often have circulating antibodies to T_3 suggesting that the patient may have immune-mediated thyroiditis. The effect of circulating antibodies on the assay for T_3 and T_4 depends upon the methodology used by the laboratory. In this case, in which a solid phase radioimmunoassay method is used, the test results are abnormally high. The same would have been true using a double antibody technique. If a nonspecific separation technique is used the T_3 or T_4 assay values are spuriously low in the presence of autoantibodies. The veterinarian should be aware of the technique utilized.

In a patient such as the one described, hypothyroidism is difficult to confirm. The hypercholesterolemia, with a history of dietary control, is compatible with hypothyroidism. Because of the interference of autoantibodies a TSH stimulation test (Chapter 9) would be of little value. Autoantibodies to thyroxine can be determined using an immunologic test for antithyroid globulins. Final confirmation of immune-mediated thyroiditis is best accomplished by a biopsy.

Creatine kinase activity is occasionally increased in patients with hypothyroidism and no evidence of muscle damage (normal AST). The reason for this is unclear.

DIAGNOSIS

Hypothyroidism caused by immune-mediated thyroiditis.

COMMENT

For academic reasons, a thyroid biopsy was completed after an immunologic test for antithyroid antibodies was found to be positive. The pathologist reported a diffuse infiltration of lymphocytes, plasma cells, and macrophages.

FINAL DIAGNOSIS

Immune-mediated thyroiditis.

Patient: Cat, domestic shorthair, neutered male, 10 years old.

Presenting Signs and Complaints: Weight loss; poor appetite; drinking more water; lethargic; diarrhea.

Physical Examination: Thin; heart rate 200 bpm with gallop rhythm ascultated; soft 2-cm mass palpated in right ventral cervical region; evidence of diarrhea in perianal area.

Problem List: 1. Weight loss. 2. Mass in right ventral cervical region. 3. Tachycardia. 4. Gallop cardiac rhythm. 5. Diarrhea. 6. Anorexia.

Hematology		Serum Chemistry	
RBC × 10⁶/μL	8.61 (8.6 × 10¹²/L)	AST (SGOT) (IU/L)	42 (42 U/L)
Hemoglobin (g/dL)	12.5 (7.8 mmol/L)	↑ **ALT (SGPT) (IU/L)**	**161 (161 U/L)**
PCV (%)	38.5 (0.385 volume fraction)	↑ **ALP (IU/L)**	**56 (56 U/L)**
MCV (fL)	48	↑ **Total bilirubin (mg/dL)**	**1.9 (32.5 μmol/L)**
MCHC (g/dL)	32.4 (20.1 mmol/L)	Total protein (g/dL)	7.3 (73 g/L)
NRBC/100 WBC	0	Albumin (g/dL)	3.4 (34 g/L)
RBC morphology	Normal	Globulin (g/dL)	3.9 (39 g/L)
WBC × 10³/μL	13.6 (13.6 × 10⁹/L)	Glucose (mg/dL)	89 (4.9 mmol/L)
		Urea nitrogen (mg/dL)	30 (10.7 mmol/L)
Myelocytes/μL	0 (0 × 10⁹/L)	Creatinine (mg/dL)	1.9 (168.0 μm/L)
Metamyelocytes/μL	0 (0 × 10⁹/L)	Calcium (mg/dL)	9.0 (2.3 mmol/L)
Band neutrophils/μL	0 (0 × 10⁹/L)	Phosphorus (mg/dL)	4.3 (1.4 mmol/L)
Segmented neutrophils/μL	8,704 (8.7 × 10⁹/L)	Sodium (mEq/L)	155 (155 mmol/L)
Lymphocytes/μL	3,672 (3.7 × 10⁹/L)	Potassium (mEq/L)	4.0 (4.0 mmol/L)
Monocytes/μL	272 (0.27 × 10⁹/L)	Na : K ratio	38.8
Eosinophils/μL	952 (0.95 × 10⁹/L)	↑ **Total T₄ (μg/dL)**	>12 (>154 nmol/L)
Basophils/μL	0 (0 × 10⁹/L)		
Toxic neutrophils	None		
Plasma estimate	Adequate		

Urinalysis (Cystocentesis)	
Appearance	Clear, yellow
Specific gravity	1.035
pH	6.0
Protein	Negative
Glucose	Negative
Ketones	Negative
↑ **Blood**	**2+**
Bilirubin	Negative
Sediment	
WBC/hpf	2–4
RBC/hpf	Negative
Casts	Negative
Crystals	Negative
Bacteria	Negative

HEMOGRAM

The hemogram is unremarkable.

BIOCHEMICAL PROFILE

The ALT is increased, indicating leakage through the hepatocellular membrane while the increased alkaline phosphatase and hyperbilirubinemia reflect cholestasis. There is also bilirubinuria, which is a reflection of hyperbilirubinemia. The presence of bilirubinuria in the cat should always be viewed with suspicion.

Examination of the biochemical data implies the presence of primary liver disease; however, the age and history of the animal and physical findings of a gallop cardiac rhythm with tachycardia are suggestive of hyperthyroidism. It has been reported that cats with hyperthyroidism can produce altered liver tests without having primary liver disease. Because of those facts a T_4 was run and was markedly increased. The mass on the neck was aspirated and found to be a reactive lymph node. The patient was managed for tachycardia and was eventually taken to surgery and the thyroid removed. A liver biopsy taken at the time of surgery indicated mild hepatocellular cholestasis with no evidence of inflammatory or vacuolar changes. Histopathology of the thyroid gland revealed a benign thyroid adenoma.

Three weeks after surgery the liver tests had returned to normal.

DIAGNOSIS

Hyperthyroidism.

COMMENT

Thyroid hormones do affect the biliary excretory process and compound the interpretation of liver tests in certain patients. The judicious approach to any patient with abnormal liver tests is to assume that the liver is a secondary problem and search for a primary disorder. If an underlying disease process cannot be identified then a primary liver disease process can be considered.

Patient: Dog, chow chow, female, 6 months old.

Presenting Signs and Complaints: Inappetence, lethargy, and reluctance to move for 5 days; vaccinated 2 to 3 weeks prior to admission.

Physical Examination: Temperature 103.5 F; very rigid neck with pain when flexed.

Hematology		Serum Chemistry	
RBC × 10⁶/μL	4.1 (4.1 × 10¹²/L)	AST (SGOT) (IU/L)	25 (25 U/L)
Hemoglobin (g/dL)	8.8 (5.46 mmol/L)	ALT (SGPT) (IU/L)	47 (47 U/L)
PCV (%)	31 (0.32 volume fraction)	↑ **ALP (IU/L)**	**210 (210 U/L)**
MCV (fL)	72	GGT (IU/L)	1 (1 U/L)
MCHC (g/dL)	33 (20.5 mmol/L)	Total bilirubin (mg/dL)	0.1 (1.7 mmol/L)
NRBC/100 WBC	0	Total protein (g/dL)	7.0 (70 g/L)
RBC morphology	Normal	Albumin (g/dL)	3.4 (34 g/L)
WBC × 10³/μL	18.5 (18.4 × 10⁹/L)	Globulin (g/dL)	3.6 (36 g/L)
		Glucose (mg/dL)	103 (5.7 mmol/L)
Band neutrophils/μL	0 (0 × 10⁹/L)	Urea nitrogen (mg/dL)	15 (5.4 mmol/L)
↑ **Segmented neutrophils/μL**	**15,580 (15.6 × 10⁹/L)**	Creatinine (mg/dL)	0.8 (70.7 μmol/L)
Lymphocytes/μL	2,405 (2.4 × 10⁹/L)	Carbon dioxide (mEq/L)	21 (21 mmol/L)
Monocytes/μL	370 (0.37 × 10⁹/L)	Chloride (mEq/L)	105 (105 mmol/L)
Eosinophils/μL	185 (0.19 × 10⁹/L)	Sodium (mEq/L)	148 (148 mmol/L)
Basophils/μL	0 (0 × 10⁹/L)	Potassium (mEq/L)	4.3 (4.3 mmol/L)
Platelets*a* × 10³/μL	136 (0.14 × 10¹²/L)	Na : K ratio	38
Plasma proteins (g/dL)	7.6 (76 g/dL)	Calcium (mg/dL)	9.9 (2.48 mmol/L)
↑ **Fibrinogen (mg/dL)**	**500 (5 g/L)**	↑ **Phosphorus (mg/dL)**	**6.6 (2.1 mmol/L)**

a Some large platelets.

Urinalysis (Cystocentesis)	
Appearance	Clear, yellow
Specific gravity	1.034
pH	7
Protein	Negative
Glucose	Negative
Ketones	Negative
Blood	Negative
Bilirubin	Negative
Sediment	
WBC/hpf	0–1
RBC/hpf	1–2
Casts	Negative
Crystals	Negative
Bacteria	Negative

Cerebrospinal Fluid	
↑ Nucleated cells/μL	(1.2 × 10⁹/L)
↑ Neutrophils, mature (%)	80
Mononuclear, small (%)	15
Mononuclear, large (%)	5
Bacteria	None
Protein (mg/dL)	(1.5 g/L)

HEMOGRAM

There is a leukocytosis due to a mature neutrophilia; this may be a reflection of stress or an inflammatory process. An inflammatory process is supported by the hyperfibrinogenemia. The mild thrombocytopenia may have been a normal finding for this patient or could be related to the vaccinations that were administered 2–3 weeks previously; modified live vaccines can cause a mild transient thrombocytopenia.

BIOCHEMICAL PROFILE

The profile is unremarkable except for a slight increase for the alkaline phosphatase and phosphorus values. These values are increased in growing patients.

CEREBROSPINAL FLUID EXAMINATION

Because of the neurologic signs cerebrospinal fluid was examined. There was a pleocytosis with increased numbers of neutrophils and mononuclear cells. The total protein was increased. These findings are compatible with a sterile inflammatory process. A postvaccinal response sometimes produces an inflammatory response of this type.

ADDITIONAL INFORMATION

The dog was treated with glucocorticoids and was clinically normal after 48 hours. A repeat hemogram revealed a normal platelet count.

DIAGNOSIS

Neurologic reaction to vaccination with modified live virus vaccine.

Patient: Dog, Maltese, spayed female, 6 years old.

Presenting Signs and Complaints: Acute onset of inappetence; and weakness of hind legs; stumbles while walking.

Physical Examination: Right sided paralysis of face; absent right sided menace response; moderately disoriented throughout the physical examination.

Problem List: Hind leg paralysis; facial nerve palsy; trigeminal nerve palsy.

Cerebrospinal Fluid	
Nucleated cells/μL	750 (0.75 × 10⁹/L)
Neutrophils, mature (%)	25
Mononuclear, small (%)	60 (lymphocytes)
Mononuclear, small (%)	15 (lymphoplasmocytic)
Bacteria	Negative
Protein (mg/dL)	280 (2.8 g/L)

The hemogram, biochemical profile, and urinalysis were all normal.

CEREBROSPINAL FLUID EXAMINATION

The CSF findings and history are supportive of granulomatous meningioencephalitis-encephalomyelitits.

ADDITIONAL INFORMATION

Patient was treated with glucocorticoids and after a week the owner elected euthanasia.

DIAGNOSIS

At necropsy, multifocal granulomatous meningioencephalitis was confirmed.

Patient: Horse, quarter horse, gelding, 12 years old.

Presenting Signs and Complaints: Two-week history of muscular weakness and incoordination.

Physical Examination: Ataxic; posterior paresis.

Problem List: 1. Ataxia. 2. Posterior paresis.

Cerebrospinal Fluid (Lumbar Puncture)	
Nucleated cells/μL	260 (0.26 × 10^9/L)
Neutrophils, mature (%)	0
Mononuclear, small (%)	93 (lymphocytes)
Mononuclear, large (%)	7 (with some vacuolar cytoplasmic change)
Bacteria	Negative
Protein (mg/dL)	25 (0.25 g/L)

Hemogram, biochemical profile, and urinalysis were unremarkable.

CEREBROSPINAL FLUID EXAMINATION

The lack of a neutrophilic response is suggestive of equine protozoal myeloencephalopathy or a viral infection. The owner requested euthanasia based on a guarded to poor prognosis.

DIAGNOSIS

Histologic examination confirmed protozoal myeloencephalopathy. Occasionally eosinophils are noted in horses with this condition.

Patient: Horse, quarter horse, male, 6 weeks old.

Presenting Signs and Complaints: Foal treated for joint illness for the past 2 weeks; now is unable to stand; will nurse from a bottle.

Physical Examination: Temperature 104.2° F; generalized weakness; unable to remain standing except with help.

Problem List: 1. Pyrexia. 2. Ataxia. 3. Weakness.

Hematology		Serum Chemistry	
RBC × 10⁶/μL	5.6 (5.6 × 10¹²/L)	↑ AST (SGOT) (IU/L)	**546 (546 U/L)**
Hemoglobin (g/dL)	11.5 (7.14 mmol/L)	ALT (SGPT) (IU/L)	12 (12 U/L)
PCV (%)	35 (0.35 volume fraction)	ALP (IU/L)	15 (15 U/L)
MCV (fL)	62.5	GGT (IU/L)	2 (2 U/L)
MCHC (g/dL)	32.8 (20.3 mmol/L)	Total bilirubin (mg/dL)	0.3 (5.1 μmol/L)
NRBC/100 WBC	0	Total protein (g/dL)	7.1 (71 g/L)
WBC × 10³/μL	25.5 (125.5 × 10⁹/L)	Albumin (g/dL)	3.6 (36 g/dL)
		Globulin (g/dL)	3.5 (35 g/L)
↑ **Band neutrophils/μL**	**3,825 (3.8 × 10⁹/L)**	Glucose (mg/dL)	86 (4.7 mmol/L)
↑ **Segmented neutrophils/μL**	**16,575 (16.6 × 10⁹/L)**	Urea nitrogen (mg/dL)	12 (4.3 mmol/L)
Lymphocytes/μL	3,825 (3.8 × 10⁹/L)	Creatinine (mg/dL)	0.6 (53.0 μmol/L)
Monocytes/μL	1,275 (1.3 × 10⁹/L)	Total carbon dioxide (mEq/L)	24 (24 mmol/L)
Eosinophils/μL	0 (0. × 10⁹/L)	Chloride (meq/L)	105 (105 mmol/L)
Basophils/μL	0 (0. × 10⁹/L)	Sodium (mEq/L)	154 (154 mmol/L)
↑ **Toxic neutrophils**	**2+**	Potassium (mEq/L)	4.5 (4.5 mmol/L)
Platelets × 10³/μL	140 (0.14 × 10¹²/L)	Calcium (mg/dL)	8.9 (2.23 mmol/L)
Plasma proteins (g/dL)	7.8 (76 g/L)	Phosphorus (mg/dL)	3.4 (1.1 mmol/L)
↑ **Fibrinogen (mg/dL)**	**700 (5 g/L)**	↑ **Creatine kinase (IU/L)**	**986 (986 U/L)**

Cerebrospinal Fluid	
↑ **Nucleated cells/μL**	**3,200 (3.2 × 10⁹/L)**
↑ **Neutrophils, mature**[a] **(%)**	**98**
Mononuclear, large (%)	2
↑ **Bacteria**	**Cocci in chains**
↑ **Protein (mg/dL)**	**350 (3.5 g/L)**
↓ **Glucose (mg/dL)**	**25 (1.38 mmol/L)**

[a] Neutrophils are karyolytic, and some contain bacterial cocci.

HEMOGRAM

The leukocytosis, neutrophilia, left shift, and toxic neutrophils are compatible with an inflammation, probably bacterial. Hyperfibrinogenemia supports an inflammatory process.

BIOCHEMICAL PROFILE

The increased AST and creatine kinase support muscle damage, probably from prolonged recumbence.

CEREBROSPINAL FLUID EXAMINATION

The presence of neutrophils, many of which are degenerate, supports bacterial meningioencephalitis. The presence of bacteria within the neutrophils confirms this diagnosis. The marked increase in total protein also supports the presence of an inflammation. Hypoglycorrachia with the CSF glucose less than 60% of the serum glucose also supports a bacterial infection.

DIAGNOSIS

Bacterial meningioencephalitis.

Part III

Algorithms

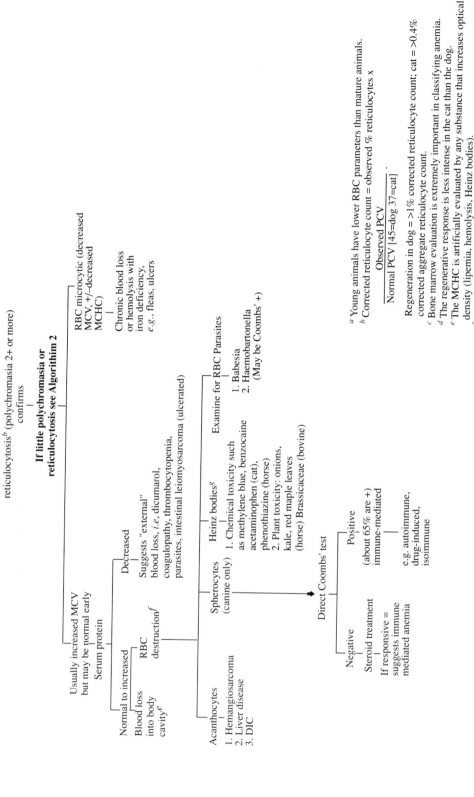

Algorithm 1

RESPONSIVE ANEMIA[a,c,d]

reticulocytosis[b] (polychromasia 2+ or more) confirms

If little polychromasia or reticulocytosis see Algorithm 2

Usually increased MCV but may be normal early
Serum protein

RBC microcytic (decreased MCV, +/–decreased MCHC)

Chronic blood loss or hemolysis with iron deficiency, e.g., fleas, ulcers

Normal to increased
Blood loss into body cavity[e]

Decreased
RBC destruction[f]

Suggests "external" blood loss, i.e, dicumarol, coagulopathy, thrombocytopenia, parasites, intestinal leiomyosarcoma (ulcerated)

Examine for RBC Parasites
1. Babesia
2. Haemobartonella (May be Coombs' +)

Acanthocytes
1. Hemangiosarcoma
2. Liver disease
3. DIC

Spherocytes (canine only)

Heinz bodies[g]
1. Chemical toxicity such as methylene blue, benzocaine acetaminophen (cat), phenothiazine (horse)
2. Plant toxicity: onions, kale, red maple leaves (horse) Brassicaceae (bovine)

Direct Coombs' test

Positive
(about 65% are +) immune-mediated

e.g. autoimmune, drug-induced, isoimmune

Negative
Steroid treatment
If responsive = suggests immune mediated anemia

---

[a] Young animals have lower RBC parameters than mature animals.

[b] Corrected reticulocyte count = observed % reticulocytes x

$$\frac{\text{Observed PCV}}{\text{Normal PCV [45=dog 37=cat]}}.$$

Regeneration in dog = >1% corrected reticulocyte count; cat = >0.4% corrected aggregate reticulocyte count.

[c] Bone marrow evaluation is extremely important in classifying anemia.

[d] The regenerative response is less intense in the cat than the dog.

[e] The MCHC is artificially evaluated by any substance that increases optical density (lipemia, hemolysis, Heinz bodies).

[f] Blood loss or hemolysis is often accompanied by a leukocytosis (see Fig. 2-1).

[g] A small % of Heinz bodies may be normal in cats; also associated with propylene glycol that is added to semimoist cat food as a preservative as well as toxins associated with gastrointestinal disorders.

Algorithm 2

POORLY RESPONSIVE OR NONRESPONSIVE ANEMIA[a,c,d]

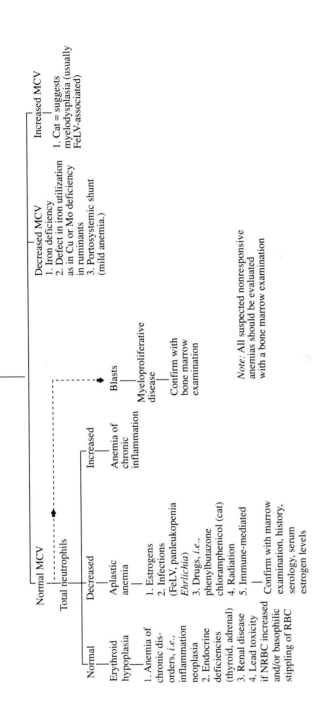

Polychromasia 1+ or less and minimal/no reticulocytosis[b]

Normal MCV — Total neutrophils

Normal — Erythroid hypoplasia
1. Anemia of chronic disorders, i.e., inflammation neoplasia
2. Endocrine deficiencies (thyroid, adrenal)
3. Renal disease
4. Lead toxicity if NRBC increased and/or basophilic stippling of RBC

Decreased — Aplastic anemia
1. Estrogens
2. Infections (FeLV, panleukopenia Ehrlichia)
3. Drugs, i.e., phenylbutazone chloramphenicol (cat)
4. Radiation
5. Immune-mediated
Confirm with marrow examination, history, serology, serum estrogen levels

Increased — Anemia of chronic inflammation

Blasts → Myeloproliferative disease → Confirm with bone marrow examination

Note: All suspected nonresponsive anemias should be evaluated with a bone marrow examination

Decreased MCV
1. Iron deficiency
2. Defect in iron utilization as in Cu or Mo deficiency in ruminants
3. Portosystemic shunt (mild anemia.)

Increased MCV
1. Cat = suggests myelodysplasia (usually FeLV-associated)

[a] Young animals have lower RBC parameters than mature animals.

[b] Corrected reticulocyte count = observed % reticulocyte x $\dfrac{\text{Observed PCV}}{\text{Normal PCV [45=dog 37=cat]}}$.

Regeneration in dog = >1% corrected reticulocyte count; cat = >0.4% corrected aggregate reticulocyte count.

[c] Bone marrow evaluation is important in classifying anemia.

[d] All cats with anemias should be tested for FeLV and FIV.

308

Algorithm 3

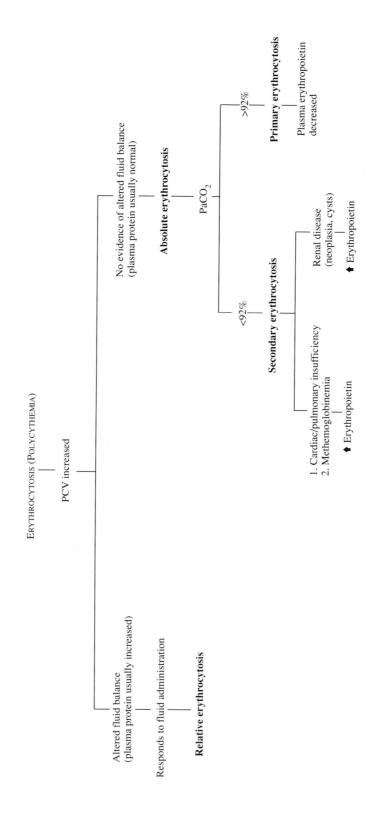

ERYTHROCYTOSIS (POLYCYTHEMIA)

PCV increased

Altered fluid balance
(plasma protein usually increased)

Responds to fluid administration

Relative erythrocytosis

No evidence of altered fluid balance
(plasma protein usually normal)

Absolute erythrocytosis

$PaCO_2$

<92%

Secondary erythrocytosis

1. Cardiac/pulmonary insufficiency
2. Methemoglobinemia

⬆ Erythropoietin

Renal disease
(neoplasia, cysts)

⬆ Erythropoietin

>92%

Primary erythrocytosis

Plasma erythropoietin
decreased

Algorithm 4

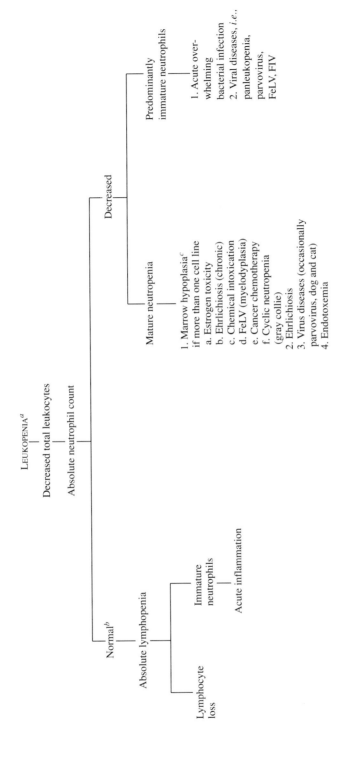

LEUKOPENIA[a]

Decreased total leukocytes
Absolute neutrophil count

Normal[b]

Absolute lymphopenia

Lymphocyte loss

Immature neutrophils

Acute inflammation

Decreased

Mature neutropenia

1. Marrow hypoplasia[c]
   if more than one cell line
   a. Estrogen toxicity
   b. Ehrlichiosis (chronic)
   c. Chemical intoxication
   d. FeLV (myelodysplasia)
   e. Cancer chemotherapy
   f. Cyclic neutropenia
      (gray collie)
2. Ehrlichiosis
3. Virus diseases (occasionally
   parvovirus, dog and cat)
4. Endotoxemia

Predominantly immature neutrophils

1. Acute overwhelming bacterial infection
2. Viral diseases, i.e., panleukopenia, parvovirus, FeLV, FIV

[a]Bone marrow examination is recommended in patients with a persistent leukopenia
[b]Occurs only in animals where absolute lymphocyte counts normally exceed absolute neutrophil counts (ruminants, occasionally horse)
[c]Marrow hypoplasia frequently involves more than one cell line. Anemia and/or thrombocytopenia are often present.

Algorithm 5

NORMAL OR INCREASED TOTAL LEUKOCYTE COUNT
WITH ABNORMAL DIFFERENTIAL COUNTS[a]

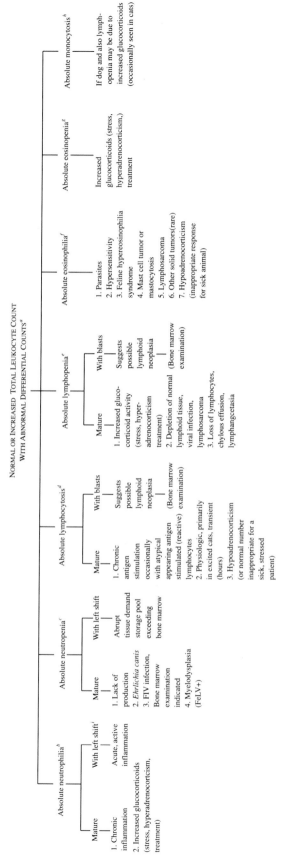

[a] Leukocytosis: Dog = 17,000; Cat = 20,000; Horse = 13,000; Cow = 12,000; Pig = 22,000; Sheep = 12,000; Goat = 13,000
[b] Neutrophilia: Dog = 12,000; Cat = 12,500; Horse = 7,000; Cow = 5,000; Pig = 10,000; Sheep = 6,000; Goat = 7,500
[c] Neutropenia: Dog = <3,000; Cat = <2,500; Horse = <2,700; Cow = <1,500; Pig = <3,200; Sheep = <700; Goat = <1,200
[d] Lymphocytosis: Dog = 5,000; Cat = 7,000; Horse = 6,000; Cow = 7,500; Pig = 13,000; Sheep = 9,000; Goat = 9,000
[e] Lymphopenia: Dog = 1,000; Cat = 1,500; Horse = 1,500; Cow = 3,000; Pig = 4,500; Sheep = 2,000; Goat = 2,000
[f] Eosinophilia: Dog = 1,500; Cat = 800; Horse = 1,000; Cow = 1,500; Pig = 2,000; Sheep = 1,000; Goat = 700
[g] Eosinopenia: Dog = 100; Cat = 100; Horse = 100; Cow = 1,100; Pig = 100; Sheep = 100; Goat = 100
[h] Monocytosis: Dog = 1,450; Cat = 800; Horse = 1,000; Cow = 1,500; Pig = 2,000; Sheep = 1,000; Goat = 700
[i] Left shift (band cells or younger): Dog = 300; Cat = 300; Horse = 100; Cow = 200; Pig = 800; Sheep = 100; Goat = 100

Algorithm 6

PLATELET/COAGULATION
FACTOR DEFICIENCIES

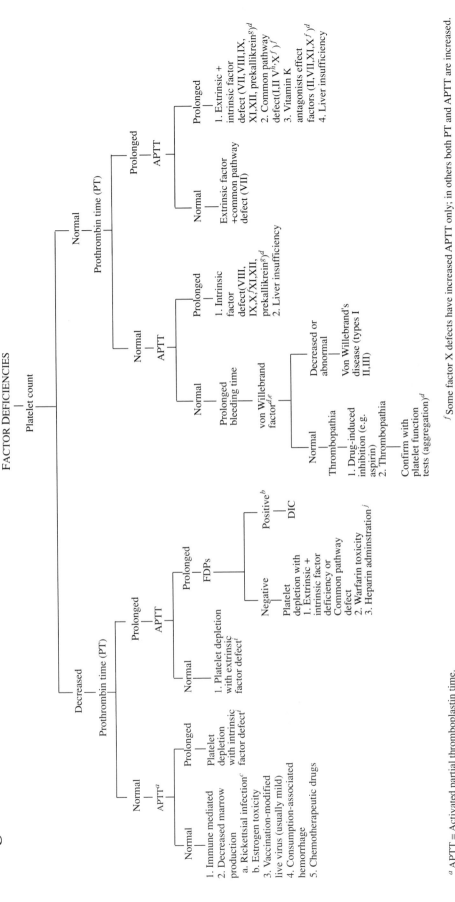

Platelet count

- **Decreased**
  - **Prothrombin time (PT)**
    - **Normal**
      - **APTT[a]**
        - **Normal**
          1. Immune mediated
          2. Decreased marrow production
             a. Rickettsial infection[c]
             b. Estrogen toxicity
          3. Vaccination-modified live virus (usually mild)
          4. Consumption-associated hemorrhage
          5. Chemotherapeutic drugs
        - **Prolonged**
          Platelet depletion with intrinsic factor defect[i]
    - **Prolonged**
      - **APTT**
        - **Normal**
          1. Platelet depletion with extrinsic factor defect[i]
        - **Prolonged**
          - **FDPs**
            - **Negative**
              Platelet depletion with
              1. Extrinsic + intrinsic factor deficiency or Common pathway defect
              2. Warfarin toxicity
              3. Heparin administration[j]
            - **Positive[b]**
              DIC
- **Normal**
  - **Prothrombin time (PT)**
    - **Normal**
      - **APTT**
        - **Normal**
          - **Prolonged bleeding time**
            - **von Willebrand factor[d,e]**
              - **Normal**
                Thrombopathia
                1. Drug-induced inhibition (e.g. aspirin)
                2. Thrombopathia
                Confirm with platelet function tests (aggregation)[d]
              - **Decreased or abnormal**
                Von Willebrand's disease (types I II,III)
        - **Prolonged**
          1. Intrinsic factor defect (VIII, IX,X,[f]XI,XII, prekallikrein[g])[d]
          2. Liver insufficiency
    - **Prolonged**
      - **APTT**
        - **Normal**
          Extrinsic factor +common pathway defect (VII)
        - **Prolonged**
          1. Extrinsic + intrinsic factor defect (VII,VIII,IX, XI,XII, prekallikrein[g])[d]
          2. Common pathway defect(I,II V[h]–X[f])[f]
          3. Vitamin K antagonists effect factors (II,VII,XI,X[f])[f]
          4. Liver insufficiency

---

[a] APTT = Activated partial thromboplastin time.

[b] Some animals with DIC will have low or undetectable levels of fibrin degradation products (FDP).

[c] Specific tests may be necessary. Ehrlichia and RMSF = serologic test. Estrogen = serum estrogen levels.

[d] Tests for these defects should be conducted at a special coagulation laboratory.

[e] Formerly called factor VIII-related antigen

[f] Some factor X defects have increased APTT only; in others both PT and APTT are increased.

[g] Fletcher factor

[h] Some factor V defects have an increased PT only, and some have increased in PT and APTT.

[i] Large platelets are often observed in blood.

[j] Especially if heparin used to keep intravenous line open and blood is taken from it.

Algorithm 7

HEPATIC TEST ABNORMALITIES WITH
MODERATE TO MARKEDLY INCREASED AMINOTRANSFERASES
(ALT,AST,SD)[a,b]
(if normal or slight increase see Algorithm 8)

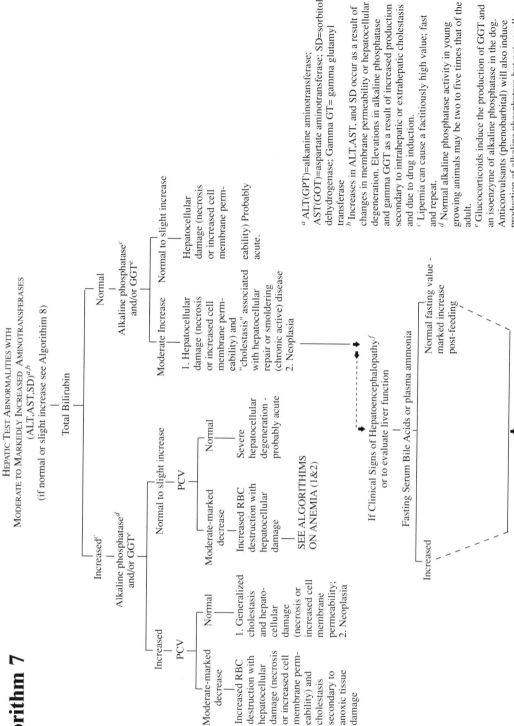

Total Bilirubin

Increased[c]

Alkaline phosphatase[d] and/or GGT[e]

- **Increased**

  PCV

  - **Moderate-marked decrease**

    Increased RBC destruction with hepatocellular damage (necrosis or increased cell membrane permeability) and cholestasis secondary to anoxic tissue damage

  - **Normal**

    1. Generalized cholestasis and hepatocellular damage (necrosis or increased cell membrane permeability)
    2. Neoplasia

- **Normal to slight increase**

  PCV

  - **Moderate-marked decrease**

    Increased RBC destruction with hepatocellular damage

    SEE ALGORITHMS ON ANEMIA (1&2)

  - **Normal**

    Severe hepatocellular degeneration - probably acute

Normal

Alkaline phosphatase[c] and/or GGT[e]

- **Moderate Increase**

  1. Hepatocellular damage (necrosis or increased cell membrane perm-eability) and "cholestasis" associated with hepatocellular repair or smoldering (chronic active) disease
  2. Neoplasia

- **Normal to slight increase**

  Hepatocellular damage (necrosis or increased cell membrane perm-eability) Probably acute.

If Clinical Signs of Hepatoencephalopathy[f] or to evaluate liver function

Fasting Serum Bile Acids or plasma ammonia

- Normal fasting value - marked increase post-feeding

- Increased

  1. Liver insufficiency
  2. Portosystemic venous anomaly-congenital or acquired

---

[a] ALT(GPT)=alkanine aminotransferase; AST(GOT)=aspartate aminotransferase; SD=sorbitol dehydrogenase; Gamma GT= gamma glutamyl transferase

[b] Increases in ALT,AST, and SD occur as a result of changes in membrane permeability or hepatocellular degeneration. Elevations in alkaline phosphatase and gamma GGT as a result of increased production secondary to intrahepatic or extrahepatic cholestasis and due to drug induction.

[c] Lipemia can cause a factitiously high value; fast and repeat.

[d] Normal alkaline phosphatase activity in young growing animals may be two to five times that of the adult.

[e] Glucocorticoids induce the production of GGT and an isoenzyme of alkaline phosphatase in the dog. Anticonvulsants (phenobarbital) will also induce production of alkaline phosphatase but not usually GGT. Drug induction is much less common in cats, but occasionally they may have a mild increase.

[f] Function test not needed if bilirubin is increased except in the horse; bile acid concentration is diagnostically helpful

Algorithm 8

HEPATIC TEST ABNORMALITIES WITH NORMAL OR SLIGHTLY INCREASED AMINOTRANSFERASES (ALT, AST, SD)[a,b]
If marked increase see Algorithm 7

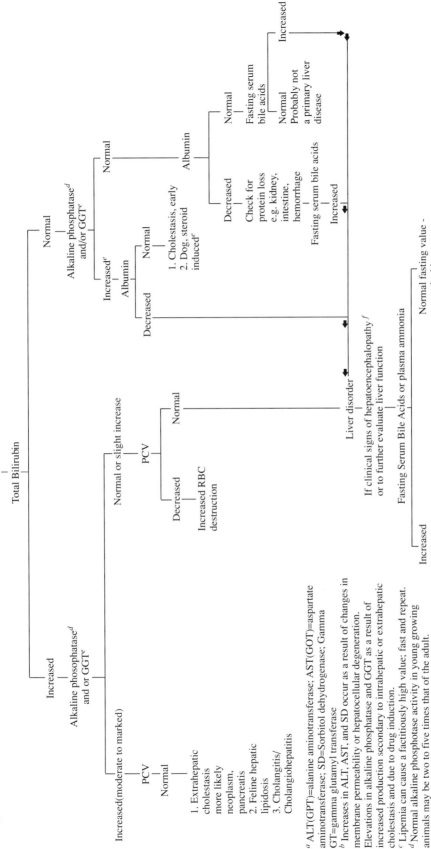

[a] ALT(GPT)=alanine aminotransferase; AST(GOT)=aspartate aminotransferase; SD=Sorbitol dehydrogenase; Gamma GT=gamma glutamyl transferase

[b] Increases in ALT, AST, and SD occur as a result of changes in membrane permeability or hepatocellular degeneration. Elevations in alkaline phosphatase and GGT as a result of increased production secondary to intrahepatic or extrahepatic cholestasis and due to drug induction.

[c] Lipemia can cause a factitiously high value; fast and repeat.

[d] Normal alkaline phosphotase activity in young growing animals may be two to five times that of the adult.

[e] Glucocorticoids induce the production of GGT and an isoenzyme of alkaline phosphatase in the dog. Anticonvulsants (phenobarbital) will also induce production of alkaline phosphatase but not GGT. Drug induction is much less common in cats, but occasionally they may have a mild increase.

[f] Function test not needed if bilirubin is increased except in the horse; bile acid concentration is diagnostically helpful.

Algorithm 9

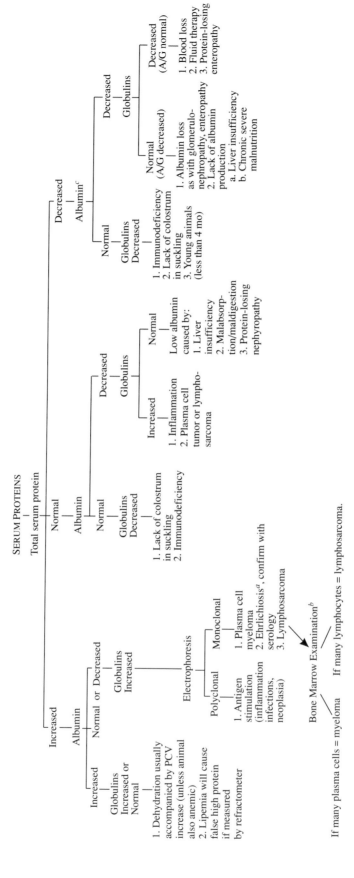

SERUM PROTEINS
Total serum protein

Increased

Albumin
— Increased
  - Globulins Increased or Normal
    1. Dehydration usually accompanied by PCV increase (unless animal also anemic)
    2. Lipemia will cause false high protein if measured by refractometer
— Normal or Decreased
  - Globulins Increased
    - Electrophoresis
      - Polyclonal
        1. Antigen stimulation (inflammation, infections, neoplasia)
      - Monoclonal
        1. Plasma cell myeloma
        2. Ehrlichiosis[a], confirm with serology
        3. Lymphosarcoma
        - Bone Marrow Examination[b]
          - If many plasma cells = myeloma   If many lymphocytes = lymphosarcoma.

Normal

Albumin
— Normal
  - Globulins Decreased
    1. Lack of colostrum in suckling
    2. Immunodeficiency
— Decreased
  - Globulins Increased
    1. Inflammation
    2. Plasma cell tumor or lymphosarcoma
  - Globulins Normal
    Low albumin caused by:
    1. Liver insufficiency
    2. Malabsorption/maldigestion
    3. Protein-losing nephyropathy

Decreased

Albumin[c]
— Normal
  - Globulins Decreased
    1. Immunodeficiency
    2. Lack of colostrum in suckling
    3. Young animals (less than 4 mo)
  - (A/G decreased)
    1. Albumin loss as with glomerulo-nephropathy, enteropathy
    2. Lack of albumin production
       a. Liver insufficiency
       b. Chronic severe malnutrition
— Decreased
  - Globulins
    - Decreased (A/G normal)
      1. Blood loss
      2. Fluid therapy
      3. Protein-losing enteropathy

---

[a] Prominent plasmacytosis may be observed in the bone marrow.

[b] Plasma cells and lymphocytes may show mild to moderate increases when there is chronic antigen stimulation elsewhere in the body; seldom exceeding 10–20% respectively.

[c] Lipemia can cause a "false low" albumin. The patient should be fasted and the sample repeated.

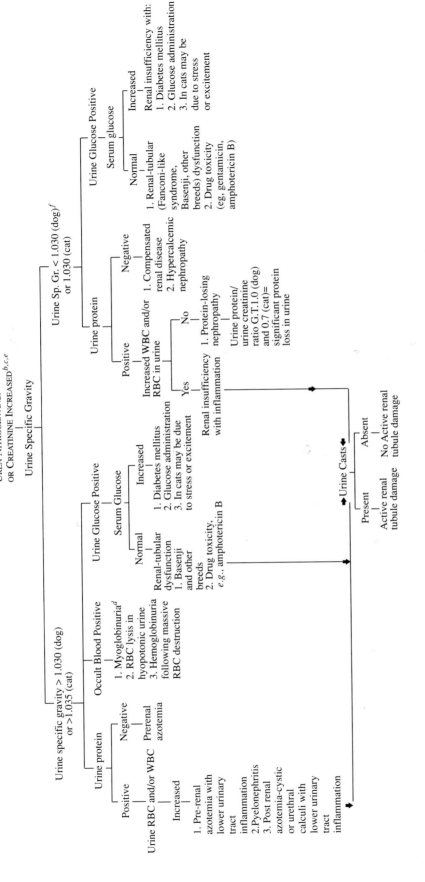

Algorithm 10

UREA NITROGEN AND/
OR CREATININE INCREASED[b,c,e]

Urine Specific Gravity

Urine specific gravity > 1.030 (dog) or >1.035 (cat)

Urine protein

- Positive
  - Urine RBC and/or WBC
    - Increased
      1. Pre-renal azotemia with lower urinary tract inflammation
      2. Pyelonephritis
      3. Post renal azotemia-cystic or urethral calculi with lower urinary tract inflammation
- Negative
  - Prerenal azotemia

Occult Blood Positive
1. Myoglobinuria[d]
2. RBC lysis in hyopotonic urine
3. Hemoglobinuria following massive RBC destruction

Urine Glucose Positive

Serum Glucose

- Normal
  - Renal-tubular dysfunction
    1. Basenji and other breeds
    2. Drug toxicity, e.g., amphotericin B
- Increased
  1. Diabetes mellitus
  2. Glucose administration
  3. In cats may be due to stress or excitement

Urine Sp. Gr. < 1.030 (dog)[f] or 1.030 (cat)

Urine protein

- Positive
  - Increased WBC and/or RBC in urine
    - Yes
      - Renal insufficiency with inflammation
    - No
      1. Protein-losing nephropathy

        Urine protein/urine creatinine ratio G.T.1.0 (dog) and 0.7 (cat)= significant protein loss in urine
- Negative
  1. Compensated renal disease
  2. Hypercalcemic nephropathy

Urine Glucose Positive

Serum glucose

- Normal
  1. Renal-tubular (Fanconi-like syndrome, Basenji, other breeds) dysfunction
  2. Drug toxicity (eg, gentamicin, amphotericin B)
- Increased

  Renal insufficiency with:
  1. Diabetes mellitus
  2. Glucose administration
  3. In cats may be due to stress or excitement

Urine Casts

- Present
  - Active renal tubule damage
- Absent
  - No Active renal tubule damage

G.T.=greater than; L.T.=less than

[a] The type of kidney disease can be confirmed only with a renal biopsy.

[b] In the dog and cat phosphate levels are also increased when there is a reduction in glomerular filtration. In the horse (occasionally in dogs) serum calcium may be increased while phosphate is normal.

[c] Azotemia may be accompanied by hyperamylasmia in dogs.

[d] Differentiate from hemoglobin by special precipitation test with ammonium sulfate.

[e] Advanced renal disease may lead to secondary hyperparathyroidism. (see Fig. 7-1).

[f] Fluid administration will decrease the urine specific gravity

316

Algorithm 11

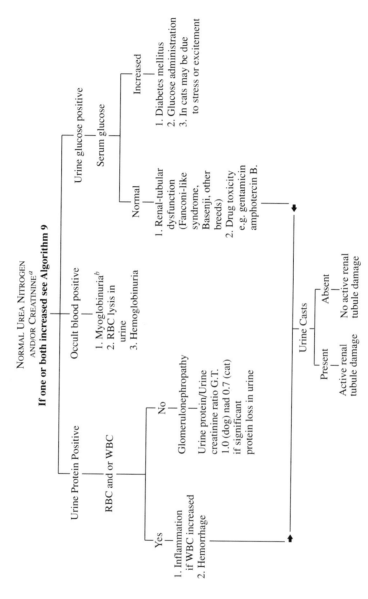

NORMAL UREA NITROGEN
AND/OR CREATININE[a]
If one or both increased see Algorithm 9

Urine Protein Positive

Occult blood positive

Urine glucose positive

RBC and or WBC

1. Myoglobinuria[b]
2. RBC lysis in urine
3. Hemoglobinuria

Serum glucose

Yes

No

Normal

Increased

1. Inflammation if WBC increased
2. Hemorrhage

Glomerulonephropathy

Urine protein/Urine creatinine ratio G.T. 1.0 (dog) nad 0.7 (cat) if significant protein loss in urine

1. Renal-tubular dysfunction (Fanconi-like syndrome, Basenji, other breeds)
2. Drug toxicity e.g. gentamicin amphotercin B.

1. Diabetes mellitus
2. Glucose administration
3. In cats may be due to stress or excitement

Urine Casts

Present

Absent

Active renal tubule damage

No active renal tubule damage

[a] The type of kidney disease can be confirmed only with a renal biopsy
[b] Differentiate from hemoglobin by precipitation test with ammonium sulfate.

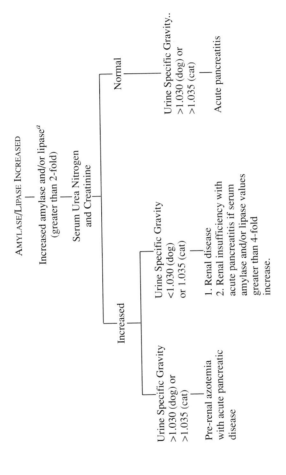

Algorithm 12

AMYLASE/LIPASE INCREASED
|
Increased amylase and/or lipase[a]
(greater than 2-fold)

Serum Urea Nitrogen
and Creatinine

Increased

Urine Specific Gravity
>1.030 (dog) or
>1.035 (cat)

Pre-renal azotemia
with acute pancreatic
disease

Urine Specific Gravity
<1.030 (dog)
or 1.035 (cat)

1. Renal disease
2. Renal insufficiency with
acute pancreatitis if serum
amylase and/or lipase values
greater than 4-fold
increase.

Normal

Urine Specific Gravity..
>1.030 (dog) or
>1.035 (cat)

Acute pancreatitis

[a] Not all cases of pancreatitis have increases of amylase and/or lipase.

Algorithm 13

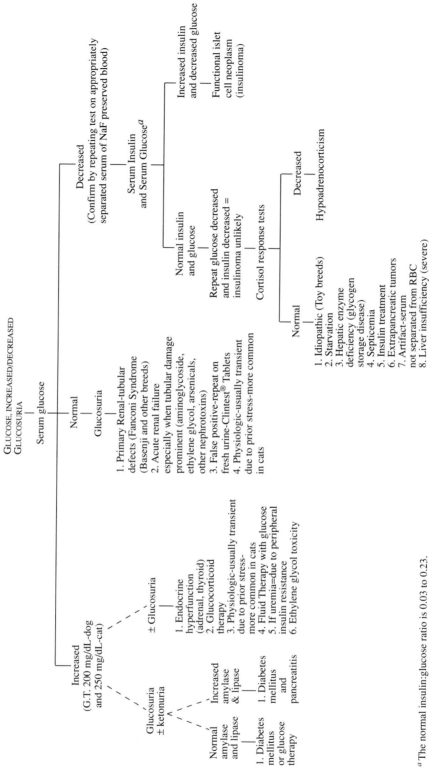

GLUCOSE, INCREASED/DECREASED
GLUCOSURIA

Serum glucose

Increased
(G.T. 200 mg/dL–dog
and 250 mg/dL–cat)

± Glucosuria

1. Endocrine
hyperfunction
(adrenal, thyroid)
2. Glucocorticoid
therapy
3. Physiologic–usually transient
due to prior stress–
more common in cats
4. Fluid Therapy with glucose
5. If uremia=due to peripheral
insulin resistance
6. Ethylene glycol toxicity

Glucosuria
± ketonuria

Increased
amylase
& lipase

1. Diabetes
mellitus
and
pancreatitis

Normal
amylase
and lipase

1. Diabetes
mellitus
or glucose
therapy

Normal

Glucosuria

1. Primary Renal-tubular
defects (Fanconi Syndrome
(Basenji and other breeds)
2. Acute renal failure
especially when tubular damage
prominent (aminoglycoside,
ethylene glycol, arsenicals,
other nephrotoxins)
3. False positive–repeat on
fresh urine–Clintest® Tablets
4. Physiologic–usually transient
due to prior stress–more common
in cats

Decreased
(Confirm by repeating test on appropriately
separated serum of NaF preserved blood)

Serum Insulin
and Serum Glucose[a]

Normal insulin
and glucose

Repeat glucose decreased
and insulin decreased =
insulinoma unlikely

Cortisol response tests

Normal

1. Idiopathic (Toy breeds)
2. Starvation
3. Hepatic enzyme
deficiency (glycogen
storage disease)
4. Septicemia
5. Insulin treatment
6. Extrapancreatic tumors
7. Artifact–serum
not separated from RBC
8. Liver insufficiency (severe)

Decreased

Hypoadrenocorticism

Increased insulin
and decreased glucose

Functional islet
cell neoplasm
(insulinoma)

[a] The normal insulin:glucose ratio is 0.03 to 0.23.

Algorithm 14

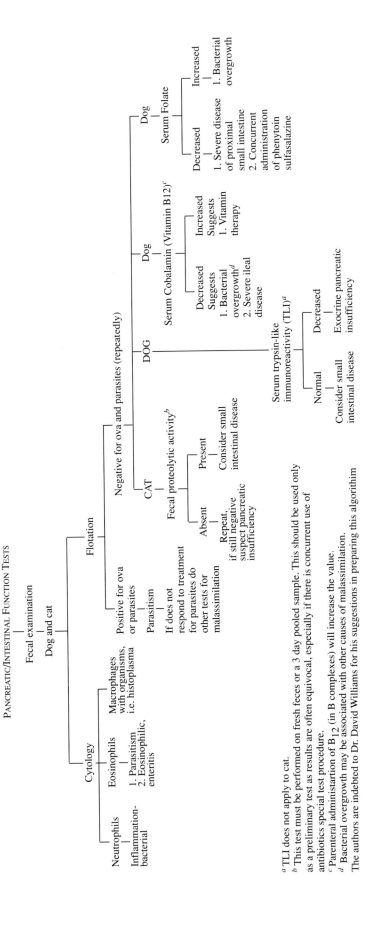

PANCREATIC/INTESTINAL FUNCTION TESTS

Fecal examination

Dog and cat

Cytology

Neutrophils
Inflammation-bacterial

Eosinophils
1. Parasitism
2. Eosinophilic, enteritis

Macrophages with organisms, i.e. histoplasma

Flotation

Positive for ova or parasites
Parasitism
If does not respond to treatment for parasites do other tests for malassimilation

Negative for ova and parasites (repeatedly)

CAT

Fecal proteolytic activity[b]

Absent
Repeat, if still negative suspect pancreatic insufficiency

Present
Consider small intestinal disease

DOG

Serum trypsin-like immunoreactivity (TLI)[a]

Normal
Consider small intestinal disease

Decreased
Exocrine pancreatic insufficiency

Serum Cobalamin (Vitamin B12)[c]
Dog

Decreased
Suggests
1. Bacterial overgrowth[d]
2. Severe ileal disease

Increased
Suggests
1. Vitamin therapy

Serum Folate
Dog

Decreased
1. Severe disease of proximal small intestine
2. Concurrent administration of phenytoin sulfasalazine

Increased
1. Bacterial overgrowth

[a] TLI does not apply to cat.
[b] This test must be performed on fresh feces or a 3 day pooled sample. This should be used only as a preliminary test as results are often equivocal, especially if there is concurrent use of antibiotics special test procedure.
[c] Parenteral administartion of B$_{12}$ (in B complexes) will increase the value.
[d] Bacterial overgrowth may be associated with other causes of malassimilation.
The authors are indebted to Dr. David Williams for his suggestions in preparing this algorithm

Algorithm 15

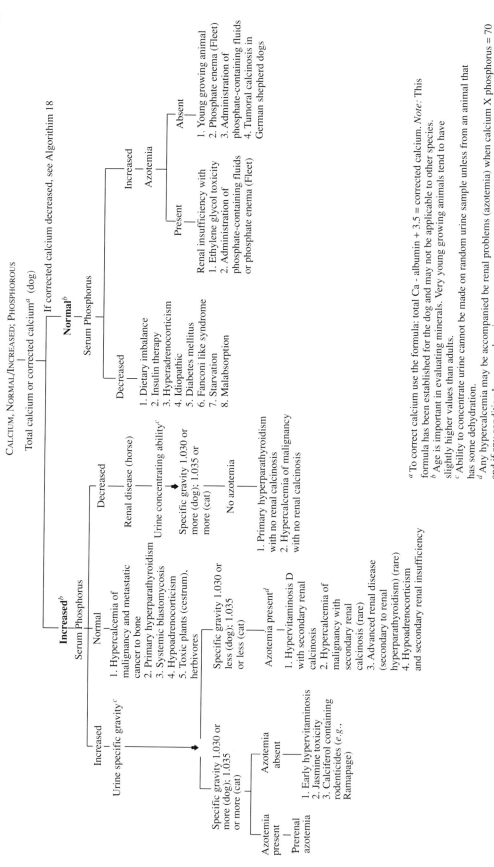

CALCIUM, NORMAL/INCREASED; PHOSPHOROUS

Total calcium or corrected calcium[a] (dog)

If corrected calcium decreased, see Algorithm 18

Increased[b]
Serum Phosphorus

Normal

Urine specific gravity[c]

Increased

Specific gravity 1.030 or more (dog); 1.035 or more (cat)

Azotemia present

Prerenal azotemia

Azotemia absent

1. Early hypervitaminosis
2. Jasmine toxicity
3. Calciferol containing rodenticides (e.g., Ramapage)

Specific gravity 1.030 or less (dog); 1.035 or less (cat)

Azotemia present[d]

1. Hypervitaminosis D with secondary renal calcinosis
2. Hypercalcemia of malignancy with secondary renal calcinosis (rare)
3. Advanced renal disease (secondary to renal hyperparathyroidism) (rare)
4. Hypoadrenocorticism and secondary renal insufficiency

1. Hypercalcemia of malignancy and metastatic cancer to bone
2. Primary hyperparathyroidism
3. Systemic blastomycosis
4. Hypoadrenocorticism
5. Toxic plants (cestrum), herbivores

Decreased

Renal disease (horse)

Urine concentrating ability[c]

Specific gravity 1.030 or more (dog); 1.035 or more (cat)

1. Primary hyperparathyroidism with no renal calcinosis
2. Hypercalcemia of malignancy with no renal calcinosis

No azotemia

Normal[b]
Serum Phosphorus

Decreased

1. Dietary imbalance
2. Insulin therapy
3. Hyperadrenocorticism
4. Idiopathic
5. Diabetes mellitus
6. Fanconi like syndrome
7. Starvation
8. Malabsorption

Increased

Azotemia

Present

Renal insufficiency with
1. Ethylene glycol toxicity
2. Administration of phosphate-containing fluids or phosphate enema (Fleet)

Absent

1. Young growing animal
2. Phosphate enema (Fleet)
3. Administration of phosphate-containing fluids
4. Tumoral calcinosis in German shepherd dogs

[a] To correct calcium use the formula: total Ca - albumin + 3.5 = corrected calcium. *Note:* This formula has been established for the dog and may not be applicable to other species.

[b] Age is important in evaluating minerals. Very young growing animals tend to have slightly higher values than adults.

[c] Ability to concentrate urine cannot be made on random urine sample unless from an animal that has some dehydration.

[d] Any hypercalcemia may be accompanied be renal problems (azotemia) when calcium X phosphorus = 70 and if any condition becomes chronic.

Algorithm 16

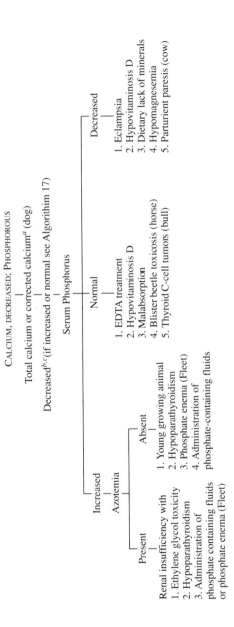

CALCIUM, DECREASED; PHOSPHOROUS

Total calcium or corrected calcium[a] (dog)

Decreased[b,c](if increased or normal see Algorithm 17)

Serum Phosphorus

Increased

Azotemia

Present

Renal insufficiency with
1. Ethylene glycol toxicity
2. Hypoparathyroidism
3. Administration of
phosphate containing fluids
or phosphate enema (Fleet)

Absent
1. Young growing animal
2. Hypoparathyroidism
3. Phosphate enema (Fleet)
4. Administration of
phosphate-containing fluids

Normal
1. EDTA treatment
2. Hypovitaminosis D
3. Malabsorption
4. Blister beetle toxicosis (horse)
5. Thyroid C-cell tumors (bull)

Decreased
1. Eclampsia
2. Hypovitaminosis D
3. Dietary lack of minerals
4. Hypomagnesemia
5. Parturient paresis (cow)

[a]To correct calcium use the formula: total calcium - albumin + 3.5 = corrected calcium. *Note:* This formula has been established for the dog and may not be applicable to other species.

[b]Age is important in evaluating minerals. Very young growing animals tend to have a slightly higher values than adults.

[c]Artifacts that may influence serum calcium include low level if sample is contaminated with EDTA, if sample is diluted, or if lipemia is present.

Algorithm 17

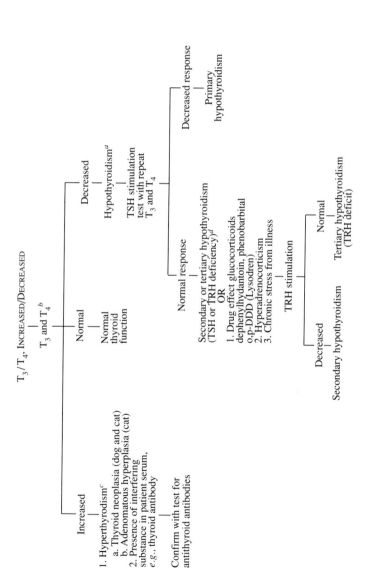

T_3/T_4, INCREASED/DECREASED

T_3 and T_4 [b]

Increased

1. Hyperthyroidism [c]
   a. Thyroid neoplasia (dog and cat)
   b. Adenomatous hyperplasia (cat)
2. Presence of interfering substance in patient serum, e.g., thyroid antibody

Confirm with test for antithyroid antibodies

Normal

Normal thyroid function

Decreased

Hypothyroidism [a]

TSH stimulation test with repeat T_3 and T_4

Normal response

Secondary or tertiary hypothyroidism (TSH or TRH deficiency) [d]
OR
1. Drug effect glucocorticoids dephenylhydantoin, phenobarbital o,p-DDD (Lysodren)
2. Hyperadrenocorticism
3. Chronic stress from illness

TRH stimulation

Decreased

Secondary hypothyroidism

Normal

Tertiary hypothyroidism (TRH deficit)

Decreased response

Primary hypothyroidism

[a] Cholesterol increased in about 2/3 of the cases of hypothyroidism
[b] T_4 is considered to be the test of choice in evaluating thyroid disease in the dog and cat.
[c] Hyperthyroidism may be accompanied by polyuria and polydipsia in the dog and cat.
[d] Secondary and tertiary hypothyroidism are rarely diagnosed.

Algorithm 18

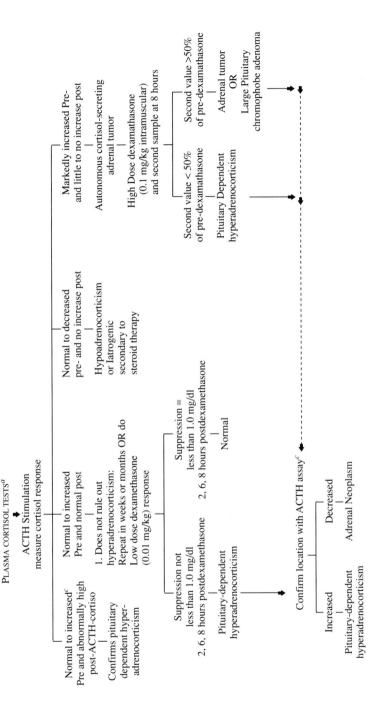

CORTISOLS, INCREASED/DECREASED
PLASMA CORTISOL TESTS[a]

ACTH Stimulation
measure cortisol response

Normal to increased[c]
Pre and abnormally high
post-ACTH-cortiso

Confirms pituitary
dependent hyper-
adrenocorticism

Normal to increased
Pre and normal post

1. Does not rule out
hyperadrenocorticism:
Repeat in weeks or months OR do
Low dose dexamethasone
(0.01 mg/kg) response

Suppression not
less than 1.0 mg/dl
2, 6, 8 hours postdexamethasone

Pituitary-dependent
hyperadrenocorticism

Suppression =
less than 1.0 mg/dl
2, 6, 8 hours postdexamethasone

Normal

Confirm location with ACTH assay[c]

Increased

Pituitary-dependent
hyperadrenocorticism

Decreased

Adrenal Neoplasm

Normal to decreased
pre- and no increase post

Hypoadrenocorticism
or Iatrogenic
secondary to
steroid therapy

Markedly increased Pre-
and little to no increase post

Autonomous cortisol-secreting
adrenal tumor

High Dose dexamethasone
(0.1 mg/kg intramuscular)
and second sample at 8 hours

Second value < 50%
of pre-dexamathasone

Pituitary Dependent
hyperadrenocorticism

Second value >50%
of pre-dexamathasone

Adrenal tumor
OR
Large Pituitary
chromophobe adenoma

[a] Opinions vary as to the sensitivity of the combined dexamethasone suppression /ACTH
stimulation tests VS the isolated ACTH or dexamethasone tests.
[b] Acute severe stress, i.e., trauma, can cause mildly high pre- and post ACTH cortisol values.
[c] ACTH assay not conveniently available at this time. Specimen must be received frozen or
value may be erroneously low.
The above information represents the opinion and experience of the authors. The diagnosis
of diseases of the endrocrine glands remains controversial and is continually the subject of new information.
The author's appreciate Dr. Michael Schaer's assistance for this algorithim.

324

Algorithm 19

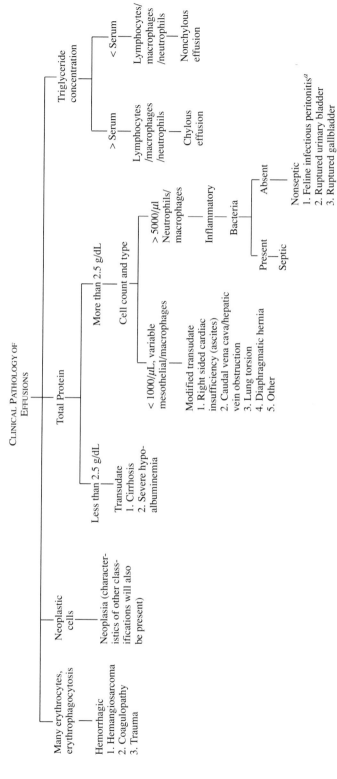

CLINICAL PATHOLOGY OF EFFUSIONS

Total Protein

Many erythrocytes, erythrophagocytosis

Hemorrhagic
1. Hemangiosarcoma
2. Coagulopathy
3. Trauma

Neoplastic cells

Neoplasia (characteristics of other classifications will also be present)

Less than 2.5 g/dL

Transudate
1. Cirrhosis
2. Severe hypo-albuminemia

More than 2.5 g/dL

Cell count and type

< 1000/μL, variable mesothelial/macrophages

Modified transudate
1. Right sided cardiac insufficiency (ascites)
2. Caudal vena cava/hepatic vein obstruction
3. Lung torsion
4. Diaphragmatic hernia
5. Other

> 5000/μl Neutrophils/macrophages

Inflammatory

Bacteria

Present

Septic

Absent

Nonseptic
1. Feline infectious peritonitis[a]
2. Ruptured urinary bladder
3. Ruptured gallbladder
4. Other

Triglyceride concentration

> Serum

Lymphocytes /macrophages /neutrophils

Chylous effusion

< Serum

Lymphocytes/ macrophages /neutrophils

Nonchylous effusion

[a]Albumin:globulin (A:G) ratio of less than 0.81 on the fluid further supports FIP.

Algorithm 20

CLINICAL PATHOLOGY OF
SYNOVIAL FLUIDS

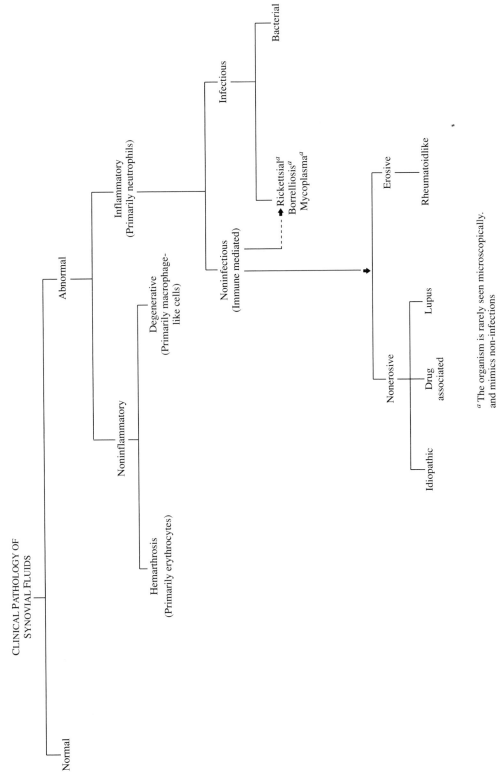

[a] The organism is rarely seen microscopically.
and mimics non-infections

Part IV

Appendix: Normal Values and Conversion Tables

TABLE 1. Normal Hematology Values of Adult Animals[a]

Laboratory Test	Dog	Cat	Horse	Cow	Pig	Sheep
RBC $\times$ $10^6/\mu$L	5.5–8.5	5.0–10.0	7.0–13	5.0–8.0	5–8	8–15
Hemoglobin (g/dL)	12.0–18.0	8.0–15.0	11.0–19	8.0–14	10–18	8–16
PCV (%)	37–55	24–45	32–52	26–42	33–50	24–49
MCV (fL)	60–72	37–49	36–50	37–54	50–67	23–48
MCHC (g/dL)	31–37	30–36	31–38	26–36	30–34	29–35
RDW (%)[b]	12–16	13–17	17–21			
WBC $\times$ $10^3/\mu$L	5.5–16.9	5.5–19.5	6–12.5	4.0–12	10–22	4.0–12.0
Band neutrophils $\times$ $10^3/\mu$L	0.0–0.299	0.0–0.299	0.0–0.09	0.0–0.19	0.0–0.8	0.0–0.1
Segmented neutrophils $\times$ $10^3/\mu$L	3.0–12.0	2.5–12.5	2.7–7.0	1.5–5.0	3.2–10	1.0–5.0
Lymphocytes $\times$ $10^3/\mu$L	1.0–4.9	1.4–7.0	1.5–6.0	3.0–7.5	4.5–13	2.0–9.0
Monocytes $\times$ $10^3/\mu$L	0.1–1.4	0.1–.79	0.1–1.0	0.1–1.5	0.1–2.0	2.0–9.0
Eosinophils $\times$ $10^3/\mu$L	0.1–1.49	0.1–.79	0.1–1.0	0.1–1.5	0.2–2.0	0.1–0.75
Basophils $\times$ $10^3/\mu$L	Rare	Rare	Rare	Rare	Rare	Rare
Platelets $\times$ $10^3/\mu$L	175–500	175–500	90–350	175–620	200–500	300–800

[a] Values used in this text. Check your own laboratory for differences.
[b] Normal RDW values are dependent on the laboratory.

TABLE 2. Normal Serum Chemistry Values for Adult Animals[a]

Laboratory Test	Dog	Cat	Horse	Cow	Pig	Sheep
Alkaline phosphatase (IU/L)	20–150	10.0–80	143–395	90–170	26–362	68–387
ALAT (IU/L)	10.0–88.0	10.0–80	34–113	14–38	32–84	60–84
Amylase (IU/L)	300–2000	500–1800	35–100	126–250		
ASAT (IU/L)	10.0–88.0	10.0–80	226–366	78–132	9–113	98–278
Bile acids (μmol/L)	<10	<5	<15			
Bile acids, postfeed (μmol/L)	<25	<15				
Bilirubin, total (mg/dL)	0.1–0.06	0.1–0.6	0–2.0	0.1–0.5	0–0.2	0–0.4
Bilirubin, conjugated (mg/dL)	0.0–0.3	0.0–0.3	0–0.4	0.04–0.14	0–0.1	0–0.3
Bilirubin, unconjugated (mg/dL)	0.1–0.3	0.0–0.5	0.2–2.0	0–0.3		
Calcium (mg/dL)	8.6–11.2	8.0–10.7	11.2–13.6	9.7–12.4	8–12	10.4–13
Carbon dioxide (mEq/L)	18–24	16–21	24–32	21–32	18–26	21–28
Chloride (mEq/L)	105–115	117–123	99–109	97–111	100–105	98–115
Cholesterol (mg/dL)	125–270	90–205	75–150	80–180	36–54	50–140
Cobalamin (vitamin B_{12}) (ng/L)	300–800	200–1680				
Cortisol, resting (μg/dL)	1.0–4.0	1.0–1.3				
Creatine kinase (IU/L)	20–200	50–450	86–140	66–120		
Creatinine (mg/dL)	0.5–1.5	0.8–1.8	1.2–1.9	1–2.0	1.0–2.7	1.2–1.9
Fibrinogen (mg/dL)	125–300	100–400	200–400	200–500	200–400	100–500
Folate (μg/L)	7.5–17.5	13.4–38				
GGT (IU/L)	1.0–10.0	1.0–10	4–13.4	11–24		
Glucose (mg/dL)	60–110	70–150	75–115	45–75	65–95	50–80
Iron (μg/L)	94–122	68–215	73–140	57–162	91–199	166–222
LDH (IU/L)	50–495	75–490	162–412	8–302	96–160	60–111
Lipase (IU/L)	25–750	25–375				
Phosphorus (mg/dL)	2.2–5.5	1.8–6.4	3.1–5.6	5.6–6.5	5.3–9.6	5.0–7.3
Potassium (mEq/L)	3.7–5.8	3.8–4.5	2.4–4.7	3.9–5.8	4.9–7.1	4.0–6.0
Protein (g/dL)	5.4–7.7	5.4–7.8	5.2–7.9	6.7–7.5	7.0–8.9	6.0–7.9
Albumin (g/dL)	2.3–3.8	2.1–3.9	2.6–3.7	3.0–3.6	1.9–3.3	2.4–3.9
Globulin (g/dL)	2.3–5.2	1.5–5.7	2.6–4.0	3.0–3.5	5.3–6.4	3.5–5.7
Sodium (mEq/L)	141–153	147–156	132–146	132–152	139–152	136–154
Sorbitol dehydrogenase (IU/L)	2.9–8.2	3.9–7.7	1.9–5.8	4.3–15.3	1–6	6–28
T_3 (ng/dL)	75–200	60–200	31–158	41–170		
T_4 (μg/dL)	1.0–4.0	1.5–5.0	1.0–2.4	3.6–8.9		
T_4 free (ng/dL)	0.7–3.3					
TLI (μg/L)	5–35					
Urea nitrogen (mg/dL)	12.0–25.0	10.0–30.0	10.0–24	20–30	8–24	18–31

[a] Values used in this text. Check your own laboratory for differences.

TABLE 3. Conversion of Conventional Units to SI Units in Serum Chemistry

Component	Conventional Units	X Factor	SI Units
ACTH	pg/mL	0.22	pmol/L
Albumin	g/dL	10	g/L
Ammonia	μg/dL	0.5872	μmol/L
Amylase	Somogyi units	1.85	U/L
Base excess	mEq/L	1	mmol/L
Bicarbonate	mEq/L	1	mmol/L
Bile acids	μg/mL	2.45	μmol
Bilirubin	mg/dL	17.1	μmol/L
BSP (dog and cat)	% retention	0.1	Fraction retention
Calcium	mg/dL	0.25	mmol/L
Carbon dioxide, total	mEq/L	1	mmol/L
Carbon dioxide, partial pressure	mmHg	0.133	kPa
Chloride	mEq/L	1	mmol/L
Cholinesterase	IU/L	1	U/L
Cholesterol	mg/dL	0.026	mmol/L
Cortisol	μg/dL	0.0276	μmol/L
Creatine kinase	IU/L	1	U/L
Creatinine	mg/dL	88.4	μmol/L
Creatinine clearance	ml/min	0.0167	ml/sec
Fibrinogen	mg/dL	0.01	g/L
GGT	IU/L	1	U/L
Globulin	g/dL	10	g/L
Glucose	mg/dL	0.055	mmol/L
Hemoglobin	g/dL	0.6206	mmol/L
Insulin	μU/L	7.175	pmol/L
Iron binding	μg/dL	0.179	μmol/L
Iron, total	μg/dL	0.179	μmol/L
Lipase	IU/L	1	U/L
Lipase	Cherry-Crandall U	278	U/L
Magnesium	mEq/L	0.5	mmol/L
Magnesium	mg/dL	0.41	mmol/L
Osmolality	Osm/kg	1	mmol/L
Phosphatase, alkaline	IU/L	1	U/L
Phosphorus	mg/dL	0.323	mmol/L
Potassium	mEq/L	1	mmol/L
Protein, total	g/dL	10	g/L
Sodium	mEq/L	1	mmol/L
T_3 (RIA)	ng/dL	0.0154	nmol/L
T_4 (RIA)	μg/dL	12.87	nmol/L
T_4, free	ng/dL	79	pmol/L
Transferases	IU/L	1	U/L
Triglycerides	mg/dL	0.011	μmol/L
Urea nitrogen	mg/dL	0.357	mmol/L
Uric acid	mg/dL	0.059	mmol/L
Xylose absorption	mg/dL	0.067	mmol/L

TABLE 4. Normal Ranges of Hematology Values for Adult Animals Expressed in SI Units

Laboratory Test	Dog	Cat	Horse	Cow	Pig	Sheep
RBC × 10^{12}/L	5.5–8.5	5.0–10.0	7.0–13.0	5.0–8.0	5–8	8–15
Hemoglobin (mmol/L)	7.5–11.1	5.0–9.3	6.8–11.8	5.0–8.7	10–18	8–16
PCV (volume fraction)	37–55	24–45	32–52	26–42	33–50	24–49
MCV (fL)	60–72	37–49	36–50	37–54	50–67	23–48
MCHC (mmol/L)	19.2–23	18.6–23.6	19.2–23.6	16.1–22.3	18.0–20.4	17.4–21
WBC × 10^9/L	5.5–16.9	5.0–19	6–12.5	4.0–12	10–22	4.0–12
Band neutrophils × 10^9/L	0.–0.299	0.–0299	0.–0.090	0.–0.190	0.0–0.8	0.0–0.1
Segmented neutrophils × 10^9/L	3.0–12.0	2.5–12.5	2.7–7.0	1.5–5.0	3.2–10	1.0–5.0
Lymphocytes × 10^9/L/L	1.0–4.9	1.4–7.0	2.0–6.0	3.0–7.5	4.5–13	2.0–9.0
Monocytes × 10^9/L	0.1–1.4	0.1–0.79	0.1–1.0	0.1–1.5	0.1–2.0	2.0–9.0
Eosinophils × 10^9/L	0.1–1.49	0.1–0.79	0.1–1.0	0.1–1.5	0.2–2.0	0.1–0.75
Basophils × 10^9/L	Rare	Rare	Rare	Rare	Rare	Rare
Platelets × 10^9/L	175–500	175–500	90–350	175–620	200–500	300–800

TABLE 5. Normal Ranges of Serum Chemistry Values for Adult Animals Expressed in International Units

Laboratory Test	Dog	Cat	Horse	Cow	Pig	Sheep
Alkaline phosphatase (U/L)	20–150	10–80	143–395	90–170	26–362	68–387
ALAT (U/L)	10–88	10–80	34–113	14–38	32–84	60–84
Amylase (U/L)	300–2000	500–1800	35–100	126–250		
ASAT (U/L)	10–88	10–80	226–366	78–132	9–113	98–278
Bile acids (μmol/L)	<10	<5	<15			
Bile acids, postfeed (μmol/L)	<25	<15				
Bilirubin, direct (μmol/L)	0.0–5.1	0.0–5.1	0–8.55	0.68–2.4	0–3.4	0–6.8
Bilirubin, indirect (μmol/L)	1.71–5.1	0.0–8.5	3.4–34.2	0–5.1	0–1.7	0–5.1
Bilirubin, total (μmol/L)	1.71–10.3	1.71–10.3	3.4–34.2	1.71–8.55		
Calcium (mmol/L)	2.15–2.8	2.0–2.7	2.8	2.4–3.1	2.00–3.00	2.6–3.25
Carbon dioxide (mmol/L)	18–24	16–21	24–32	21–32	18–26	21–28
Chloride (mmol/L)	105–115	117–123	99–109	97–111	100–105	98–115
Cholesterol (mmol/L)	3.3–7.0	2.3–5.3	1.9–3.9	2.1–4.7	36–54	1.3–3.6
Cortisol, resting (μmol/L)	0.03–0.011	0.014–0.1				
Creatine kinase (U/L)	20–200	50–450	86–140	66–120		
Creatinine (μmol/L)	35.4–133	71–159	106–168	88–177	88–239	106–168
Fibrinogen (g/L)	1.25–3.0	1.0–4.0	2.0–4.0	2.0–5.0	2.0–4.0	1.0–5.0
GGT (U/L)	1.0–10.0	1.0–10	4–13.4			
Glucose (mmol/L)	3.3–6.0	3.9–8.3	4.1–55.8	2.5–4.1	3.6–5.2	2.8–4.4
Iron (μmol/L)	16.8–21.8	12.2–38.5	13.1–25.1	10.2–29.0	16.3–35.6	29.7–39.7
LDH (U/L)	50–495	75–490	162–412	8–302	96–160	60–111
Lipase (U/L)	25–750	25–375				
Phosphorus (mmol/L)	0.7–1.8	0.58–2.07	1	1.81–2.1	1.7–3.1	1.6–2.4
Potassium (mEq/L)	3.7–5.8	3.8–4.5	2.4–4.7	3.9–5.8	4.9–7.1	4.0–6.0
Protein (g/L)	54–77	54–78	52–79	67–75	70–89	60–79
Albumin (g/L)	250–370	210–390	260–370	300–360	19–33	24–39
Globulin (g/L)	23–52	15–57	26–41	30–35	53–64	35–57
Sodium (mEq/L)	141–153	147–156	132–146	132–152	139–152	136–154
T_3 (nmol/L)	1.16–3.08	0.9–3.1	0.48–2.4	0.6–2.62		
T_4 (nmol/L)	12.9–55.5	19.3–64.3	12.9–30.9	46–114		
T_4, free (ng/dL)	0.7–3.3					
Urea nitrogen (mmol/L)	4.3–8.9	3.6–10.7	3.6–8.6	7.1–10.7	2.9–8.6	6.4–11.1

TABLE 6. Variations in Serum Chemistry Values by Age: Beagle Dogs, 2 to 52 Weeks Old[a]

Laboratory Test	2 Weeks	4 Weeks	6 Weeks	8 Weeks	12 Weeks	24 Weeks	36 Weeks
Alkaline phosphatase (IU/L)	81–215	40–145	56–168	47–203	85–201	56–125	29–108
ALAT (IU/L)	1.4–16.6	0.1–24.1	1.0–33.8	0–43.1	10.1–37.7		
ASAT (IU/L)	6–26	8–20	7–26	8–30	12–28	19–39	16–40
Bilirubin, total (mg/dL)	0.0–2.0	0.0–0.9	0.0–0.8	0.0–0.8	0.1–0.5		
Calcium (mg/dL)	8.8–15.9	10.6–15.3	10.6–14.2	10.9–15.1	10.2–13.8	10.0–14.4	9.7–13.7
Cholesterol (mg/dL)	158–333	97–379	65–296	69–220	105–188		
Creatinine (mg/dL)	0.2–0.7	0.2–0.6	0.2–0.6	0.3–0.7	0.4–0.8	0.6–1.1	0.7–1.1
GGT (IU/L)	0–29.6	0–1.4	0.0	0.0	0.0		
Glucose (mg/dL)	107–159	104–175	97–154	94–137	83–127		
LDH (IU/L)	0–253	0–247	0–127	7–102	14–54		
Phosphorus (mg/dL)	6.8–10.8	5.7–10.5	6.8–10.0	7.4–10.6	6.2–10.8	5.1–8.8	4.1–6.9
Protein (g/dL)	3.4–4.4	3.2–4.6	3.5–5.1	3.6–5.2	4.2–5.1	4.7–6.0	5.0–6.6
T$_4$ (μg/dL)	5.5–14.3	3.0–13.8	0–12.2	1.3–6.5	1.6–4.0		
Triglycerides	0–217	12–163	3–127	29–107	17–50		

[a] Mean ± 2 standard deviations. (Loweth, Lisa A., *et al.*: The effects of aging on hematology and serum chemistry values in the beagle dog. *Vet. Clin. Pathol., 19:*13, 1990. Wolford, S. T., *et al.*: Effect of age on serum chemistry profile, electrophoresis and thyroid hormones in beagle dogs two weeks to one year of age. *Vet. Clin. Pathol. 17:*35, 1988.)

TABLE 7. Variations in Serum Chemistry Values by Age: Beagle Dogs, 3 to 14 Years Old

Laboratory Test[a]	3 Years	6 Years	9 Years	12 Years	14 Years
Alkaline phosphatase (IU/L)	40–75	39–115	51–140	58–112	44–143
ALAT (IU/L)	35–61	30–55	27–51	58–141	41–68
ASAT (IU/L)	24–32	21–29	24–40	30–50	25–34
Bilirubin, total (mg/dL)	0–0.1	0.1–0.1	0.05–0.1	0.05–0.1	0.05–0.1
Calcium (mg/dL)	10–11	10–10	9–10	10–11	10–11
Chloride (mEq/L)	109–114	103–110	107–112	105–108	107–111
Cholesterol (mg/dL)	139–171	154–224	126–300	156–248	159–231
Triglycerides (mg/dL)	23–36	24–54	19–87	34–102	26–38
Creatinine (mg/dL)	0.8–1.0	0.6–1.0	0.5–0.7	0.7–0.9	0.5–0.8
GGT (IU/L)	0–17	0–2	2–4	0–7	0–5
Glucose (mg/dL)	91–102	89–104	92–104	80–95	83–100
Iron (μg/L)	137–285	187–276	41–233	119–189	91–192
LDH (IU/L)	74–112	58–145	134–261	179–360	91–216
Phosphorus (mg/dL)	3.9–5.1	3.2–4.4	3.9–5.0	3.7–5.2	3.9–4.5
Potassium (mEq/L)	4.6–5.0	4.5–5.1	4.6–5.2	5.0–5.5	4.7–5.3
Protein (g/dL)	5.4–5.9	6.0–6.3	5.8–6.6	6.0–6.6	5.8–6.7
Albumin (g/dL)	3.3–3.6	3.1–3.5	3.0–3.5	3.0–3.3	2.7–3.4
Globulin (g/dL)	2.2–2.6	2.5–2.9	2.6–3.3	3.1–3.5	2.9–3.5
Sodium (mEq/L)	150–154	143–149	149–151	145–149	145–149
Urea nitrogen (mg/dL)	19–22	9–16	10–13	10–18	10–19

[a] Limits represent the 10th and 90th percentile values. (Loweth, Lisa A., *et al.*: The effects of aging on hematology and serum chemistry values in the beagle dog. *Vet. Clin. Pathol. 19:*13, 1990.)

TABLE 8. Variations in Hematology Values by Age: Beagle Dogs, 3 to 14 Years Old

Laboratory Test[a]	3 Years	6 Years	9 Years	12 Years	14 Years
RBC × $10^6/\mu L$	6.6–7.8	6.5–7.6	5.9–7.4	6.1–7.3	5.7–7.1
Hemoglobin (g/dL)	15–18	16–18	14–18	14–17	14–17
PCV (%)	43–50	44–49	38–50	40–49	40–47
Band neutrophils/μL	0	0	0–63	0–68	0–54
Segmented neutrophils/μL	3944–9287	3605–7724	4207–7217	4724–9587	4464–10,255
Lymphocytes/μL	2185–3318	1334–2467	1667–2702	1676–2658	1628–2453
Monocytes/μL	101–769	173–626	149–620	181–521	189–688
Eosinophils/μL	208–1010	217–500	275–711	99–721	201–408
Basophils/μL	0	0–70	0–102	0	0

[a] Limits represent the 10th and 90th percentile values. (Loweth, Lisa A., *et al.*: The effects of aging on hematology and serum chemistry values in the beagle dog. *Vet. Clin. Pathol., 19:*13, 1990.)

TABLE 9. Erythrocyte Changes During Pregnancy in Beagles, Brittany Spaniels, and Labrador Retrievers

	Gestation Week 1			Gestation Week 8			Lactation Week 8		
	Beagles	*Brittany Spaniels*	*Labrador Retrievers*	*Beagles*	*Brittany Spaniels*	*Labrador Retrievers*	*Beagles*	*Brittany Spaniels*	*Labrador Retrievers*
RBC × $10^6/\mu L$									
Mean	7.2	6.2	7.3	5.1	5.0	5.6	7.0	5.6	6.7
Range[a]	6.2–9.2	5.2–7.2	5.5–9.1	4.1–6.1	4.1–6.0	4.4–6.8	5.8–8.2	4.4–6.8	5.7–7.7
PCV (%)									
Mean	47	43.3	50	34.3	33.0	38.2	46.6	40.8	44.1
Range[a]	38.4–54.6	38.5–48.1	42.4–57.6	39.2–50.8	25.2–40.8	30.4–46.0	39.2–54.0	32.8–48.8	36.1–52.1
Hemoglobin (g/dL)									
Mean	17.2	15.9	18.1	12.3	11.8	13.9	16.5	14.7	15.9
Range[a]	15.2–19.2	14.1–17.7	15.3–20.9	10.3–14.3	9.2–14.4	11.7–16.1	13.9–19.1	11.7–17.7	13.1–18.7
MCV (fl)									
Mean	66.6	70.3	69.2	67.3	72.6	67.9	67.3	73.3	65.9
Range[a]	59.2–76	59.7–80.9	50.6–87.8	60.7–73.6	58.6–86.6	52.9–82.9	60.7–73.6	63.1–83.4	55.8–76.0
MCHC (g/dL)									
Mean	36.8	36.6	36.2	36	36.4	36.8	35.5	36	36.1
Range[a]	30.6–43	34.4–38.8	34.2–38.2	31.2–40.8	34.6–38.2	31.8–41.4	31.7–39.4	33.0–39.0	32.7–39.5

[a] Range is mean ± 2 standard deviations. (Allard, R. L., Carlos, A. D., and Faltin, E. C.: Canine hematological changes during gestation and lactation. *Comp. Anim. Pract., 19:*3–6, 1989.)

TABLE 10. Hematologic Values of Growing Healthy Beagle Dogs from Birth to 8 Weeks of Age: Range and (Median)

Hematology Parameter	Birth	1 Week	2 Weeks	3 Weeks	4 Weeks	6 Weeks	8 Weeks
RBC × $10^6/\mu L$	4.7–5.6 (5.1)	3.6–5.9 (4.6)	3.4–4.4 (3.9)	3.5–4.3 (3.8)	3.6–4.9 (4.1)	4.3–5.1 (4.7)	4.5–5.9 (4.9)
Hemoglobin (g/dL)	14–17 (15.2)	10.4–17.5 (12.9)	9–11 (10.0)	8.6–11.6 (9.7)	8.5–10.3 (9.5)	8.5–11.3 (10.2)	10.3–12.5 (11.2)
PCV (%)	45–52.5 (47.5)	33–52 (40.5)	29–34 (31.8)	27–37 (31.7)	27–33.5 (29.9)	26.5–35.5 (32.5)	31–39 (34.8)
MCV (fl)	93.0	89.0	81.5	83.0	73.0	69.0	72.0
MCH (pg)	30.0	28.0	25.5	25.0	23.0	22.0	22.5
MCHC (g/dL)	32.0	32.0	31.5	31.0	32.0	31.5	32.0
NRBC/100 WBC	0–13 (2.3)	0–11 (4.0)	0–6 (2.0)	0–9 (1.6)	0–4 (1.2)	0–0	0–1 (0.2)
WBC × $10^3/\mu L$	6.8–18.4 (12.0)	9–23 (14.1)	8.1–15.1 (11.7)	6.7–15.1 (11.2)	8.5–16.4 (12.9)	12.6–26.7 (16.3)	12.7–17.3 (15)
Band neutrophils/×$10^3 \mu L$	0–1.5 (0.23)	0–4.8 (0.50)	0–1.2 (0.21)	0–0.5 (0.09)	0–0.3 (0.06)	0–0.3 (0.05)	0–0.3 (0.08)
Segmented neutrophils/×$10^3 \mu L$	4.4–15.8 (8.6)	3.8–15.2 (7.4)	3.2–10.4 (5.2)	1.4–9.4 (5.1)	3.7–12.8 (7.2)	4.2–17.6 (9.0)	6.2–11.8 (8.5)
Lymphocytes/×$10^3 \mu L$	0.5–4.2 (1.9)	1.3–9.4 (4.3)	1.5–7.4 (3.8)	2.1–10.1 (5.0)	1.0–8.4 (4.5)	2.8–16.5 (5.7)	3.1–6.9 (5.0)
Monocytes/×$10^3 \mu L$	0.2–2.2 (0.9)	0.3–2.5 (1.1)	0.2–1.4 (0.7)	0.1–1.4 (0.7)	0.3–1.5 (0.8)	0.5–2.7 (1.1)	0.5–2.7 (1.1)
Eosinophils/×$10^3 \mu L$	0–1.3 (0.4)	0.1–2.8 (0.8)	0.08–1.8 (0.6)	0.07–0.9 (0.3)	0–0.7 (0.25)	0.1–1.9 (0.5)	0–1.2 (0.4)
Basophils/×$10^3 \mu L$	0.0	0–0.2 (0.01)	0.0	0.0	0.015 (0.01)	0.0	0.0

(Melvegar, B. A., and Wilson, R. L.: The hemogram and bone marrow profile of normal neonatal and weanling beagle dogs. *Lab. Anim. Sci.,* 23:630, 1973.)

TABLE 11. Hematologic Values of Growing Healthy Kittens from Birth to 17 Weeks of Age: Mean (± 2 Standard Deviations)

Hematology Parameter	0–2 Weeks	2–4 Weeks	4–6 Weeks	6–8 Weeks	8–9 Weeks	12–13 Weeks	16–17 Weeks
RBC × 10^6/μL	5.29 (4.81–5.77)	4.67 (4.47–4.87)	5.89 (5.43–6.35)	6.57 (6.05–7.09)	6.95 (6.77–7.13)	7.43 (6.97–7.89)	8.14 (7.60–8.68)
Hemoglobin (g/dL)	12.1 (10.9–13.3)	8.7 (8.3–9.1)	8.6 (8.0–9.2)	9.1 (8.5–9.7)	9.8 (9.4–10.2)	10.1 (9.5–10.7)	11.0 (10.2–11.9)
PCV (%)	35.3 (31.9–38.7)	26.5 (24.9–28.1)	27.1 (25.5–28.7)	29.8 (27.2–32.4)	33.3 (31.9–34.7)	33.1 (29.9–36.3)	34.9 (32.7–37.1)
MCV (fl)	67.4 (63.6–71.2)	53.9 (51.5–56.3)	45.6 (43.0–48.2)	45.6 (43.6–47.6)	47.8 (46.0–49.6)	44.5 (40.9–48.1)	43.1 (40.1–46.1)
MCH (pg)	23.0 (21.8–24.2)	18.8 (17.2–20.4)	14.8 (13.7–16.0)	13.9 (13.3–14.5)	14.1 (13.7–14.5)	13.7 (12.9–14.5)	13.5 (12.7–14.3)
MCHC (g/dL)	34.5 (32.9–36.1)	33.0 (31.0–34.0)	31.9 (30.7–33.1)	30.9 (29.9–31.9)	29.5 (28.7–30.3)	31.3 (29.5–32.1)	31.6 (30.0–33.2)
WBC × 10^3/μL	9.67 (8.53–10.81)	15.31 (12.89–17.73)	17.45 (14.71–20.19)	18.07 (14.19–21.95)	23.68 (19.9–27.46)	23.10 (16.48–29.92)	19.7 (17.46–21.94)
Band neutrophils/× 10^3 μL	0.06 (0.02–0.10)	0.11 (0.03–0.19)	0.20 (0.08–0.32)	0.22 (0.06–0.38)	0.12 (0.0–0.30)	0.15 (0.01–0.27)	0.16 (0.020–0.30)
Neutrophils/× 10^3 μL	5.96 (4.60–7.32)	6.92 (5.38–8.46)	9.57 (6.27–12.87)	6.75 (4.69–8.81)	11.0 (8.18–13.82)	11.0 (7.46–14.54)	9.74 (7.90–11.58)
Lymphocytes/× 10^3 μL	3.73 (2.69–4.77)	6.56 (5.38–7.74)	6.41 (4.87–7.95)	9.59 (6.45–12.73)	10.17 (6.75–13.59)	10.46 (5.24–15.68)	8.7 (6.58–10.82)
Monocytes/× 10^3 μL	0.01 (0.0–0.03)	0.02 (0.0–0.06)	0.0	0.01 (0.0–0.03)	0.11 (0.0–0.23)	0.0	0.02 (0.0–0.06)
Eosinophils/× 10^3 μL	0.96 (0.10–1.82)	1.40 (1.08–1.72)	1.47 (0.97–1.97)	1.08 (0.68–1.48)	2.28 (1.66–2.90)	1.55 (0.85–2.25)	1.00 (0.62–1.38)
Basophils/× 10^3 μL	0.02 (0.0–0.04)	0	0	0.02 (0.0–0.06)	0	0.03 (0.0–0.09)	0

(Meyers-Wallen, V. N., Haskins, M. E., and Patterson, D. F.: Hematologic values in healthy neonatal, weanling and juvenile kittens. *Am. J. Vet. Res.*, 45:1322, 1984.)

TABLE 12. Normal Values for Biochemical Indicators of Hepatobiliary Disorders in Young Dogs and Cats: Median and (Range)

Test[a]	Puppies					Kittens		
	1–3 Days	2 Weeks	4 Weeks	8 Weeks	Adult	2 Weeks	4 Weeks	Adult
BSP (%, 30 min)	<5	<5	<5	<5	0–5	ND[b]	ND	0–3
Bile acids (μmol/L)	<15	<15	<15	<15	0–15	ND	<10	0–10
Bilirubin (mg/dL)	0.5 (0.2–1.0)	0.3 (0.1–0.5)	0 (0–0.1)	0.1 (0.1–0.2)	(0–0.04)	0.3 (0.1–1.0)	0.2 (0.1–0.2)	(0–0.2)
ALT (IU/L)	69 (17–337)	15 (10–21)	21 (20–22)	21 (9–24)	(12–94)	18 (11–24)	17 (14–26)	(25–91)
AST (IU/L)	108 (44–194)	20 (10–40)	18 (14–23)	22 (10–32)	(13–56)	18 (8–48)	17 (12–24)	(9–42)
ALP (IU/L)	3845 (618–8760)	236 (176–541)	144 (135–210)	158 (144–177)	(4–107)	123 (68–269)	111 (90–135)	(10–77)
GGT (IU/L)	1111 (163–3558)	24 (4–77)	3 (2–7)	1 (0–7)	(0–7)	1 (0–3)	2 (0–3)	(0–4)
Protein (g/dL)	4.1 (3.4–5.2)	3.9 (3.6–4.4)	4.1 (3.9–4.2)	4.6 (3.9–4.8)	(5.4–7.4)	4.4 (4.0–5.2)	4.8 (4.6–5.2)	(5.8–8.0)
Albumin (g/dL)	2.1 (1.5–2.8)	1.8 (1.7–2.0)	1.8 (1.0–2.0)	2.5 (2.1–2.7)	(2.1–2.7)	2.1 (2.0–2.4)	2.3 (2.2–2.4)	(2.5–3.0)
Cholesterol (mg/dL)	136 (221–204)	282 (223–344)	328 (266–352)	155 (111–258)	(103–299)	229 (164–443)	361 (222–434)	(150–270)
Glucose (mg/dL)	88 (52–127)	129 (111–146)	109 (86–115)	145 (124–272)	(65–110)	117 (76–129)	110 (99–112)	(63–144)

[a] The abbreviations used are: BSP, sulfobromophthalein; ALT, alanine aminotransferase; AST, aspartate aminotransferase; ALP, alkaline phosphatase; GGT, γ-glutamyltranspeptidase.
[b] ND, not determined. (Center, S. A., Hornbuckle, W. E., and Hoskins, J. D.: The liver and pancreas. *In* Hoskins, J. D.: Veterinary Pediatrics: Dogs and Cats from Birth to Six Months, Philadelphia, W. B. Saunders, 1990, Chapter 8.)

TABLE 13. Age-related Changes in Plasma and Urine Values in Young Cats: Mean and (Range)

Laboratory Test	4–6 Weeks	7–12 Weeks	13–19 Weeks	20–24 Weeks
Plasma sodium (mEq/L)	152 (147–158)	151 (144–160)	154 (148–161)	155 (149–162)
Plasma potassium (mEq/L)	4.7 (3.7–5.6)	4.9 (3.6–7.1)	4.7 (3.3–6.5)	4.4 (3.5–6.0)
Plasma chloride (mEq/L)	122 (118–127)	122 (113–128)	123 (118–130)	124 (117–129)
Plasma protein (g/dL)	4.6 (4.2–5.1)	5.2 (4.2–6.7)	5.9 (4.8–6.8)	6.2 (5.4–7.1)
Plasma calcium (mg/dL)	9.7 (8.4–11.0)	9.9 (8.8–11.2)	10.1 (8.8–11.1)	9.9 (8.9–10.9)
Plasma phosphorus (mg/dL)	7.4 (5.0–9.9)	8.2 (6.0–10.5)	7.8 (6.4–9.7)	7.1 (4.9–9.8)
Endogenous creatinine clearance (mL/min/kg)	2.19 (0.1–4.2)	4.1 (2.4–5.7)	3.96 (2.6–5.9)	3.38 (2.1–4.7)
FE[a] sodium (%)	0.25 (0.02–0.46)	0.50 (0.01–1.08)	0.57 (0.34–0.79)	0.55 (0.32–0.75)
FE potassium (%)	12.84 (2.37–25.15)	22.56 (12.61–41.51)	22.64 (11.91–37.64)	23.21 (13.51–31.26)
FE chloride (%)	0.62 (0.25–1.13)	1.10 (0.54–1.79)	1.14 (0.6–1.73)	1.16 (0.76–1.62)
FE calcium (%)	0.39 (0.04–2.11)	0.32 (0.04–2.01)	0.12 (0.02–0.50)	0.06 (0.01–0.13)
FE phosphorus (%)	17.10 (1.51–43.76)	27.43 (9.30–48.88)	30.14 (13.95–53.84)	36.20 (12.35–96.19)
24-Hour urinary protein excretion (mg/dL)	4.62 (0.23–16.43)	9.09 (2.54–27.57)	7.34 (3.15–27.93)	6.80 (2.55–17.28)
Plasma osmolality (mOsm/kg)	307 (275–334)	316 (277–343)	313 (187–333)	309 (264–333)
Urine osmolality (mOsm/kg)	1424 (618–2680)	2432 (1214–3474)	2792 (1408–3814)	2383 (918–3384)
Urine production (ml/kg/24 hours)	25.3 (10.4–66.2)	32.1 (4.3–62.3)	26.2 (12.6–53.4)	20.9 (10.2–30.9)

[a] FE, urinary fractional excretion. (Crawford, M. A.: The urinary system. *In* Hoskins, J. D.: Veterinary Pediatrics: Dogs and Cats from Birth to Six Months, Philadelphia, W. B. Saunders, 1990, Chapter 10.)

TABLE 14. Erythrogram of Foals Up to One Year of Age[a]

Age	PCV (%)	Hemoglobin (g/dL)	RBC × 10⁶/µL	MCV (fl)	MCHC (g/dL)
<12 hours	43 ± 3	15.4 ± 1.2	10.7 ± 0.8	40 ± 2	36 ± 2
1 day	40 ± 3	14.2 ± 1.1	9.9 ± 0.6	41 ± 3	35 ± 2
3 days	38 ± 3	14.1 ± 1.3	9.6 ± 0.7	39 ± 2	37 ± 1
1 week	35 ± 3	13.3 ± 1.2	8.8 ± 0.6	39 ± 2	38 ± 1
2 weeks	34 ± 3	12.6 ± 1.4	8.9 ± 0.9	38 ± 2	38 ± 1
3 weeks	34 ± 3	12.6 ± 1.2	9.2 ± 0.6	37 ± 2	37 ± 1
1 month	34 ± 4	12.5 ± 1.2	9.3 ± 0.8	36 ± 1	37 ± 1
2 months	37 ± 4	13.6 ± 1.5	10.8 ± 1.7	35 ± 2	37 ± 1
3 months	36 ± 2	13.4 ± 0.9	10.5 ± 0.9	35 ± 1	37 ± 2
4 months	36 ± 3	13.4 ± 1.1	10.4 ± 0.9	34 ± 1	38 ± 2
5 months	35 ± 3	12.7 ± 1.2	10.2 ± 0.6	35 ± 2	37 ± 2
6 months	34 ± 2	12.2 ± 0.8	9.5 ± 0.7	36 ± 2	36 ± 1
9 months	36 ± 3	12.6 ± 1.0	9.4 ± 0.8	39 ± 2	35 ± 1
12 months	36 ± 3	13.3 ± 1.0	9.5 ± 0.7	38 ± 2	37 ± 2

[a] Values are mean ± 1 standard deviation. (Harvey J. W., *et al.*: Haematology of foals up to one year old. *Equine Vet. J., 16*:347, 1984.)

TABLE 15. Hemostasis Values for Healthy Horses

Laboratory Test	Mean ± S.D.	Range
Prothrombin time (seconds)	9.8 ± 0.34	9.2–10.5
APPT (seconds)	46.5 ± 9.2	31–93
Antithrombin III (%)	193 ± 28	115–239
Plasminogen (%)	110 ± 23	63–146
Fibrinogen (mg/dL)	192 ± 80	120–490
Fibrin(ogen) degradation products (µg/dL)	24 ± 19	0–64
Platelet count × 10⁵/µL	1.33 ± 0.34	0.89–2.32

(Prasse K.W., *et al.*: Evaluation of coagulation and fibrinolysis during the prodromal stages of carbohydrate-induced acute laminitis in horses. *Am. J. Vet. Res., 51*:1950, 1990.)

TABLE 16. Leukograms of Foals Up to One Year of Age

Age	Total WBC × 10³/μL	Neutrophils × 10³/μL	Lymphocytes × 10³/μL	Monocytes × 10³/μL	Eosinophils × 10³/μL	Basophils × 10³/μL
<12 hours	9.5 ± 2.44	7.94 ± 2.22	1.34 ± 0.60	0.19 ± 0.12	0	0.002 ± 0.007
1 day	8.44 ± 1.77	6.80 ± 1.72	1.43 ± 0.42	0.19 ± 0.10	0.11 ± 0.027	0.003 ± 0.010
3 days	7.55 ± 1.50	5.70 ± 1.44	1.45 ± 0.36	0.32 ± 0.13	0.045 ± 0.062	0.032 ± 0.046
1 week	9.86 ± 1.79	7.45 ± 1.55	2.10 ± 0.63	0.27 ± 0.11	0.028 ± 0.042	0.058 ± 0.069
2 weeks	8.53 ± 1.68	6.00 ± 1.54	2.22 ± 0.45	0.24 ± 0.013	0.063 ± 0.063	0.012 ± 0.021
3 weeks	8.57 ± 1.90	5.66 ± 1.64	2.59 ± 0.63	1.22 ± 0.10	0.078 ± 0.066	0.026 ± 0.032
1 month	8.14 ± 2.2	5.27 ± 2.00	2.46 ± 0.45	0.29 ± 0.17	0.121 ± 0.148	0.016 ± 0.032
2 months	9.65 ± 2.13	5.70 ± 1.88	3.46 ± 0.63	0.31 ± 0.015	0.092 ± 0.092	0.018 ± 0.039
3 months	11.69 ± 2.51	6.43 ± 1.96	4.73 ± 1.21	0.38 ± 0.019	0.184 ± 0.181	0.018 ± 0.028
4 months	10.18 ± 1.99	4.78 ± 1.36	4.70 ± 1.31	0.32 ± 0.17	0.353 ± 0.319	0.018 ± 0.027
5 months	10.17 ± 2.29	4.60 ± 1.90	4.92 ± 1.48	0.27 ± 0.12	0.272 ± 0.152	0.010 ± 0.027
6 months	9.03 ± 1.13	4.00 ± 0.84	4.53 ± 0.74	0.23 ± 0.11	0.247 ± 0.150	0.014 ± 0.024
9 months	8.68 ± 1.19	3.82 ± 0.78	4.39 ± 1.10	0.22 ± 0.10	0.234 ± 0.232	0.021 ± 0.024
12 months	9.19 ± 1.36	4.28 ± 0.81	4.27 ± 1.13	0.20 ± 0.12	0.339 ± 0.221	0.19 ± 0.37

(Harvey J. W., *et al.*: Haematology of foals up to one year old. *Equine Vet. J.*, *16*:347, 1984.

TABLE 17. Per Cent Fractional Urinary Excretion of Electrolytes in Cows: Mean and (Standard Error)

Electrolyte	Summer	Autumn	Winter	Spring
Sodium	1.3 (0.13)	0.68 (0.09)	0.63 (0.13)	0.33 (0.06)
Potassium	55.16 (4.12)	47.41 (3.80)	32.44 (3.15)	21.65 (3.41)
Chloride	2.12 (0.11)	2.25 (0.12)	1.80 (0.17)	0.68 (0.12)
Osmolality	4.70 (0.25)	3.84 (0.19)	3.71 (0.16)	1.82 (0.18)

(Itoh, N.: Fractional electrolyte excretion in adult cows: Establishment of reference ranges and evaluation of seasonal variations. *Vet. Clin. Pathol.*, *18*:86–87, 1989.)

TABLE 18. Normal Per Cent Fractional Urine Creatinine/Electrolyte Clearance of Domestic Animals[a]

Electrolyte	Dog	Cat	Horse	Cow	Sheep
Sodium	0–0.7	0.24–0.1	0.02–1.0	0.2–1.43	0–0.071
Potassium[b]	0–20	6.7–23.9	15–65	15–63	80–180
Chloride	0–0.8	0.41–1.3	0.04–1.6	0.4–2.3	0–4.7
Phosphorus	3–39	17–73	0–0.2		0–0.53

[a] Calculated using the formula:

$$\% \ CrCl(Fc)(E) = \frac{Cr \ serum}{Cr \ urine} \times \frac{E \ urine}{E \ serum} \times 100.$$

[b] The Fc for potassium in herbivorous animals is largely dependent upon the diet.

INDEX

Page numbers in *italics* indicate a figure; (t) indicates a table; **bold** indicates a case history.

337

BILE ACIDS
USEFUL IN DIAGNOSIS
OF PORTOSYSTEMIC SHUNTS
AND NON ICTERIC PATIENTS.